Obstetrics and Gynecology

2nd edition

Board Review Series

Obstetrics and Gynecology
2nd edition

Elmar P. Sakala, M.D., M.A., M.P.H.
Professor of Gynecology and Obstetrics
Department of Gynecology and Obstetrics
School of Medicine
Loma Linda University
Loma Linda, California

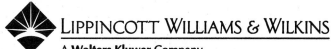

LIPPINCOTT WILLIAMS & WILKINS
A **Wolters Kluwer** Company
Philadelphia · Baltimore · New York · London
Buenos Aires · Hong Kong · Sydney · Tokyo

Editor: Elizabeth Nieginski
Development Editor: Emilie Linkins
Managing Editor: Marette D. Magargle-Smith

Printed in the United States of America

First Edition, 1977

Library of Congress Cataloging-in-Publication Data

Sakala, Elmar P.
    Obstetrics and gynecology / Elmar P. Sakala.—2nd ed.
        p.   cm. — (Board review series)
    Includes index.
    ISBN 0-683-30743-6
    1. Gynecology—Examinations, questions, etc.   2. Obstetrics—Examinations, questions, etc.   I. Title.   II. Series.
    [DNLM: 1. Obstetrics—Examination   Questions.   2. Obstetrics—Outlines. 3. Genital Diseases, Female—Examination Questions.   4. Genital Diseases, Female—Outlines. WQ 18.2 S158o 2000]
RG111.S35 2000
61 821—dc21   99-040829

The publishers have made every effort to trace the copyright holders for borrowed material. If they have inadvertently overlooked any, they will be pleased to make the necessary arrangements at the first opportunity.

To purchase additional copies of this book, call our customer service department at **(800) 638-3030** or fax orders to **(301) 824-7390**. International customers should call **(301) 714-2324**.

99 00 01 02 03
1 2 3 4 5 6 7 8 9 10

Dedication

To my wife who has graciously shared her husband's after-hours and weekends with the seemingly limitless demands of the word-processor. Darilee, without your characteristic understanding, this volume would never have been conceived, gestated, or birthed.

Contents

Preface

This book is designed primarily for the medical student or physician who is preparing to sit for the United States Medical Licensing Examination (USMLE) Step 2, or a similar clinical science examination. Its purpose is to present the content of obstetrics and gynecology in a concise, tightly organized format. This publication cannot replace the many fine medical student–level textbooks in obstetrics and gynecology that furnish the degree of detail and comprehensive background that medical students need. However, it does provide readers with a concise summary of clinical information that refreshes the memory, enabling the student to recall information that had been thoroughly learned previously.

Preparation for the United States Medical Licensing Examination (USMLE) Step 2 is challenging. The volume of information that the generalized undifferentiated medical practitioner (GUMP) is required to know is awesome. Particularly for the third-year student physician, the magnitude of the task of preparing for the USMLE Step 2 can seem overwhelming. Because students benefit when they have a framework on which to hang the endless list of seemingly unconnected facts, *BRS Obstetrics and Gynecology* seeks to provide an academic "skeleton" for obstetrics and gynecology; one on which the student can place the "muscles" and "fat" of clinical information.

As a medical student, I learned best by organizing information into visual patterns and constructing tables and charts that showed the relationships among a myriad of details. On the assumption that many readers are visual learners, I've made an effort to ensure that *BRS Obstetrics and Gynecology* contains scores of tables that bring together a wealth of data (including information about risk factors, mechanisms of disease, and pathophysiology).

To further foster understanding of the material, each chapter is followed by a series of questions accompanied by answers and complete explanations, allowing readers to assess their mastery of the material they have just reviewed. The comprehensive examination at the end of the book can serve as either a practice examination or a self-assessment tool to help students diagnose their weaknesses before beginning a review of the subject.

Changes to the second edition include an expanded discussion of the medical complications of pregnancy, a new chapter on sexually transmitted diseases, and charts that summarize the effects of numerous drugs in pregnant women, as well as updated clinical information reflecting the changes in the field that have occurred since the first edition was published.

It is my hope that this book will facilitate the successful completion of this important step in your medical career. Best wishes for successful learning!

Elmar P. Sakala

Acknowledgments

I want to recognize a number of individuals who have influenced me in my medical career by their teaching, example, and encouragement.

William Holmes Taylore, M.D., former professor of anatomy and surgery when I was a student at Loma Linda University School of Medicine, exemplified in his unrivaled and outstanding pedagogy that the teaching of medicine could be not only engaging but also fun.

Leon Speroff, M.D., my former department chairman and mentor when I was a resident at the University of Oregon, has been a role model of superb teaching. He possesses a singular talent for making ordinary tedious data come alive.

William Patton, M.D., friend and colleague at Loma Linda University, is a superb clinician and teacher with a unique gift for taking complex issues and simplifying them for the struggling medical student.

Victor Gruber, M.D., Executive Director of National Medical School Review, has been tenacious in his encouragement to me while developing this material into a format suitable for publication.

A large debt of thanks is due to the many hundreds of junior student physicians on the Gynecology & Obstetrics service at Loma Linda University School of Medicine as well as attendees at the National Medical School Review courses. They have supplied me with valuable feedback and suggestions from the previous drafts of these topics in a review-note format.

Finally, I was to sincerely thank gracious colleagues at Loma Linda University who provided me with insightful suggestions: Jeffrey Hardesty, M.D., Ibrahim Seraj, M.D., and Robert Wagner, M.D.

Elmar P. Sakala

1

Female Reproductive Tract

I. FUNCTIONAL ANATOMY OF THE FEMALE REPRODUCTIVE TRACT

A. Uterus

1. **Major structures** (Figure 1-1)
   a. The **corpus** is the larger, upper body of the uterus above the isthmus.
   b. The **isthmus** is the transverse constriction between the corpus and the cervix.
   c. The **cornu** is the upper, lateral part of the uterus at the point of entry of the fallopian tubes.
   d. The **cervix** is the smaller, lower portion of the uterus below the isthmus.
      (1) The **internal cervical os** separates the proximal cervix from the corpus.
      (2) The **external cervical os** separates the distal cervix from the vagina.

2. **Internal layers of the corpus** (see Figure 1-1)
   a. **Mesometrium (serosa)** is a reflection of visceral peritoneum and covers the uterine outer surface.
   b. **Myometrium (smooth muscle).** These fibers increase 10- to 20-fold in length during pregnancy. The layers include:
      (1) An outer longitudinal layer that is contiguous with the muscle layers of the oviduct and vagina
      (2) A middle layer composed of interlacing oblique and spiral layers
      (3) An inner longitudinal layer
   c. **Endometrium (mucosa).** The two layers of uterine inner lining undergo changes during the menstrual cycle (see Figure 1-6).
      (1) **Zona functionalis** is the layer that is shed with each menstrual cycle.
      (2) **Zona basalis** is the layer from which regeneration of the endometrium occurs.

1

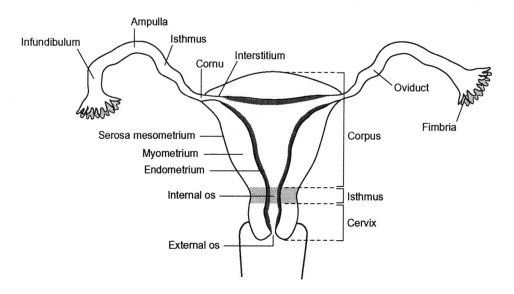

Figure 1-1. Anatomy of the female reproductive tract. (After Scott JR, DiSaia PJ, Hammond CB, et al (eds): *Danforth's Obstetrics and Gynecology,* 6th ed. Philadelphia, J.B. Lippincott, 1990, p 988.)

3. **Attachments**
   a. **Broad ligaments** are reflections of peritoneum and extend from the uterus and pelvic organs to the lateral pelvic walls.
   b. **Round ligaments** are reflections of the same peritoneum that covers the broad ligaments and extend from the fundus to the pelvic wall and into the inguinal canal.
   c. **Cardinal ligaments** are a condensation of subserous fascia extending from the uterus to the lateral pelvic wall. **Functions** of the cardinal ligaments include:
      (1) **Containing uterine blood supply** (from hypogastric vessels) and encasing the ureter.
      (2) **Providing support** for the middle and the upper thirds of the vagina and cervix.
   d. **Uterosacral ligaments** are condensations of subserous fascia that extend from the sacrum around the rectum to the cervix.
   e. **Uterovesical ligaments** are connective tissue that attach the bladder to the lower uterine segment.
4. **Positions** (Figure 1-2). All of the following positions are normal variations.
   a. **Anteverted.** The uterus is tipped **forward** in more than 50% of women.
   b. **Retroverted.** The uterus is tipped **backward** in approximately 25% of women.
   c. **Midposition.** The uterus is in the **midposition** in the remainder of women.
5. **Blood supply**
   a. The **uterine artery** is a direct branch from the hypogastric artery.

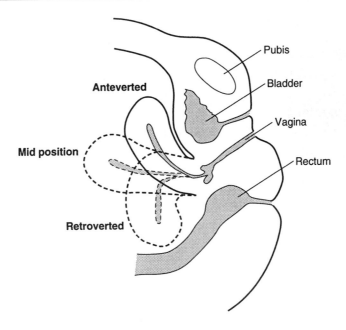

Figure 1-2. Variations in the position of the uterus.

    b. The **ovarian artery** is a direct branch from the aorta.

    c. An **anastomosis** exists between the two arteries.

  6. Lymphatic drainage is through the aortic, lumbar, and internal iliac lymph nodes.

  7. Innervation passes through the uterosacral ligaments.

    a. Afferent pain fibers (T11–T12) account for the perception of referred pain from the uterus in the lower abdomen.

    b. Sympathetic innervation arises from the **hypogastric and ovarian plexus.**

    c. Parasympathetic innervation involves the **pelvic nerve (S2–S4).**

  8. Functions

    a. Facilitates **sperm transport** from the cervix to the oviduct

    b. Provides a rich vascular environment for **nourishment of the developing embryo**

    c. Provides a **safe location for the growing fetus** throughout pregnancy

    d. Expels the mature fetus by means of **myometrial contractions** to outside the body

B. Fallopian tubes or oviducts

  1. Segments

    a. The **interstitium** is a 1-cm segment that penetrates the myometrial wall into the uterine cavity.

    b. The **isthmus** is the narrow proximal end with simple mucosal folds and a thick muscular wall.

c. The **ampulla** is the relatively dilated lateral half of the tube with a wide lumen and complex mucosal folds.

d. The **infundibulum** is the distal segment that terminates in mobile tentacle-like fimbriae that become turgid at ovulation, entrapping the ovum.

2. Attachments

   a. **Medially,** the oviducts are attached to the **uterine cornu.**

   b. **Laterally,** the oviducts are attached to the **pelvic side wall.**

   c. **Inferiorly,** the oviducts are attached to the **broad ligament** by the **mesalpinx.**

3. **Layers** (vary in size and thickness from interstitium to ampulla)

   a. **Serosa** is derived from the visceral peritoneal folds of the broad ligament.

   b. **Loose adventitia** contains lymphatics and blood vessels.

   c. **Smooth muscle** is mingled among the outer longitudinal and the inner circular layers and spiral bands. Muscle contractions move the ovum toward the uterus.

   d. **Lamina propria** is composed of vascular connective tissue elements.

   e. **Ciliated columnar epithelium** produces tubal fluid and secretions that nourish the dividing morula. Cilia beat in the direction of the uterus.

4. **Dual blood supply** through the mesosalpinx is from the **ascending uterine artery** and the **ovarian artery.**

5. Functions

   a. **Facilitate sperm migration** from the uterus to the ampulla for fertilization of the ovum

   b. **Transport the fertilized ovum** toward the uterus

C. Ovaries

1. Attachments

   a. **Medially,** the ovaries are attached to the **uterine fundus** by the **ovarian ligament.**

   b. **Laterally,** the ovaries are attached to the **pelvic side wall** by the **suspensory ligament.**

   c. **Inferiorly,** the ovaries are attached to the **broad ligament** by the **mesovarium.**

2. Vascular supply

   a. **Ovarian arteries** (branches from the aorta) traverse retroperitoneally into the mesosalpinx. **Uterine arteries** anastomose with ovarian arteries in the mesosalpinx.

   b. **Ovarian veins** drain on the right side to the inferior vena cava and on the left side to the left renal vein.

   c. **Ovarian lymphatic drainage** is through the infundibulopelvic ligaments to the pelvic and para-aortic nodes.

3. Functions

   a. **House** the **oocytes** within the follicles

   b. **Produce** reproductive and sexual **hormones**

D. Ureters cross the lateral pelvic wall at the bifurcation of the internal and external iliac arteries. The ureters are inferior and posterior to the pelvic blood supply and traverse the entire route retroperitoneally.

E. Vagina

1. **Location.** The vagina is a tubular structure extending from the introitus to the cervix. It traverses the urogenital diaphragm and extends through the genital hiatus of the levator ani. The anterior wall, which has an average length of 8 cm, is usually shorter than the posterior wall, which has an average length of 9 cm.

2. **Blood supply**
   a. **Hypogastric artery** (directly)
   b. **Uterine arteries**
   c. **Middle rectal artery**
   d. **Inferior vaginal artery** (from internal pudendal artery)

3. **Innervation**
   a. **Sympathetic** innervation involves the **hypogastric plexus.**
   b. **Parasympathetic** innervation involves the **pelvic nerve (S2–S4).**

4. **Support**
   a. The **lower third of the vagina** is supported by the pelvic diaphragm, the urogenital diaphragm, and the perineal body.
   b. The **middle third of the vagina** is supported by the pelvic diaphragm and the cardinal ligaments.
   c. The **upper third of the vagina** is supported by the cardinal ligaments and the uterosacral ligaments.

5. **Functions**
   a. Acts as the **female copulatory organ** in heterosexual intercourse
   b. Serves as the **distal outflow tract** to transport menstrual flow out of the body
   c. Forms the **birth canal** in parturition

F. The **hymen** is a perforated fold of mucosal-covered connective tissue located between the distal vagina and the vestibule.

G. Structures within the urogenital triangle arise in both genders from common embryonic origins. In the female, these structures include the vulva and external genitalia (Figure 1-3).

1. The **mons pubis** is created by a fat pad that lies anterior and superior to the symphysis pubis. The skin is covered by hair distributed in a triangular area **(escutcheon)** with the base at the pubis.

2. The **labia majora** (homologue of male scrotum) arise from the labioscrotal folds and are inferior extensions of the mons fat pad.
   a. **Characteristics**
      (1) The amount of fat determines individual appearance among women.
      (2) The labia majora are less prominent in multiparas.
      (3) The labia majora involute after menopause.

Female   **Male**

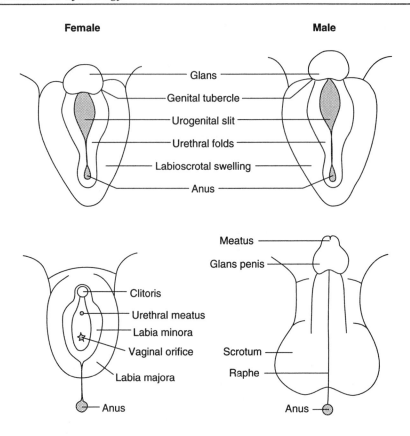

Figure 1-3. Comparison of development of female and male external genitalia differentiation in the embryo and in the fully developed individual. (Reprinted with permission from Speroff L, Glass RH, Kase NG: *Clinical Endocrinology and Infertility,* 5th ed. Baltimore, Williams & Wilkins, 1994, p 327.)

    b. Anatomy
        (1) The labia majora are covered by thick skin, coarse hair follicles, and sweat and sebaceous glands that respond to sex hormone changes at puberty.
        (2) A rich plexus of veins is present. This may rupture with trauma and form a hematoma.
        (3) The labia majora extend to the posterior fourchette.
        (4) The round ligaments terminate in the upper borders of the labia majora.
  3. The **labia minora** (homologue of penile urethra and skin of penis in male) are thin folds of stratified squamous epithelium that arise from the urethral folds.
    a. These structures are continuous with the epithelium of the **vestibule,** which is between the vaginal opening and the labia majora.
    b. They vary greatly in size and shape, superiorly forming the **prepuce** and **frenulum** of the clitoris.
    c. They contain sebaceous glands but no hair follicles.
  4. The **clitoris** (homologue of male penis) is an erectile organ that arises from the **genital tubercle.**
    a. Located superior to the vaginal vestibule, this structure usually mea-

sures 0.5 cm × 2 cm. It is attached to the pubic periosteum by two **crura.**

    b. Its sponge-like system of vascular spaces is richly supplied by sympathetic and parasympathetic nerves.

  5. The **urethra,** a membranous tube 3–5 cm long, is for the passage of urine.

    a. The proximal two thirds of this structure are lined with stratified transitional epithelium, and its distal one third is lined with stratified squamous epithelium.

    b. An estrogen-dependent paraurethral venous plexus contributes to urethral pressure, maintaining urinary continence in the premenopausal female.

  6. **Skene's glands** (homologue of the male prostate gland) are **paraurethral** glands adjacent to the distal urethra that empty into the urethra and vaginal vestibule. Their principal function is lubrication.

  7. **Bartholin's glands** (homologue of male Cowper's glands) lie within the gluteal fat pad under the posterolateral surface of the vagina. These glands are covered with cuboidal epithelium; the duct has transitional epithelium.

H. Pelvic diaphragm. This muscular layer forms the inferior border of the abdominal-pelvic cavity and extends from the pubic bone to the coccyx and between the pelvic walls. The primary muscle is the **levator ani,** which forms the floor of the pelvis and the roof of the perineum.

  1. Functions of the levator ani muscle include flexing the coccyx, raising the anus, and constricting the rectum and vagina.

  2. The **pubococcygeus,** the **most significant component** of the levator ani muscle (Figure 1-4), has attachments to the urethra, rectum, vagina, and the perineal body. Structures that pass through the pubococcygeus include the urethra, vagina, and rectum. Other components are the **pubovaginalis muscle,** the **puborectalis muscle,** and the **iliococcygeus muscle.**

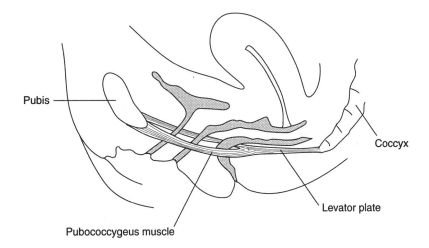

Pubis

Coccyx

Levator plate

Pubococcygeus muscle

Figure 1-4. Relationship of the pubococcygeus muscle and the levator plate. The pubococcygei unite posterior to the rectum and continue to the coccyx as the levator plate, which is normally oriented in a horizontal position. The empty vagina sits on the empty rectum, which rests on the levator plate, as shown. (Reprinted with permission from Scott JR, DiSaia PJ, Hammond CB, et al (eds): *Danforth's Obstetrics and Gynecology,* 6th ed. Philadelphia, J.B. Lippincott, 1990, p 889.)

II. FUNCTIONAL HISTOLOGY OF THE FEMALE REPRODUCTIVE TRACT

A. Cervical epithelium

1. **Embryonic development in utero.** The cervix and upper vagina are initially covered with columnar epithelium. Vaginal columnar epithelium is gradually replaced by stratified squamous epithelium.

2. **At birth**
   a. **Region of columnar epithelium**
      (1) In most normal girls, the columnar epithelium is limited to the endocervix and the central ectocervix.
      (2) In 4% of normal girls and 30% of diethylstilbestrol (DES) daughters, the cervical columnar epithelium extends onto the vaginal fornices **(adenosis).**
      (3) Because the columnar epithelium is only one cell-layer thick, blood vessels in the underlying stroma show through, giving an orange-red appearance.
   b. The **original squamocolumnar (SC) junction** is formed by a boundary between original (native) squamous and columnar epithelia.

3. **During adolescence and first pregnancy,** a new SC junction is formed through squamous metaplasia.
   a. The **new SC junction** is more proximal to the external os than is the original SC junction.
   b. The **transformation zone (T-zone)** is an area of squamous metaplasia between the original and the new SC junctions (Figure 1-5). **Approximately 90% of cervical dysplasia develops within the T-zone.**

B. Endometrium

1. **Layers in the late luteal phase are hormonally responsive.**
   a. The **zona functionalis** sheds from the entire endometrium after each menstruation.
      (1) **Layers**
         (a) **Zona compacta** is the superficial layer at the mouth of the glands.
         (b) **Zona spongiosa** is the deeper layer in which glands are tortuous and dilated.
      (2) **Vascular supply** is via spiral arterioles, which alternately constrict and relax in response to progesterone withdrawal, producing endometrial ischemia and sloughing in the latter part of the menstrual cycle.
   b. The **zona basalis** is the deepest layer from which zona functionalis regenerates by outgrowth of gland epithelium.

2. **Endometrial changes during the menstrual cycle** (Figure 1-6; Table 1-1)
   a. The **proliferative (follicular) phase** depends on **estrogen** produced by the granulosa cells of the ovarian follicles under the

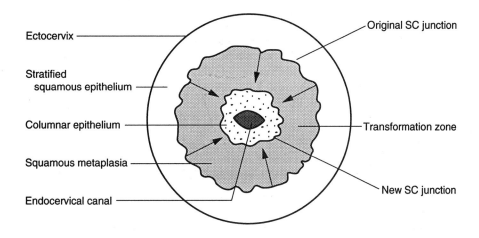

Figure 1-5. Development of the transformation zone of the cervix between the original squamocolumnar (SC) junction and the new SC junction.

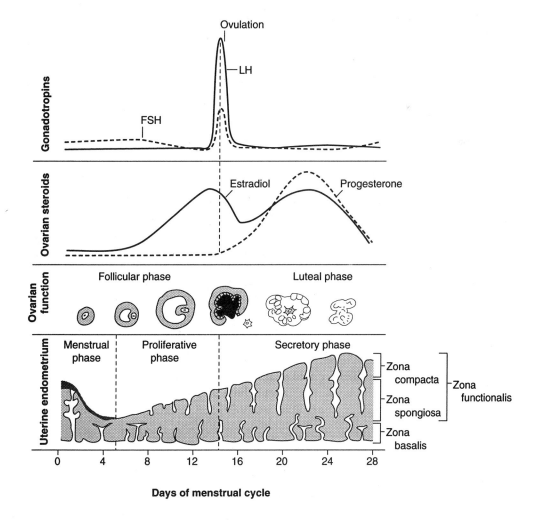

Days of menstrual cycle

Figure 1-6. The menstrual cycle: pituitary, ovarian, endometrial correlations.

Table 1-1. Phases of the Menstrual Cycle

	Preovulatory Phase	Postovulatory Phase
Name by phase of ovarian cycle	Follicular phase	Luteal phase
Name by findings on histology	Proliferative phase	Secretory phase
Length	Variable (7–21 days)	Constant (14 days)
Begins	Day 1 of menses	Day of ovulation
Ends	Day of ovulation	Start of mensus
Basal body temperature	Low-basal	Elevated over baseline
Dominant hormone	Estrogen	Progesterone
Hormone source	Follicular granulosa cells	Corpus luteum
Histology	Straight tubular glands	Tortuous glands with secretions
Cervical mucus	Thin and watery	Thick and sticky

stimulation of follicle-stimulating hormone (FSH). Glands and epithelium show **intense mitotic activity,** as well as:

(1) Tall, columnar epithelium
(2) Straight, tubular glands
(3) Compact stroma

    b. The **secretory (luteal) phase** depends on **progesterone** produced by the luteal cells of the corpus luteum. Tortuous, sinuous glands with a saw-tooth pattern are visible, with glycogen appearing in the gland lumen. The stroma becomes edematous.

    c. The **menstrual phase** depends on **withdrawal of progesterone,** assuming pregnancy does not occur. Alternating contraction and relaxation of spiral arterioles produces dehydration, hemorrhage, and bleeding. The entire endometrial zona functionalis layer sheds. This contrasts with the random bleeding from isolated locations that occurs with dysfunctional uterine bleeding from unopposed estrogen stimulation.

C. Vagina

    1. The **vagina** is lined by **stratified squamous, nonkeratinizing epithelium.** There are no glands in the vaginal mucosa.

    2. The **lamina propria** is connective tissue rich with blood vessels and lymphatics. Moisture transudates the epithelium with sexual arousal, producing the physiologic lubrication response.

D. Ovarian follicular development

    1. **Origin and migration of germ cells** (Figure 1-7)

       a. Germ cells arise from **yolk sac endoderm** and migrate caudally by ameboid motion along the hindgut into genital ridges.

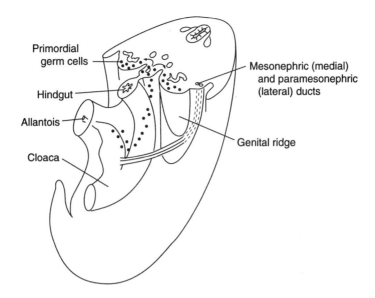

Figure 1-7. Migratory path of primordial germ cells from the yolk sac along the hindgut mesentery to the urogenital ridge. (Reprinted with permission from Hacker NF, Moore JG (eds): *Essentials of Obstetrics and Gynecology,* 2nd ed. Philadelphia, W.B. Saunders, 1992, p 320.)

    b. By 5 weeks' gestation, a few hundred germ cells are present in the genital ridges.

        (1) Germ cells not reaching their final destination usually undergo **atresia.**

        (2) If germ cells outside the ovary do not become atretic, they may survive to form **germ cell tumors.**

    c. After germ cells undergo **rapid mitosis,** they begin an ongoing process of **involution,** which continues until menopause when all follicles are gone.

        (1) By 20 weeks' gestation, the germ cell population is 7 million.

        (2) By term, the number has declined to 1.5 million (see Figure 12-1).

2. Eggs in postnatal ovary

    a. Primary oocytes are arrested in meiotic prophase of the **first maturational division.**

    b. After puberty, with each menstrual cycle, a group of primary oocytes begins to mature under **FSH stimulation.**

    c. Follicle recruitment

        (1) Six or more follicles begin growth and maturation in any cycle, producing increasing levels of estrogen.

        (2) Only one follicle undergoes the preovulatory swelling and develops into the **dominant follicle.** The **length of the first part of the follicular phase** of the menstrual cycle is determined by how long selection of the dominant follicle takes.

        (3) Ovulation of the dominant follicle occurs as a result of stimulation by a **luteinizing hormone (LH)** surge that is triggered by escalating estrogen levels.

3. **Layers surrounding the oocyte of the dominant follicle** (from inner to outer)

   a. **Zona pellucida** is a highly refractory membrane.

   b. **Avascular granulosa cells** rest on a well-marked basement membrane; the inner layer of cells forms the **cumulus oophorus** surrounding the ovum.

   c. **Vascular theca interna cells,** which arise from the stroma, undergo marked hypertrophy as the follicle matures.

   d. **Relatively avascular theca externa cells** form a connective tissue capsule.

4. **Completion of oocyte meiosis**

   a. **Just before ovulation,** under the influence of the LH surge, a primary oocyte becomes **a secondary oocyte** by completing **first reduction division**. This division produces the **first polar body** and results in a reduction of the number of chromosomes from 46 to 23.

   b. **Second reduction division** does not occur until **after fertilization,** producing a **second polar body.** The number of chromosomes remains 23.

5. **Follicular atresia.** Of the six to ten follicles that begin growth, only one follicle completes ovulation. The rest undergo **follicular atresia.**

6. **Development of the corpus luteum** (Figure 1-8)

   a. Following follicular rupture, the **antral cavity** collapses and contains extravasated blood.

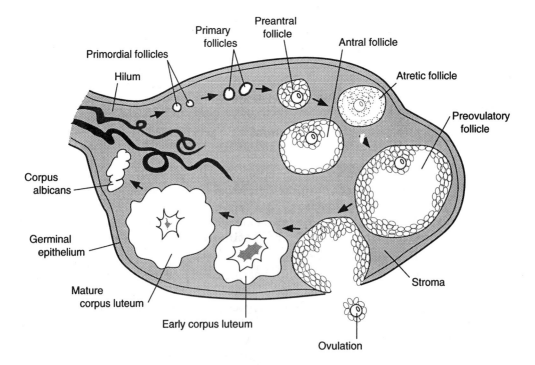

Figure 1-8. Diagram of the ovary that shows the stages of follicle development leading to maturation, rupture, luteinization, and corpus luteum involution. (Reprinted with permission from Speroff L, Glass RH, Kase NG: *Clinical Endocrinology and Infertility,* 5th ed. Baltimore, Williams & Wilkins, 1994, p 105.)

    b. Granulosa cells proliferate by mitosis, undergoing steady hypertrophy and growth into **luteal cells.**

    c. Theca interna connective tissue invades the granulosa cell layer.

    d. Larger **granulosa cells** and smaller **theca cells** become closely intermingled.

        (1) Granulosa cells and theca cells transform into **luteal cells** and form around a central cavity in radial cords.

        (2) Because luteal cells are highly vascular, they bleed heavily.

    e. The **luteal cells** resemble steroid-secreting adrenal cortex cells in appearance; they secrete **progesterone** (dominant secretory phase hormone).

    f. The **luteotropic stimulus** that maintains the corpus luteum initially is anterior **pituitary LH.** It is withdrawn if conception does not occur.

    g. The **corpus albicans** results from shrinkage and hyalinization of the former corpus luteum.

    h. If pregnancy occurs, the corpus luteum is maintained by **human chorionic gonadotropin (hCG)** from the syncytiotrophoblast.

III. DEVELOPMENT OF THE EMBRYO, FETUS, AND PLACENTA

    A. First week: ovulation to implantation

        1. Fertilization usually occurs in the ampullae (widest part) of the distal oviduct. Only one of the 200 to 300 million spermatozoa deposited in the female reproductive tract is needed for fertilization.

        2. Sperm must undergo two changes to fertilize the ovum.

            a. Capacitation allows the spermatozoon to lose part of its acrosomal membrane.

            b. The **acrosomal reaction** releases enzyme contents of the acrosome to penetrate the **corona radiata** cells and the oocyte.

        3. After fertilization the zona pellucida must change to prevent the entrance of a second sperm.

            a. The **zona reaction** renders the zona pellucida impenetrable to additional sperm.

            b. Zona sperm receptors are inactivated, and cross-linking of zona proteins harden the zona.

        4. Within 36 hours of conception, the two pronuclei fuse, and one cell divides into two cells through the process of **cleavage.** Within 3 days of fertilization, the two cells have transformed into a solid mass of 12–16 cells known as the **morula.**

        5. With continuing cleavage, the blastocyst, a hollow ball of cells composed of two parts, appears.

            a. The outer cells of the blastocyst, known as the **trophoblast,** become the **placenta.**

            b. The inner cell mass of the blastocyst, known as the **embryoblast,** becomes the **embryo.**

6. **Implantation.** The developing conceptus takes 6–7 days to journey down the oviduct to the uterine cavity. When it reaches the uterine cavity, the blastocyst orients itself so that the trophoblast overlying the embryoblast implants within the endometrium. The implantation site is usually along the **anterior** and **posterior uterine walls.**

B. **Second week: formation of the bilaminar germ disc**

1. **Within a few hours after implantation,** the trophoblast invades the endometrium, producing two layers.
   a. The proliferating **Langhans' cells** form the **cytotrophoblast,** which is an inner layer of mononucleated cells.
   b. The **syncytiotrophoblast,** which is an outer multinucleated zone without distinct cell boundaries that **produces β-hCG,** forms from this layer. The syncytiotrophoblast is the front line of invading fetal tissue.

2. The **embryoblast differentiates** into a flat, bilaminar disc composed of two germ layers.
   a. The **hypoblast** has small cuboidal cells.
   b. The **epiblast** has high columnar cells.

3. **Two spaces** appear on either side of the bilaminar disc, each of which develops into a significant cavity.
   a. The **amniotic cavity** appears as a space between the epiblast and the cytotrophoblast.
   b. The **exocoelomic cavity,** or primitive yolk sac, appears as a space between the hypoblast and the cytotrophoblast.

4. **As the blastocyst becomes embedded in the endometrial stroma,** the surface epithelium grows over the original defect. The enlarging syncytiotrophoblast develops interconnecting **lacunae space.** Maternal **sinusoids** are invaded by the trophoblast, extravasating blood into the lacunae and beginning the **intervillous space,** which develops into the **uteroplacental circulation.** Entry of β-hCG into the maternal circulation results in a pregnancy test being positive for the first time.

5. The **cytotrophoblast** forms **branching projections** that become the **primary stem villi** of the primitive placenta.

C. **Third week: formation of the trilaminar germ disc**

1. The **primitive streak** develops on the surface of the epiblast with the **primitive node** on its cephalic end. Through a process of **invagination,** surface cells migrate to the primitive streak, detach from the epiblast, and slip underneath the epiblast to form the **mesoderm.** The establishment of this third germ layer is known as **gastrulation.**

2. The **primary stem villi** undergo a series of branching steps, forming **secondary** and **tertiary villi** of the placenta. The **mesoblast** (from the original trophoblast) forms a central stromal core that invades the villi, from which capillaries develop. These vessels communicate with the intra-embryonic circulatory system as it develops to form the **fetoplacental circulation.**

D. **Fourth to eighth weeks: the embryonic period.** All major organs and organ systems are formed during the embryonic period. During this period, the embryo is most susceptible to factors that result in congenital malformations.

1. The **crown–rump length (CRL)** is used to measure the growth of the embryo. Development advances:
   a. **Cranially,** then proceeds **caudally**
   b. **Proximally,** then continues **distally**

2. **Derivatives of the ectoderm** are those organs and structures that maintain external contact such as:
   a. Central and peripheral nervous systems
   b. Sensory epithelia of the ear, eye, and nose
   c. Skin, hair, and nails
   d. Pituitary, mammary, and sweat glands

3. **Derivatives of the mesoderm** include:
   a. All **supporting tissues** of the body derived from the somites
      (1) Muscle tissue arises from the **myotome.**
      (2) Cartilage and bone arise from the **sclerotome.**
      (3) Subcutaneous tissue arises from the **dermatome.**
   b. **Cardiovascular and lymphatic systems** (including blood and lymph cells)
   c. **Urogenital system** (kidneys, gonads, and their respective ducts) **but not the bladder**

4. **Derivatives of the endoderm** include:
   a. **Epithelial lining** of the gastrointestinal (GI) tract, respiratory tract, and urinary bladder
   b. **Parenchyma** of the tonsils, thyroid and parathyroid glands, thymus, liver, and pancreas

5. **Lack of closure of the ectomesodermal folds** in the various locations leads to the following anomalies:
   a. **Ectopia cordis** with lack of **cephalad** closure
   b. **Omphalocele** with lack of **lateral** closure
   c. **Bladder exstrophy** with lack of **caudad** closure

E. **Relationship of fetal membranes to the uterine wall**

1. The chorionic villi arise from the trophoblast. In early pregnancy, the villi cover the entire surface of the chorion. This changes rapidly with time.
   a. Villi on the **embryonic pole** of the trophoblast form the **chorion frondosum,** the portion of the placenta attached to the uterine wall where the branching villi resemble a leafy tree.
   b. Villi on the **opposite pole (abembryonic)** degenerate to form the denuded **chorion laeve,** which fuses with the amniotic membrane later to form the **fetal membranes.**

2. The differences in the embryonic and abembryonic poles of the chorion are reflected in the parts of the decidua.
   a. The **decidua basalis** is the endometrium in contact with the chorion frondosum. It forms the basal plate of the placenta. **Nitabuch's layer** is a zone of fibrinoid degeneration in which the trophoblast meets the

decidua, preventing the placenta from invading too deeply. **Placenta accreta** occurs when this layer is absent.

    b. The **decidua capsularis** is the endometrium covering the chorion laeve.

    c. The **decidua vera** (parietalis) is the endometrium that is not in contact with any portion of the chorion. The space between the decidua vera and the decidua capsularis is obliterated by the fourth month. The two layers fuse as they meet.

F. **Fetal circulation. Three in-utero shunts,** vital for fetal life, **close in the neonatal period.**

    1. Deoxygenated fetal blood flows to the placenta from the hypogastric arteries via the **two umbilical arteries.**

    2. Oxygenated, nutrition-bearing blood from the placenta is returned to the fetus through a **single umbilical vein.**

    3. Blood from the umbilical vein enters the liver **shunting through the ductus venosus** on its way to the inferior vena cava (IVC).

    4. Highly oxygenated blood from the IVC enters the right atrium, **shunting through the foramen ovale** into the left heart, from which it enters the ascending aorta to preferentially perfuse the coronary and cerebral circulations.

    5. Less oxygenated blood from the superior vena cava (SVC) flows through the right heart into the pulmonary artery **shunting through the ductus arteriosus** to the descending aorta to preferentially perfuse the lower part of the body.

IV. PHYSIOLOGIC CHANGES OF PREGNANCY (Table 1-2)

A. Alimentary tract

    1. Appetite

        a. Appetite is usually normal throughout pregnancy.

        b. Pica describes dietary cravings or aversions for nonnutritional substances.

            (1) In rural areas of the southern United States, women affected by pica often crave clay or starch.

            (2) In England, women with pica usually crave coal.

            (3) Other substances that are craved by women with pica include soap, toothpaste, ice, and newspaper.

    2. Mouth

        a. Saliva. The pH and rate of production probably does not change.

        b. Ptyalism is the rare, excessive loss of saliva (1–2 L/day) and is usually associated with nausea of pregnancy.

        c. Dentition. There is no evidence of increased caries or acceleration of the development of caries.

        d. Gums usually become soft and edematous and may bleed with brushing.

        e. Epulis gravidarum/pyogenic granuloma describes tumorous

Table 1-2.　Physiologic Changes of Pregnancy

	Values Increased	Values Decreased	Values Unchanged
Liver function tests	Alkaline phosphatase Fibrinogen Steroid-binding hormones Cholesterol and other serum lipids All gamma globulins	Albumin	ALT AST Bilirubin GGT 5′ Nucleotidase Prothrombin time
Lung volumes	Tidal volume (TV)	All lung volumes except TV Inspiratory reserve volume (IRV) Expiratory reserve volume (ERV) Residual volume (RV)	—
Lung capacities	Inspiratory capacity (IC)	Functional residual capacity (FRC) Total lung capacity (TLC)	Vital capacity (VC)
Arterial blood gas	pH Po_2	Pco_2	HCO_3^- Base express Base deficit
Renal function tests	Glomerular filtration rate (GFR) Renal blood flow Creatinine clearance (Cr cl)	Blood urea nitrogen (BUN) Serum creatinine Serum uric acid	—
Complete blood count	White blood cell count (WBC) Erythrocyte sedementation rate (ESR) Left shift	Hemoglobin Hematocrit	Platelet count Mean corpuscular volume (MCV) Red cell distribution width (RDW)
Thyroid tests	Thyroid-binding globulin (TBG) Total T_3 Total T_4	T_3 resin uptake	Thyrotropin-releasing hormone (TRH) Thyroid-stimulating hormone (TSH) Free T_3 Free T_4

ALT = alanine aminotransferase; *AST* = aspartate aminotransferase; *GGT* = gamma glutamyltransferase; T_3 = triiodothyronine; T_4 = thyroxine

gingivitis with pedunculated lesions that may bleed profusely and seldom require excision. They usually regress 1–2 months after delivery.

3. Stomach

　　a. **Tone and motility** decrease because of:

　　　　(1) The smooth muscle–relaxing effect of progesterone

　　　　(2) Decreased levels of **motilin,** a gut hormone that stimulates smooth muscle

　　　　(3) Nausea of pregnancy (possible cause)

    b. Emptying half-time after a 750-ml watery test meal increases from 11 minutes in the nonpregnant state to 18 minutes during pregnancy.

    c. Residual volume 30 minutes after a test meal increases from 186 ml in the nonpregnant state to 275 ml during pregnancy and 393 ml during labor.

    d. Gastroesophageal junction sphincter tone decreases from the smooth muscle effect of progesterone. Decreased tone leads to acid reflux into the esophagus, causing heartburn.

    e. Gastric acid secretion decreases in the first and second trimesters but is increased in the third trimester.

    f. Peptic ulcer disease decreases because of:

        (1) Decreased gastric acid secretion

        (2) Decreased gastric emptying

        (3) Increased gastric mucous secretion

        (4) The protective effect of prostaglandins on gastric mucosa

4. Small bowel

    a. Motility decreases. The stomach-to-cecum transit time increases from 52 hours in a nonpregnant state to 58 hours in pregnancy.

    b. Nutrient absorption, except for increased iron absorption, does not change.

5. Colon

    a. Motility decreases, resulting in **constipation** caused by:

        (1) Smooth muscle relaxation from progesterone

        (2) Mechanical obstruction of the enlarging uterus

        (3) Water absorption increase of 60%

        (4) Sodium absorption increase of 45% (from increased aldosterone level)

    b. Hemorrhoidal veins dilate, leading to **hemorrhoids.** An increase in portal venous pressure is transmitted through all portosystemic anastomoses.

6. Gallbladder

    a. Emptying time increases.

    b. Fasting and residual volumes double.

    c. Biliary cholesterol saturation increases, predisposing to gallstone formation.

7. Liver

    a. Size, blood flow, and histology do not change.

    b. Laboratory tests. See Table 1-2 for a review of results. Albumin normally decreases in pregnancy. Liver enzymes remain unchanged (the rise in alkaline phosphatase is from placental not liver production). All hormone-binding proteins, gamma globulins, and serum lipids increase in pregnancy.

    c. Signs of normal pregnancy that may **mimic liver disease** include:

        (1) Spider angiomata and palmar erythema from increased estrogen levels

        (2) Decreased albumin

        (3) Increased alkaline phosphatase and cholesterol

8. **Nausea and vomiting** ("morning sickness") occurs in up to 70% of all pregnancies. The usual onset is at 4–8 weeks of pregnancy, normally lasting to 14–16 weeks of pregnancy.

   a. The **mechanism** is unclear; nausea and vomiting may be caused by decreased stomach tone or increased hCG level.

   b. **Treatment** is supportive and involves reassurance and frequent small meals.

   c. **Hyperemesis gravidarum** results in severe nausea and vomiting, which may be pernicious and persistent, requiring hospitalization with intravenous (IV) hydration and nutrition. Weight loss, ketonemia, and electrolyte disturbances are characteristic. This severe type frequently occurs in women with a **molar pregnancy.**

B. **Respiratory system—upper respiratory tract**

   1. Nasopharyngeal mucosa is hyperemic and edematous. Mucous secretion is increased from increased capillary dilation throughout the respiratory tract. **Nasal stuffiness** and epistaxis are common, and **nasal polyposis** may develop.

   2. **Mechanical changes**

      a. The subcostal angle increases from 68 to 103 degrees.

      b. The transverse chest diameter increases 2 cm.

      c. Chest circumference increases 5–7 cm.

      d. The diaphragm level is pushed up 4 cm.

      e. Diaphragmatic excursion increases 1–2 cm.

   3. **Lung volume and pulmonary function** (Figure 1-9). Tidal volume (TV) increases, but all other lung volumes decrease. Inspiratory capacity increases and vital capacity decreases, but other lung capacities remain unchanged.

   4. **Gas exchange**

      a. Oxygen consumption is increased by 20%.

      b. TV is increased 40%, whereas respiratory rate (RR) remains unchanged.

      c. Minute ventilation (TV × RR) is increased 40%.

      d. Alveolar and arterial PO_2 levels increase.

      e. Alveolar and arterial PCO_2 levels decrease. The fetal-maternal gradient increases, which facilitates CO_2 transfer.

      f. Arterial pH increases, reflecting a partially compensated respiratory alkalosis.

   5. **"Dyspnea of pregnancy"** describes an increased awareness of a desire to breathe (in 60%–70% of normal women) stimulated via the brain stem respiratory center (from decreased PCO_2 and increased TV).

C. **Skin**

   1. **Vascular changes** result from increased **estrogen** levels and regress after delivery.

      a. **Spider angiomata** are seen in 70% of white women and 10% of black women. They are most common on the face, upper chest, and arms.

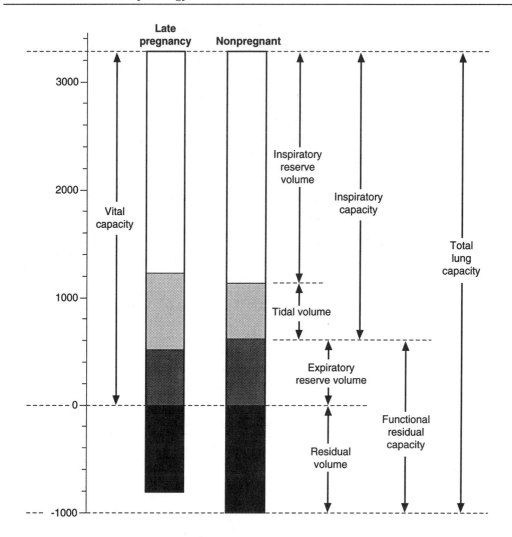

Figure 1-9. Changes in lung volume and lung capacities with pregnancy. (Reprinted with permission from Hytten FE, Lind T: *Diagnostic Indices in Pregnancy.* Summit, NJ, CIBA-GEIGY Corporation, Medical Education Division, 1973, p 26.)

    b. Palmar erythema, from increased skin blood flow to the hands, is seen in 60% of women.

2. **Striae gravidarum** is seen in 50% of women, usually on their breasts, lower abdomen, and upper thighs. The color is pink-purple and becomes silvery white. Striae are caused by normal stretching of the skin in genetically predisposed women. There is no relationship to weight gain, and there is no effective prophylactic treatment.

3. **Pigmentation changes.** Increased **melanocyte-stimulating hormone** is stimulated by increased estrogen and progesterone. Pigmentation changes are more common in brunettes than in blondes. Darkening may fade but may never disappear completely. Changes include:

    a. Darkening of nipples, areolae, umbilicus, axillae, perineum, and linea nigra

  b. Melasma (chloasma or "mask of pregnancy"), which describes blotchy irregular lesions on the forehead, cheeks, nose, and upper lip (seen also with oral contraceptives)

  c. Pigmented nevi, which may darken and enlarge with increased junctional activity and tend to reverse after pregnancy

 4. Hair changes. During pregnancy, the amount of scalp hair in **telogen** (resting phase) decreases from 20% to 10%. Postpartum, the amount of hair in telogen phase increases to 30%. Thus, there is a marked increase in scalp hair loss 2–4 months after delivery.

 5. Abdominal wall. Separation of the rectus muscles in the midline caused by the enlarging uterus is called **diastasis recti.**

D. Urinary system

 1. Anatomic changes

  a. Kidneys increase in both length and weight, with the right kidney enlarging more than the left kidney.

   (1) The **renal pelves** increase in size, which results in **physiologic hydronephrosis.**

   (2) Up to 200 ml of residual urine is found in each dilated collecting system.

  b. Ureters dilate to 2 cm in diameter beginning by 8 weeks' gestation.

   (1) The right ureter is larger than the left in 90% of women. The mechanism may involve uterine dextrorotation, compressing the right ureter with sigmoid colon cushioning of the left ureter.

   (2) The dilated ureters cause **hydroureter** and **urinary stasis.** The urine volume of each ureter is 20–50 ml.

   (3) Ureteric dilation is seen mostly above the pelvic brim. The mechanism is unclear but may possibly be the smooth muscle–relaxing effect of progesterone or may be mechanical.

  c. Consequences of the changes in the kidneys and ureters include:

   (1) Increased risk of **pyelonephritis** if **asymptomatic bacteriuria** occurs

   (2) Alteration of the "normal" nonpregnant intravenous pyelogram (IVP) appearance

 2. Tests of renal function produce the following results.

  a. Renal plasma flow, glomerular filtration rate (GFR), and creatinine clearance (CrCl) are all increased more than 50%.

  b. Serum blood urea nitrogen (BUN), creatinine, and uric acid are all decreased by 25%.

 3. Urinary excretion of nutrients

  a. Glucosuria is common in normal pregnancy with poor correlation between blood and urine glucose levels.

   (1) The **increased urinary excretion** in pregnant women results from the filtered tubular glucose load being increased by a higher GFR and the decreased tubular reabsorptive capacity.

   (2) Consequences of glucosuria with normal blood glucose levels include a higher risk of urinary tract infections (UTIs).

  b. Proteinuria is not normal in pregnancy.

    c. Aminoaciduria with certain amino acids (i.e., glycine, histidine, threonine, serine, alanine) may contribute to a higher risk of UTIs.

    d. Water-soluble vitamin excretion increases (e.g., folate, vitamin B_{12}).

E. Cardiovascular system

    1. Heart. The **position** of the heart in the chest is more horizontal. Elevation of the diaphragm from the enlarging uterus displaces the heart upward and to the left. The heart is rotated on the long axis, moving the apex and point of maximal impulse laterally. A straightened left heart border gives the appearance of cardiomegaly.

      a. Cardiothoracic ratio is unchanged.

      b. Normal changes in **heart sounds** include:

        (1) Exaggerated splitting of S_1; no change in S_2

        (2) S_3 or S_3 gallop (in 90% of normal pregnant women)

        (3) Systolic ejection murmur along the left sternal border (in 95% of normal pregnant women) from an increased flow across the aortic and pulmonary valves due to increased blood volume and cardiac output (CO).

        (4) Mammary souffle, a bilateral continuous murmur in the second, third, or fourth intercostal space, occurs in 10% of pregnant women and increases blood flow through the mammary vessels supplying the breasts **(NOTE: Diastolic murmurs are never normal.)**

      c. Electrocardiogram (EKG) is unchanged except for a slight axis deviation to the left.

    2. Cardiac output (CO) is the product of stroke volume (SV) and heart rate (HR) [CO = SV × HR].

      a. By 20 weeks' gestation, the CO has risen 35% (Figure 1-10).

        (1) SV increases early in pregnancy by 10% (to 75 ml/stroke) and returns to normal by term. Heart size also increases by 10%.

        (2) HR increases gradually to term (15–20 beats/min higher than nonpregnant rate).

      b. CO is dependent on maternal position.

        (1) CO is lowest when the pregnant woman is supine (30% lower at term).

          (a) Mechanism. Low CO when supine results from **IVC occlusion;** blood returns via the paravertebral collaterals.

          (b) Compensation involves a rise in peripheral vascular resistance (PVR).

        (2) Supine hypotensive syndrome exists in 5% of women. Symptoms include dizziness, lightheadedness, nausea, and syncope.

        (3) Optimal CO occurs when the woman is in the **left lateral position;** the IVC is not compressed.

      c. Distribution of CO changes from the first to third trimesters. The **CO percentage:**

        (1) Increases in the uterus (2%–17%) and the breasts (1%–2%).

        (2) Decreases in the splanchnic bed and skeletal muscle (absolute blood flow is unchanged).

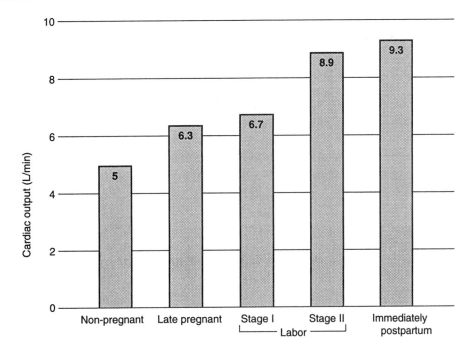

Figure 1-10. Changes in cardiac output during pregnancy. Note that the highest output is immediately after the removal of the placenta.

  (3) Remains unchanged in the kidneys, skin, brain, and coronary arteries (absolute blood flow is increased 20%, 10%, 10%, and 5%, respectively).
 d. Effect of labor and immediate puerperium
  (1) First stage of labor. CO increases by 40% largely as a result of pain and anxiety, which can be moderated by regional anesthesia. With each contraction, an autotransfusion of 300–500 ml uterine blood from the intervillous space and placental sinuses moves in and out of the systemic circulation.
  (2) Second stage of labor. Maternal expulsive efforts **increase CO** further.
  (3) Third stage of labor. CO increases immediately by 15% because of rapid infusion of uteroplacental blood into the peripheral circulation. PVR increases as a result of the loss of a low-resistance arteriovenous shunt (i.e., the placenta). Blood must then pass through the peripheral capillary beds.
 3. Arterial blood pressure (BP) is dependent on **maternal position.** It is lowest when the woman is on her side, it is in the middle range when the woman is supine, and it is highest when the woman is seated. **(NOTE: In normal pregnancy, BP is never higher than nonpregnant values.)**
  a. A progressive **decrease** in both systolic (5–10 mm Hg) and diastolic (10–15 mm Hg) pressures occurs.
  b. After 24 weeks, systolic and diastolic pressures **gradually increase** and return to nonpregnancy levels by term.

4. **Venous pressure**
    a. **Central** venous pressure remains **unchanged** (10 cm H_2O).
    b. **Antecubital** venous pressure remains **unchanged.**
    c. **Lower extremity** pressure
        (1) **Femoral** venous pressure **increases** twofold to threefold by term (2–3 cm H_2O higher on the side where the placenta is implanted).
        (2) **Clinical syndromes resulting** from this pressure include dependent lower extremity edema, varicosities of the legs and the vulva, and hemorrhoids.
        (3) **Contributing factors** include venous stasis, increased venous pressure, and decreased intravascular oncotic pressure.
5. **PVR** equals BP divided by CO (BP ÷ CO).
    a. PVR markedly **decreases** in pregnancy, because BP decreases and CO increases.
    b. The PVR decrease is **mediated by** the smooth muscle–relaxing effect of **progesterone,** as well as heat production of the fetus.
6. **Control of vascular reactivity to pressor agents**
    a. Normal pregnant women **remain normotensive** despite a marked increase in plasma renin, angiotensin II, and aldosterone.
    b. Normal pregnant women are **refractory to the pressor effects of infused angiotensin II.** This blunted response is mediated by a relative increase in progesterone and prostacyclin along with a decrease in thromboxane.
    c. This **normal refractoriness is lost with preeclampsia,** a pregnancy-induced hypertension. This condition, which is unique to pregnant human females, is characterized by diffuse vasospasm that affects most organ systems (see Chapter 4 I).
        (1) **Clinical onset** is usually after 24 weeks' gestation.
        (2) **Incidence** is eight times higher in primigravidas.
        (3) The **triad of clinical findings** includes:
            (a) Persistent **hypertension** (increased systolic pressure ≥ 30 mm Hg, diastolic pressure ≥ 15 mm Hg, or ≥ 140/90 mm Hg on two or more occasions 6 hours apart or longer)
            (b) **Proteinuria** (≥ 300 mg/24 hr collection)
            (c) Clinically evident **edema** of the upper extremities and/or face.

F. **Hematologic changes** (Figure 1-11)
    1. **Plasma volume** increases 50% by term. The increase begins by 10 weeks' gestation and plateaus at 30 weeks' gestation. The increase is greater with multiple fetuses or larger fetuses.
    2. **Red blood cell (RBC)** mass increases 30% by term. The increase begins by 10 weeks' gestation and continues to term. The change results from greater erythrocyte production, not increased RBC life span. Mean corpuscular volume (MCV) increases slightly, with cells becoming more spherical (decreased diameter and increased thickness). The increase in RBC mass is smaller if iron is not supplemented.
    3. **Physiologic "anemia"** is a decreased hemoglobin value that results from a smaller increase in red blood cells than in plasma volume. This

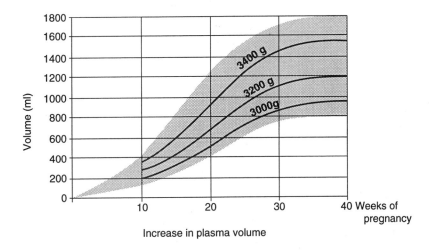

Figure 1-11. Increase in plasma volume during pregnancy. Note that the greater the plasma volume increase, the larger the fetal size. (Reprinted with permission from Hytten FE, Lind T: *Diagnostic Indices in Pregnancy.* Summit, NJ, CIBA-GEIGY Corporation, Medical Education Division, 1973, p 36.)

dilution effect reaches its nadir at 30 weeks' gestation, when plasma volume plateaus. It is not a true anemia because the oxygen-carrying capacity is increased (Figure 1-12).

4. **Benefits of increased blood volume** include:
   a. Meeting the physiologic demands of increased vascular system capacity and increased oxygen requirements of the fetus and placenta
   b. Offsetting the effects of decreased venous return with standing and supine positions
   c. Safeguarding the mother from blood loss during delivery, which can be > 500 ml with a vaginal delivery and > 1000 ml with a cesarean delivery
   d. Facilitating the dissipation of fetal heat production
   e. Providing for increased renal filtration of metabolic wastes

5. **Leukocytes and platelets**
   a. **White blood cells (WBCs),** mostly polymorphonuclear granulocytes, increase progressively during pregnancy.
      (1) During the **first trimester,** the mean WBC count is 9500/mm^3 (3000–15,000/mm^3).
      (2) During the **second and third trimesters,** the mean WBC count is 10,500/mm^3 (6000–16,000/mm^3).
      (3) During the **intrapartum period,** the WBC count may increase to 30,000/mm^3.
      (4) **By 1 week postpartum,** the levels have returned to normal nonpregnant values.
   b. **Platelets** slightly decrease from 275,000/mm^3 (< 20 weeks) to 260,000/mm^3 (> 35 weeks) because of increased peripheral destruction, although they remain in the normal range.

6. **Coagulation mechanism**
   a. **Pregnancy is a hypercoagulable state.**

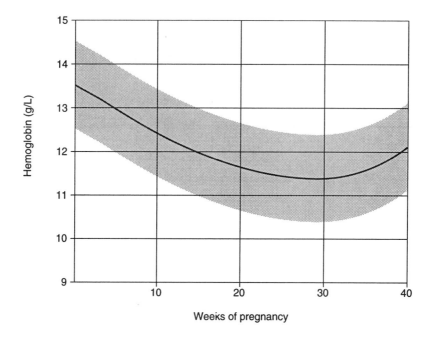

Figure 1-12. Hematologic changes during pregnancy: Decrease in the whole blood hemoglobin concentration. (Reprinted with permission from Hytten FE, Lind T: *Diagnostic Indices in Pregnancy*. Summit, NJ, CIBA-GEIGY Corporation, Medical Education Division, 1973, p 36–37.)

  (1) Fibrinogen (factor I) increases by 50% from 300 to 450 mg/dl.
  (2) Factors VII, VIII, IX, and X increase progressively throughout pregnancy.
 b. Thromboembolism is the number one cause of maternal mortality in the United States. The **relative risk** of thromboembolism, which changes over time, is:
  (1) **1.0 in the nonpregnant state**
  (2) **1.8 during pregnancy**
  (3) **5.5 during puerperium**
 c. Pathophysiology of increased thromboembolism risk in pregnancy, especially postpartum, involves:
  (1) **Increases in clotting factors**
  (2) **Venous stasis**
  (3) **Vessel wall injury**
7. Iron metabolism
 a. Iron is absorbed primarily from the proximal duodenum.
  (1) **Ferric** iron (from vegetable sources) must be converted to **ferrous** iron, which passes into mucosal cells and then is selectively released into the circulation.
  (2) The iron is bound to **transferrin** and is carried to the liver, spleen, and bone marrow, where it is incorporated into hemoglobin/myoglobin or stored as ferritin/hemosiderin.
  (3) Unabsorbed iron is excreted in sloughed-off mucosal cells.
 b. Variation in efficiency of iron absorption from mucosal cells.

The percentage of iron absorbed from a woman's GI tract varies depending on pregnancy and state of bone marrow iron stores.

(1) 10% in the normal nonpregnant state

(2) 20% in the normal pregnant state

(3) 40% in the iron-deficient pregnant state

c. **Iron requirements of pregnancy**

(1) The **mean daily requirement of elemental iron** for a normal pregnant woman is **3.5 mg.**

(2) The **total pregnancy iron requirement** is **1000 mg.** In pregnancy, iron is needed for **several purposes:**

(a) **500 mg** for **increased RBC mass**

(b) **300 mg** for **fetoplacental unit growth**

(c) **200 mg** for **daily iron losses**

(3) Most women have 500 mg of iron stored in their **bone marrow.**

(4) Most pregnant women benefit from **iron supplementation.**

(a) A **single dose of 60 mg** elemental iron per day (325 mg $FeSO_4$) **prevents** development of maternal iron-deficiency anemia but does not maintain or raise hemoglobin to nonpregnant values.

(b) Maternal iron deficiency does not jeopardize fetal iron stores because **active iron transport** occurs across a high placental concentration gradient **to the fetus.**

G. **Endocrine and metabolic changes**

1. **Thyroid gland** (Table 1-3)

a. The **size** of the **thyroid gland increases 15%** during pregnancy as a result of glandular hyperplasia and increased vascularity. The increase is usually not clinically detectable.

b. **Thyroid-binding globulin (TBG) increases** from estrogen stimulation of hepatic production. The increase results in the elevation of total and bound forms of triiodothyronine (T_3) and total thyroxine (T_4). However, the active unbound hormone forms remain unchanged (i.e., free T_3 and T_4, free T_4 index).

c. **Thyrotropin-releasing hormone (TRH) and thyroid-stimulating hormone (TSH)** are unchanged.

d. The following thyroid hormones **do not cross the placenta:** TBG, T_3, T_4, and TSH.

e. The following thyroid-related substances **do cross the placenta:**

(1) **Thyroid-stimulating immunoglobulin,** which can cause neonatal thyrotoxicosis

(2) **Antithyroid medications,** including propylthiouracil (PTU) and methimazole, which can cause neonatal hypothyroidism or goiter

(3) **TRH,** which can stimulate the fetal thyroid as well as enhance fetal pulmonary surfactant production

2. **Adrenal gland**

a. The **size** of the **adrenal gland does not** change in pregnancy.

b. **Total and free cortisol increase twofold to threefold.** Transcortin (cortisol-binding globulin) increases from estrogen-mediated increases in hepatic synthesis.

Table 1-3. Change in Thyroid-Related Moieties During Pregnancy

Thyroid Hormone	Changes in Pregnancy?	Crosses Placenta?
Free triiodothyronine (T₃)	No	No
Free thyroxine (T₄)	No	No
Total T₃	Increases	No
Total T₄	Increases	No
Free T₄ index	No	N/A
Thyroid-stimulating hormone (TSH)	No	No
Thyrotropin-releasing hormone (TRH)	No	Yes
Thyroxine-binding globulin (TBG)	Increases	No
Thyroid-stimulating immunoglobulin (TSI)	N/A	Yes
Propylthiouracil (PTU)	N/A	Yes
Methimazole	N/A	Yes

    c. Aldosterone secretion is markedly increased to offset the natriuretic effect of progesterone.

    d. Deoxycorticosterone levels markedly increase, largely from extra-adrenal conversion of progesterone in the kidney, the skin, and the blood vessels.

  3. Pancreas and fuel metabolism

    a. Hypertrophy, hyperplasia, and hypersecretion of β-cells occur.

    b. The **maternal response to fasting is accelerated starvation.** Fasting blood glucose is 15 mg/dl lower in pregnant women than in nonpregnant women because of the constant drain on maternal glucose by the fetoplacental unit.

      (1) Fasting insulin levels increase.

      (2) The starvation ketosis response is exaggerated. Levels of β-hydroxybutyric acid and acetoacetic acid increase.

    c. The **maternal responses to feeding** are prolonged hyperglycemia, hyperinsulinemia, and hypertriglyceridemia. These responses ensure a sustained supply of nutrients to the fetus.

      (1) Peripheral tissue resistance to insulin is suggested by:

        (a) Increased insulin response to glucose

        (b) Decreased peripheral uptake of glucose

        (c) Decreased glucagon response

      (2) The **mechanism of insulin resistance** includes:

        (a) Human placental lactogen (hPL)

        (b) Placental insulinase

        (c) Increased free cortisol

        (d) Increased progesterone

    d. Fetoplacental transport. Glucose is the primary metabolic fuel for the fetus. Fetal plasma glucose is 20 mg/dl lower than maternal values. **Hyperglycemia during embryogenesis is teratogenic.**

      (1) Insulin and glucagon do not cross the placenta.

      (2) The following substances **do cross the placenta:**

        (a) Glucose crosses by **facilitated diffusion,** which does not require energy but is carrier mediated.

        (b) Ketones cross by **simple diffusion.** Excessive levels of ketones may pose a fetal hazard.

        (c) Amino acids cross by **active transport.**

        (d) Free fatty acids cross by **simple diffusion.**

4. Pituitary gland

    a. The **increase in size** of the pituitary gland during pregnancy is caused by the proliferation of chromophobe cells in the anterior pituitary gland. The pituitary gland size increases from 45% by 12 weeks of pregnancy to 100% by term.

    b. Sheehan's syndrome is postpartum **ischemic necrosis of the anterior pituitary gland,** which is caused by hypotensive shock from severe postpartum hemorrhage. There are varying degrees of hypopituitarism. The characteristic clinical picture is **failure to lactate** because of decreased prolactin production. Late onset may occur, with a mean delay of 7 years.

Review Test

Directions: Each of the numbered items or incomplete statements in this section is followed by answers or by completions of the statement. Select the ONE lettered answer or completion that is BEST in each case.

1. The sensory pain fibers to the uterus pass through which one of the following ligaments?

(A) Broad ligament
(B) Round ligament
(C) Cardinal ligament
(D) Uterosacral ligament
(E) Uterovesical ligament

2. The relative orientation of the ureter to the uterine artery (at the point where they meet) is which of the following positions?

(A) Superior and posterior
(B) Lateral and deep
(C) Inferior and posterior
(D) Medial and superficial
(E) Superior and anterior

3. Which one of the following muscles is the most significant component of the female levator muscle sling?

(A) Pubococcygeus
(B) Puborectalis
(C) Iliococcygeus
(D) Pubovaginalis
(E) Piriformis

4. Which one of the following statements regarding the transformation zone (T-zone) is correct?

(A) It is covered by columnar epithelium
(B) It normally extends onto the vaginal fornices
(C) It forms in the second month of fetal development
(D) It is histologically described as adenosis
(E) It develops through the process of squamous metaplasia

5. The regeneration of the endometrial lining arises from which one of the following layers?

(A) Zona basalis
(B) Zona pellucidum
(C) Zona compacta
(D) Zona functionalis
(E) Zona spongiosa

6. The follicular phase of the menstrual cycle is characterized by

(A) predictable length
(B) progesterone dominance
(C) edematous endometrial stroma
(D) intense endometrial mitotic activity
(E) tortuous endometrial glands

7. At which time in prenatal female development are the gonadal germ cells the maximum number?

(A) 5 weeks
(B) 10 weeks
(C) 20 weeks
(D) 30 weeks
(E) 40 weeks

8. Which of the following statements regarding first and second reductional divisions of the female germ cells is true? They

(A) involve only primary oocytes
(B) result in a chromosome number of 23
(C) occur prior to fertilization
(D) produce the second polar body
(E) are dependent on rising progesterone levels

9. Which of the following statements regarding the gastrointestinal (GI) tract in pregnancy is correct? It results in

(A) increased motilin levels
(B) decreased gastric residual volume
(C) increased gastroesophageal sphincter tone
(D) increased peptic ulcer disease
(E) increased reflux esophagitis

10. Which of the following statements regarding changes in the venous system in pregnancy is true?

(A) Central venous pressure increases slightly
(B) Femoral venous pressure increases markedly
(C) Intravascular oncotic pressure increases
(D) Femoral venous flow increases
(E) Vulvar varicosities improve

Directions: Each of the numbered items or incomplete statements in this section is negatively phrased, as indicated by a capitalized word such as NOT, LEAST, or EXCEPT. Select ONE lettered answer or completion that is BEST in each case.

11. Which of the following structures does NOT derive at least partial blood supply from the uterine artery?

(A) Oviduct
(B) Bladder
(C) Ovary
(D) Cervix
(E) Fundus

12. All of the following statements about the ovarian vessels are true EXCEPT

(A) the left ovarian artery originates from the descending aorta
(B) the left ovarian vein drains into the left renal vein
(C) the blood supply to the ovaries is solely from the ovarian artery
(D) the ovarian arteries course through the infundibulopelvic ligament
(E) the right ovarian vein drains into the inferior vena cava

13. All of the following provide support to the vagina EXCEPT the

(A) perineal body
(B) pelvic diaphragm
(C) cardinal ligament
(D) uterosacral ligament
(E) infundibulopelvic ligament

14. All of the following statements about the corpus luteum are true EXCEPT that it

(A) is the primary source of progesterone in nonpregnant women
(B) is initially stimulated by anterior pituitary luteinizing hormone (LH)
(C) may result in a functional ovarian cystic structure
(D) is maintained by human chorionic gonadotropin (hCG) if pregnancy occurs
(E) can occur independently of ovulation

15. All of the following regarding respiratory gas exchange in pregnancy are true EXCEPT

(A) decrease in oxygen consumption
(B) increase in alveolar/arterial PO_2
(C) decrease in alveolar/arterial PCO_2
(D) increased pH
(E) increase in minute ventilation

16. All of the following statements regarding the anatomy and physiology of the heart in pregnancy are true EXCEPT

(A) the heart is displaced upward and to the left in the chest
(B) the baseline heart rate (HR) is increased
(C) the stroke volume (SV) is increased
(D) there is a normal diastolic murmur along the left sternal border
(E) there is normal left axis deviation on electrocardiogram

17. All of the following statements are true regarding the beneficial effects of increased blood volume in pregnancy EXCEPT

(A) it meets physiologic demands of increased vascular system capacity
(B) it offsets the effects of decreased venous return while in standing posture
(C) it safeguards the mother from delivery blood loss
(D) it facilitates dissipation of fetal heat production
(E) it enhances renal reabsorption of metabolic wastes

Directions: The set of matching questions in this section consists of a list of four to twenty-six lettered options (some of which may be in figures) followed by several numbered items. For each numbered item, select ONE lettered option that is most closely associated with it. To avoid spending too much time on matching sets with large numbers of options, it is generally advisable to begin each set by reading the list of options. Then, for each item in the set, try to generate the correct answer and locate it in the option list, rather than evaluating each option individually. Each lettered option may be selected once, more than once, or not at all.

Questions 18–22

For each of the female genital structures listed, select the most closely associated male homologue.
(A) Penis
(B) Prostate
(C) Scrotum
(D) Penile urethra
(E) Cowper's glands
(F) Vas deferens
(G) Seminiferous tubules

18. Labia majora

19. Labia minora

20. Clitoris

21. Skene's glands

22. Bartholin's glands

Answers and Explanations

1. The answer is D [I A 3, 7].

Provision of satisfactory obstetric and gynecologic anesthesia is predicated on understanding the nervous innervation of the pelvic organs. The uterosacral ligaments contain the sensory fibers to the uterus. The uterosacral ligaments are located posterior and inferior to the uterocervical junction, dividing to pass on either side of the rectum. They are derived from inferior posterior folds of peritoneum from the broad ligaments. The afferent pain fibers from the uterus pass through the uterosacral ligaments and involve the T10–L1 nerve roots. These nerves consist primarily of nerve bundles from the inferior hypogastric plexus.

2. The answer is C [I D].

The ureter passes inferiorly and posteriorly under the uterine artery as it courses toward the bladder. The uterine artery is like a "bridge" over the "water" of the ureter. This relationship is important to remember when performing pelvic surgery.

3. The answer is A [I H].

The pubococcygeus muscle is the predominant muscle of the levator muscle sling. The levator ani muscles form the floor of the pelvis and the roof of the perineum. Two to four components arise from different origins along the sides of the pelvis, but all insert in either the sacrococcygeal ligament or the fusion of fibers posterior to the organ they support. The most important is the pubococcygeus that extends from the pubis all the way to the coccyx and serves to flex the coccyx bone. The puborectalis functions as a sling to constrict the rectum, and the pubovaginalis does the same for the vagina. The iliococcygeus forms the lateral and more posterior aspect of the pelvic diaphragm. The pyriformis muscle is not part of the pelvic diaphragm.

4. The answer is E [II A 3].

The transformation zone (T-zone) is the area between the original squamocolumnar (SC) junction and the new SC junction. The original columnar epithelium is being replaced by stratified squamous epithelium through the process of squamous metaplasia. The T-zone normally is found only on the cervix (not on the vaginal fornices), and it develops postnatally. Adenosis refers to persistent areas of columnar epithelium that remain on the vagina.

5. The answer is A [II B 1 b].

The new endometrial lining arises from the zona basalis. Zona functionalis is incorrect, because it refers to the superficial endometrium that sloughs off with each menstrual cycle. Zona pellucidum is incorrect, because it is part of the follicle unrelated to the endometrium. Zona compacta and zona spongiosa are incorrect, because they are the two specific layers that constitute the zona functionalis.

6. The answer is D [II B 2 a].

The initial part of the cycle after the menses is the proliferative or follicular phase. The histologic finding of the follicular phase is intense endometrial mitotic activity. The follicular phase is of variable length not predictable length, and it is characterized by dominance of estrogen, not progesterone. Histologically, the endometrial glands of the follicular phase are straight and tubular with compact stroma rather than being tortuous with edematous stroma.

7. The answer is C [II D 1 c].

The germ cells reach their maximum number of 7 million by 20 weeks' gestation. The germ cells that migrate from the yolk sac have barely reached the genital ridge by 5 weeks' gestation. At 10 weeks, the germ cells are rapidly multiplying. The germ cells gradually undergo involution until 1.5 million are left at term.

8. The answer is B [II D 4 a].

The first reductional division occurs just prior to ovulation, with 46 chromosomes becoming 23 after producing the first polar body. The second reductional division occurs after fertilization, producing a second polar body with the number of chromosomes remaining at 23. The reductional divisions involve only secondary oocytes.

9. The answer is E [IV A 3 d].

The incidence of reflux esophagitis increases during pregnancy because of the effect of gastric acid entering and irritating the esophagus through the incompetent gastroesophageal sphincter. Motilin levels, gastroesophageal sphincter tone, and peptic ulcer disease all decrease in pregnancy, and gastric residual volume increases. Many of these changes are mediated by the smooth muscle–relaxing effect of the high levels of progesterone in pregnancy.

10. The answer is B [IV E 4].

The increased blood volume, along with vascular dilation from the smooth muscle–relaxing effect of progesterone on the blood vessel walls, results in a venous stasis and an increase in lower extremity and lower body venous pressure. Thus, marked increase in femoral venous pressure is the correct answer. The central venous pressure remains unchanged, whereas the intravascular oncotic pressure and femoral venous flow decrease. Vulvar varicosities almost always predictably worsen. Vulvar varicosities and hemorrhoids are common sequelae in pregnancy.

11. The answer is B [I C 2].

The arterial blood supply to the oviduct and ovary involve an anastomosis from the ascending branch of the uterine artery. The cervix derives its blood supply from the descending branch of the uterine artery. The fundus of the uterus receives its blood supply from the main branch of the uterine artery. Therefore, all of the organs, with the exception of the bladder, derive (at least in part) from the uterine artery. The blood supply to the bladder arises from the superior, middle, and inferior vesicle arteries coming from branches of the hypogastric artery.

12. The answer is C [I C 2].

The ovarian arterial blood supply is dual from both the ascending branch of the uterine artery and from the ovarian artery passing through the infundibulopelvic ligament. The ovarian artery is the chief source of blood for the ovary. All of the other statements are true. The veins follow the course of the arteries to a great extent.

13. The answer is E [I C, E 4].

Pelvic prolapse, particularly of the vagina, is a common problem addressed by pelvic surgeons. The infundibulopelvic ligament provides support only to the ovary, not the vagina. The vagina is supported in its lower third by the pelvic diaphragm, urogenital diaphragm, and perineal body; in its middle third by the pelvic diaphragm and cardinal ligaments; and in its upper third by the cardinal ligaments and uterosacral ligaments.

14. The answer is E [II D 6].

The corpus luteum develops in the ovary at the site of the extrusion of the egg at ovulation. Initially the ovulation site fills with blood forming a corpus hemorrhagicum. The corpus hemorrhagicum is then invaded by proliferating granulosa and theca cells, which form the corpus luteum. Therefore, the corpus luteum is dependent on ovulation; it does not arise independently. The corpus luteum is the main site of progesterone production both in the nonpregnant state as well as during the first 8 weeks of pregnancy until the placental production is adequate. Ovulation, and subsequently the appearance of the corpus luteum, is initially triggered by the luteinizing hormone (LH) surge. Maintenance of function in early pregnancy is from human chorionic gonadotropin (hCG) produced by the early trophoblast.

15. The answer is A [IV B 4 d].

The respiratory exchange of gases in pregnancy undergoes significant change. Oxygen consumption increases during pregnancy, primarily because of the increased demands of the fetoplacental unit. With the increased tidal volume (TV) and minute ventilation in pregnancy, the PO_2 levels increase, and the PCO_2 levels decrease. This results in a partially compensated respiratory alkalosis and a slightly increased pH. These changes are adaptations to the increased need for oxygen, and they allow optimum oxygenation of the fetoplacental unit.

16. The answer is D [IV E 1 b].

Pregnancy brings about major changes in the work load of the heart. Diastolic murmurs are never normal in pregnancy. However, a mid-cycle, diamond-shaped systolic flow murmur along the left sternal border is normal because of increased blood volume. The elevation of the diaphragm from the enlarging uterus results in a displacement of the heart upward and to the left in the chest. This can result in a physiologic left axis deviation on an electrocardiogram. The rise in heart rate (HR) and stroke volume (SV) are necessary to allow the cardiac output (CO) to increase appropriately to meet the increased metabolic demands of pregnancy.

17. The answer is E [IV F 1].

Plasma volume increases up to 50% in pregnancy, with the changes occurring early in the first trimester. This serves many important physiologic functions. The increased plasma volume and cardiac output (CO) result in increased renal blood flow and increased glomerular filtration and clearance (not reabsorption) of metabolic wastes.

18–22. The answers are: 18-C [I G 2], **19-D** [I G 3], **20-A** [I G 4], **21-B** [I G 6], **22-E** [I G 7].

The labia majora are the female homologue of the male scrotum. Labia minora are the female homologue of the male penile urethra. The clitoris is the female homologue of the male penis. The Skene's glands are the female homologue of the male prostate. The Bartholin's glands are the female homologue of the male Cowper's glands.

2
Pregnancy: Prenatal Care and Assessment

I. PRENATAL CARE

A. Purposes

1. **General.** Prenatal care aims to have every wanted pregnancy result in the delivery of a healthy infant by a healthy mother.

2. **Specific.** Prenatal care aims to prevent or manage conditions that cause poor pregnancy outcomes.

   a. **Premature delivery is the most significant cause of perinatal morbidity and mortality** (see Chapter 6 V).

   b. Intrauterine growth restriction (IUGR) [see IV B]

   c. Congenital malformations and birth defects (see III)

   d. Hypertensive disorders of pregnancy (see Chapter 4 I)

   e. Glucose intolerance in pregnancy (see Chapter 4 VIII)

   f. Perinatal infections (see Chapter 5)

   g. Postdates pregnancy (see V)

B. Definitions of perinatal vital statistics. (For each statistic, note whether the denominator is **live** or **total** births.)

1. **Birth rate** is the number of live births per 1000 **total** population.

2. **Fertility rate** is the number of live births per 1000 women between the ages of 15 and 44 years.

3. **Maternal mortality** is the death of a woman from any cause during pregnancy or within 90 days of delivery (Figure 2-1). **The most common cause is thromboembolism.**

4. **Maternal mortality rate** is the number of maternal deaths per 100,000 **live** births.

5. **Fetal mortality (stillborn) rate** is the number of fetal deaths ($\geq$ 20 weeks) per 1000 **total** births.

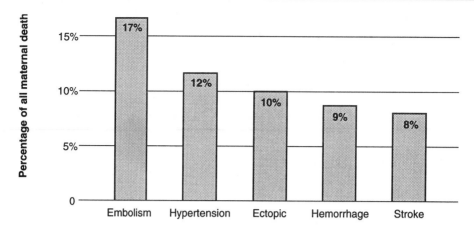

Figure 2-1. Major causes of maternal deaths in the United States. (Reprinted with permission from Cunningham FG, MacDonald PC, Gant NF, et al (eds): *Williams' Obstetrics,* 19th ed. East Norwalk, CT, Appleton & Lange, 1993, p 4.)

6. **Neonatal mortality rate** is the number of newborn deaths during the first 28 days of life per 1000 **live** births.

7. **Perinatal mortality rate** is the combination of fetal and neonatal death rates per 1000 **total** births (Figure 2-2).

8. **Infant mortality rate** is the number of infant deaths during the first year of life per 1000 **live** births.

C. **Review of clinical approach**

1. **Thorough obstetric history**

a. Identify **previous pregnancies** in chronologic order, noting complications and the following specific details:

(1) **Date and location**

(2) **Duration of pregnancy in weeks**

(3) **Pregnancy outcome**

(a) Spontaneous abortion (i.e., miscarriage < 20 weeks)

(b) Induced abortion (i.e., intentional pregnancy termination < 20 weeks)

(c) Spontaneous vaginal delivery (i.e., without forceps or vacuum extractor)

(d) Operative vaginal delivery (i.e., forceps or vacuum extractor used)

(e) Cesarean delivery (note the type of uterine incision)

(4) **Analgesia/anesthesia:** narcotics, epidural/caudal, local, pudendal, and general anesthesia

(5) **Newborn information**

(a) Gender

(b) Weight

(c) **Apgar score.** This system utilizes a five-point scoring system in which scores range from 0 to 10 points total, with 0, 1, or 2

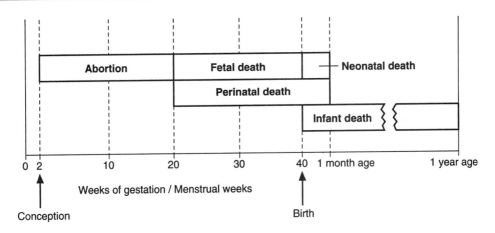

Figure 2-2. Perinatal mortality terminology.

points for each of the five following parameters: **skin color, heart rate, respirations, grimace, and muscle tone.** The lowest score is 0, and the highest score is 10. Points are assigned at 1 minute and 5 minutes. The 1-minute score indicates the type of resuscitation needed. The 5-minute score correlates with long-term outcome.

(d) Occurrence of anomalies. The organ systems most commonly involved are the central nervous system (CNS), genitourinary (GU), and gastrointestinal (GI) systems.

(e) Length of hospital stay

b. Menstrual history should be obtained. Estimated delivery date (EDD) is obtained using **Naegele's rule:** EDD = LMP − 3 months + 7 days, where LMP = last menstrual period. For example, if the LMP is July 20, 1999, then the EDD is April 27, 2000. Naegele's rule assumes a 28-day cycle, so the EDD must be adjusted according to the duration of the preovulatory phase.

(1) The EDD is **earlier** if the woman has a shorter preovulatory phase.

(2) The EDD is **later** if the woman has a longer preovulatory phase.

c. Contraceptive history. The woman should be asked the following questions:

(1) Was the pregnancy planned or unplanned?

(2) Did the patient ever have complications using oral contraceptives or an intrauterine device (IUD)?

d. Medical history. The woman should be asked if she currently has or has ever had any of the following disorders:

(1) Seizure disorder. Determine the onset, workup, type of seizures, medications, and dosage.

(2) Diabetes mellitus (DM). Determine whether the woman has type I or type II, if there is end-organ disease, and judge the degree of glycemic control.

(3) Hypertension. Determine the onset, workup, antihypertensive medications, and whether there is renal or retinal involvement.

(4) Renal disease. Determine the onset, workup, and status of renal function studies.

e. Surgical history. Ask the woman whether she has had any abdominal or pelvic procedures (e.g., resulting in pelvic adhesions) or pelvic fractures (e.g., resulting in a contracted pelvis).

f. Social history should be determined.

(1) Lifestyle habits

(a) Smoking. How long has the woman been smoking, and how many cigarettes does she smoke per day?

(b) Alcohol. How long has the woman has been drinking alcohol, how many drinks per day, and what type of beverages does she normally consume? Also determine what, if any, and how many drinks the mother consumed around the time of conception.

(c) Controlled substances. Does the woman use any medications or illegal drugs? What is the duration and extent of the use or abuse?

(2) Social support/marital status. Is the woman married? Is she a victim of domestic violence or abuse? What is the duration, extent, and nature of that abuse?

(3) Employment/occupation

(a) Physical work demands. Does the woman have to do any heavy lifting or prolonged standing at work? Is she exposed to loud noises?

(b) Exposure to teratogens. Is the woman exposed to radiation (e.g., x-rays) or chemicals at work?

(4) Educational level. How many years did the woman attend school?

2. Thorough physical and pelvic examination

a. General physical examination

(1) The following **baseline parameters** should be obtained:

(a) Prepregnancy weight (PPW)

(b) Current weight

(c) Height

(d) Blood pressure (BP)

(2) Specific organ systems are evaluated through the following examinations.

(a) Funduscopic examination of eyes

(b) Breast examination

(c) Cardiac examination

(d) Lung examination

(e) Abdominal examination

b. Pelvic examination

(1) The **external genitalia, vagina, and cervix** should be inspected.

(2) Bacterial vaginosis (BV) screening should be performed by:

(a) Assessing if vaginal pH exceeds 4.5

(b) Examining vaginal discharge for "clue cells" (see Chapter 8 IV C 5)

(3) Papanicolaou (Pap) smear of exfoliated cells from the ecto-cervix and endocervix should be obtained.

(4) Screening culture/specimens should be obtained and tested for the following:

  (a) Gonorrhea from the endocervix

  (b) Chlamydia from the endocervix

  (c) Group B β-hemolytic streptococcus from the vagina (controversial; see Chapter 5 VIII)

(5) The **cervix, uterus, and adnexae should be palpated.** Uterine diameter (in cm) on bimanual pelvic examination should approximate the number of weeks' gestation up to 12 weeks.

(6) Clinical pelvimetry can be performed, although it is not done universally (Figure 2-3).

  (a) The **pelvic inlet** is assessed by measuring the **diagonal conjugate.** The lower pubic border to the sacral promontory is measured.

  (b) The **midpelvis** is assessed by measuring the **bi-ischial diameter.** The ischial spines, sacrospinous ligaments, and sacrosciatic notch are palpated.

  (c) The **pelvic outlet** is assessed by measuring the angle of the **pubic arch.** The subpubic arch should be assessed, and the ischial tuberosities should be palpated.

  c. Abdominal examination and fundal measurement. After 20 weeks, the fundus should measure (in cm) the number of gestational weeks (Figure 2-4).

3. Four Leopold maneuvers are performed through careful palpation of the fetus through the maternal abdominal wall. They are designed to answer the following questions (Figure 2-5):

  a. First maneuver: What fetal part is in the fundus?

  b. Second maneuver: On which side are the fetal back or small parts located?

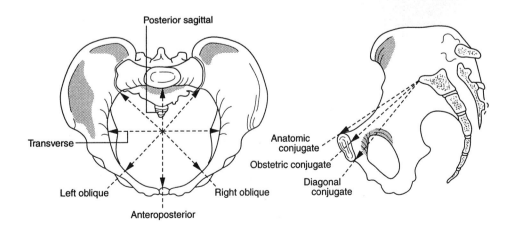

Figure 2-3. Pelvic inlet with diameters. (Reprinted with permission from Hacker NF, Moore JG (eds): *Essentials of Obstetrics and Gynecology,* 2nd ed. Philadelphia, W.B. Saunders, 1992, p 113.)

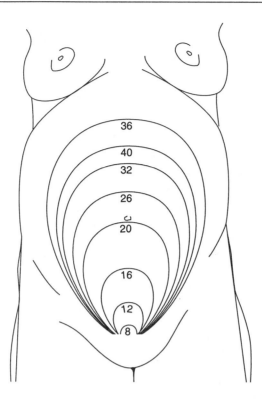

Figure 2-4. Fundal measurement and number of weeks gestation. (After Scott JR, DiSaia PJ, Hammond CB, et al (eds): *Danforth's Obstetrics and Gynecology,* 6th ed. Philadelphia, J.B. Lippincott, 1990, p 135.)

    c. Third maneuver: To what degree has the presenting part descended into the pelvis?

    d. Fourth maneuver: On which side is the cephalic prominence located?

4. **Prenatal laboratory tests** (Table 2-1) are designed to improve the pregnancy outcome of both mother and fetus/neonate.

    a. Identify and correct conditions that could jeopardize maternal well-being: anemia (cell profile); urinary tract infection (UTI) [urinalysis and culture]; sickle cell disease (sickle cell prep); tuberculosis (TB) [TB skin test]

    b. Identify and treat conditions that could jeopardize fetal well-being: isoimmunization (atypical antibody screen); gestational diabetes (glucose screen); syphilis (serology); human immunodeficiency virus (HIV) [HIV screen]

    c. Identify opportunities for primary prevention of diseases through immunization of mother and/or neonate: Rh isoimmunization (blood type and Rh status); rubella (rubella antibody screen); hepatitis B carrier (hepatitis B surface antigen screen)

    d. Screen for fetal anomalies: maternal serum α-fetoprotein (MSAFP); triple marker screen

5. **Diagnosis of pregnancy**

    a. Presumptive signs include the following:

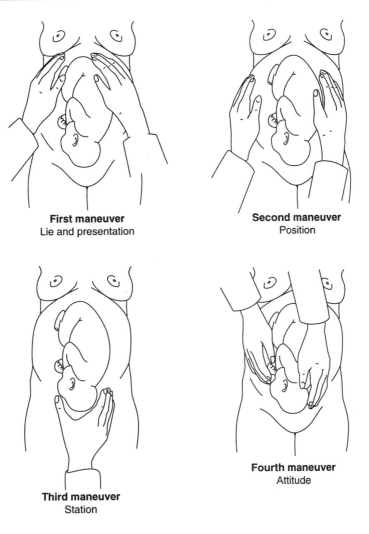

Figure 2-5. Leopold maneuvers and the specific aspect of fetal orientation in the uterus that can be determined. (Reprinted with permission from Beckmann CR, Ling FW, Barzansky BM, et al (eds): *Obstetrics and Gynecology,* 2nd ed. Baltimore, Williams & Wilkins, 1995, p 171.)

(1) Cessation of menses

(2) Breast tenderness and swelling

(3) Nausea and vomiting

(4) Changes in the skin and mucous membranes

    (a) Chadwick's sign, which is discoloration of the vulva, vaginal walls, and cervix

    (b) Increased skin pigmentation

    (c) Development of abdominal striae

b. Probable signs include the following:

    (1) Physical changes in the uterus

        (a) Uterine enlargement

        (b) Hegar's sign, which is softening between the fundus and the cervix

        (c) Uterine contractions

Table 2-1. Prenatal Laboratory Testing

Test	When Performed	Purpose of Test	Normal Finding	Management of Abnormal
ROUTINE*				
Pap smear	First prenatal visit[†]	Early diagnosis of CIN	No dysplasia (repeat at scheduled routine interval)	Colposcopy (with possible biopsy) to rule out invasive CA
Cell profile	First prenatal visit[†]	Early diagnosis of anemia	Hgb ≥ 10 mg/dl (routine iron supplementation)	Identify etiology and treat
Urine screen	First prenatal visit	Diagnosis of asymptomatic bacteriuria	Negative culture (observation)	Treat with appropriate antibiotics, then reculture
Blood type and Rh	First prenatal visit	Identify if at risk for Rh isoimmunization	Rh+ (no further testing)	Administer RhoGam as indicated
Atypical antibody screen	First prenatal visit	Identify if isoimmunization has taken place	Negative (repeat before RhoGam at 28 weeks)	Identify antibody type Assess if father is antigen + Titer the antibody
Syphilis serology	First prenatal visit	Identify possible maternal syphilis	Nonreactive (no further testing)	Perform treponema specific test (FTA-ABS or MHA-TP), then initiate appropriate antibiotic treatment
Rubella antibody titer	First prenatal visit[†]	Identify if susceptible to rubella infection	> 1:8 or > 1.0 (no further testing needed)	Avoid exposure to known/ suspected rubella Postpartum active rubella immunization
Glucola screen (1 hr 50 g)	First prenatal visit (if meet criteria) otherwise at 24–28 wks	Identify possible gestational diabetes	< 140 mg/dl (no further testing)	Administer 3-hr, 100-g OGTT
Hepatitis B surface antigen	First prenatal visit	Identify HBV carriers and those with possible active hepatitis	Negative HBsAg (repeat at 28 weeks if risk factors present)	Obtain liver function tests Obtain complete hepatitis panel Offer vaccination to household members and sexual contacts Neonatal active and passive immunization
COMMONLY PERFORMED				
Maternal Serum α-fetoprotein (MS-AFP)	15–19 weeks	Screen for neural tube defect and Down syndrome	> 0.8 MoM < 2.5 MoM	Sonogram to assess gestational age, fetal number, and structural anomalies
Triple marker screen	15–19 weeks	Screen for Down syndrome	All values within expected range for gestational age	Sonogram to assess gestational age, fetal number, and structural anomalies
Tuberculin skin test	First prenatal visit[†]	Screen for TB	Induration < 10 mm	Chest radiograph to identify active disease, then antibiotic if TB is present
SELECTED				
Sickle cell test	First prenatal visit[†]	Screen for sickle cell disease	Negative	Hemoglobin electrophoresis
Toxoplasmosis antibody	Maternal mononucleosis-like syndrome	Evaluate for toxoplasmosis susceptibility	No evidence of seroconversion	Fetal blood sampling, then pyrimethamine and sulfadiazine if infection is confirmed

CIN = cervical intraepithelial neoplasia; *CA* = carcinoma; *Hgb* = hemoglobin; *OGTT* = oral glucose tolerance test; *FTA-ABS* = fluorescent antibody absorption test; *MHA-TP* = microhemagglutination assay for *T. pallidum; MoM* = multiple of median; *HBV* = hepatitis B virus, *HBsAg* = hepatitis B surface antigen; *TB* = tuberculosis.

(2) Palpation of "fetal parts"

c. **Positive signs** include the following:

(1) Auscultation of **fetal heart tones**

(2) Recognition of **fetal movement** by external examiner

(3) Imaging of fetus by **radiograph**

(4) Imaging of fetus by **sonogram**

6. **Subsequent prenatal care**

a. **Weight gain** should be monitored.

(1) **Recommendations** are based on a percentage of the mother's PPW relative to her ideal body weight (IBW). IBW is calculated by starting with 100 pounds for the first 5 feet of height, then adding or subtracting 5 pounds for each inch above or below 100 pounds.

(a) **Low PPW** (< 90% IBW): **gain of 30–40 pounds**

(b) **Average PPW** (90%–135% IBW): **gain of 25–30 pounds**

(c) **High PPW** (> 135% IBW): **gain of 15–20 pounds**

(2) **Failure to gain weight** suggests:

(a) **Dehydration** (e.g., from severe hyperemesis)

(b) Severe anorexia or bulimia

(c) Fetal death

(d) Fetal growth restriction

(e) Oligohydramnios

(3) **Excessive weight gain** suggests:

(a) **Fluid retention** (e.g., from preeclampsia)

(b) Gestational diabetes

b. **Urine glucose and protein measurements,** although frequently performed routinely, are of questionable value.

c. **BP** normally decreases early in pregnancy. However, an upward trend may signify preeclampsia.

d. **Fundal measurement.** After 20 weeks, the fundus is measured in centimeters from the symphysis pubis. If the measurement is 3 cm (or more) greater or less than expected, further evaluation is needed (see IV).

e. **Fetal heart rate (FHR)** is normally 110–160 beats/min.

f. **Frequency of return visits for normal pregnancy**

(1) Every 4 weeks up to less than 32 weeks

(2) Every 2 weeks between 32–36 weeks

(3) Every 1 week after 36 weeks to delivery

7. **Patient education**

a. **Exercise.** The woman may continue exercise at her prepregnancy level, but she should not begin aggressive activities once pregnant. Concerns exist regarding the teratogenic effects of maternal hyperthermia and the shunting of blood away from the uterus to vital organs.

b. **Work.** Heavy physical work should be limited, and stress should be minimized.

c. **Sexual intercourse** is generally **safe in pregnancy** without restriction unless there is risk of incompetent cervix, preterm labor, premature membrane rupture, or placenta previa.

    d. Danger signs that the patient should be aware of include:

      (1) Pelvic complaints

        (a) Vaginal bleeding, which could signify spontaneous abortion, placenta previa, or abruptio placentae

        (b) Vaginal leakage of fluid, which could signify rupture of membranes

      (2) Abdominal complaints

        (a) Epigastric pain, which occurs in women who have severe preeclampsia

        (b) Uterine cramping, which occurs in women undergoing preterm labor

        (c) Decreased fetal movements, which occur when the fetus is in jeopardy

        (d) Persistent vomiting (i.e., hyperemesis)

      (3) Swelling (fingers or face), which occurs in women who have preeclampsia

      (4) Cerebral disturbances (e.g., dizziness, mental confusion, visual disturbances, persistent headache), which occur in women who have severe preeclampsia

      (5) Urinary complaints (e.g., painful urination, decreased urine output), which may signify cystitis or pyelonephritis

      (6) Chills or fever, which can occur in women who have pyelonephritis or chorioamnionitis

    e. Seatbelt use. Wearing seatbelts, with or without the shoulder harness, **is recommended,** with the lap belt low under the uterine fundus. In motor vehicle accidents during pregnancy, fetal outcome is equally poor with or without seatbelts, but maternal outcome is significantly improved with seatbelt use.

II. ANTEPARTUM FETAL ASSESSMENT

  A. General purposes of fetal monitoring

    1. Identifying potential fetal compromise to avoid morbidity or mortality and allow successful intervention

    2. Assessing fetal well-being in high-risk conditions such as:

      a. Insulin-dependent DM

      b. Postdates pregnancy

      c. Chronic hypertension

      d. IUGR

      e. Previous unexplained stillbirth

  B. Fetal movement counting

    1. Assumptions

      a. An adequately **oxygenated** fetus moves its body and limbs.

      b. As the fetus becomes **compromised,** fetal movements gradually diminish.

      c. The mother's **perception** of fetal movement is accurate.

  d. Identification of decreased movement occurs early enough to allow **intervention.**

 2. Method. When the gestational age of **fetal viability** is reached (approximately 24 weeks), the mother is instructed to keep daily records of fetal movement. Starting at 8 A.M., the mother notes the time required for 10 fetal movements. The count is abnormal if 10 movements do not occur in 12 hours, or if it takes twice as long for 10 movements to occur as it did 1 week earlier.

 3. Interpretation

  a. Normal fetal movement counts are highly reassuring of fetal well-being.

  b. Abnormal counts are **poor predictors** of fetal compromise. A non-compromised fetus is found in 80% of cases. However, in 20% of cases, a fetus is identified that eventually dies if there is no intervention. In 50% of those cases, fetal compromise is revealed with further testing. Tests that are performed include the nonstress test (NST; see II C), the contraction stress test (CST), and the biophysical profile (BPP) [Table 2-2].

 4. Recommendation

  a. The **next step in management** with abnormal fetal movements is to perform an **NST.**

  b. Fetal movement counting is helpful for **adjunctive fetal assessment in normal patients.** It is not adequate for primary fetal screening in high-risk populations.

Table 2-2. Antepartum Fetal Testing

	Fetal Kick Count	Nonstress Test (NST)	Contraction Stress Test (CST)	Biophysical Profile (BPP)
Technology required	None	EFM	EFM	Ultrasound
Parameter observed	Maternal perception of fetal movement	FHR accelerations	Late decelerations	Breathing movements Gross body movements Flexion-extension Amniotic fluid NST
Normal test (reassuring)	Adequate movements	Reactive	Negative	Negative
Abnormal test (nonreassuring)	Decreased movements	Nonreactive	Positive	Positive
% Tests falsely abnormal	80%	80%	50%	30%

EFM = electronic fetal monitor; *FHR* = fetal heart rate; *acceleration* = rise in baseline FHR of ≥ 15 beats/minute and lasting ≥ 15 seconds; *late deceleration* = gradual drop in FHR with gradual FHR return to baseline after end of contraction.

C. **Nonstress test (NST).** Any electronic fetal monitor strip with a FHR tracing can be evaluated for NST criteria.

1. **Assumptions** are based on the presence or absence of FHR accelerations.

   a. An adequately **oxygenated** fetus moves its body and limbs.

   b. **FHR accelerations** are associated with fetal movements **after 30 weeks'** gestation and indicate a normally functioning uteroplacental unit. A **lack of FHR accelerations** may occur with any of the following:

      (1) Too early a gestational age (< 30 weeks)

      (2) Fetal sleeping

      (3) Fetal CNS anomalies

      (4) Maternal sedative or narcotic administration

      (5) Fetal hypoxia in a minority of cases

2. **Method.** The external fetal cardiotocograph and contraction monitor is placed on the mother's abdomen, and the mother is positioned to **avoid supine hypotension.** Fetal movements and FHR are recorded (see Table 2-2). **FHR accelerations** are defined as an **increase of 15 beats/min or more over baseline** and an acceleration **duration of 15 seconds or more.**

3. **Interpretation.** NSTs can be interpreted as **reactive, nonreactive,** or **unsatisfactory** (Figure 2-6).

   a. **Reactive** (see Figure 2-6A). Two accelerations noted in a 20-minute interval are reassuring for fetal well-being. The fetal death rate is 3 per 1000 within 1 week after a reactive NST.

   b. **Nonreactive** (see Figure 2-6B). If any of the following criteria are met, fetal well-being cannot be assured. However, a nonreactive NST is a poor predictor of fetal compromise, because there is an 80% false-nonreactive rate. The criteria for **nonreactivity** may include any or all of the following:

      (1) Number of accelerations too few

      (2) FHR < 15 beats/min

      (3) Duration of accelerations < 15 seconds

   c. **Unsatisfactory.** The quality of the FHR tracing is technically inadequate to assess the criteria.

4. **Recommendations**

   a. **If the NST is reactive, fetal well-being is assured.** The test should be repeated weekly or biweekly.

   b. **If the NST is nonreactive, fetal well-being is questionable.** Any of the following options may be chosen:

      (1) **Vibroacoustic stimulation** should be considered. A healthy fetus accelerates its heart rate in response to sound stimulation that is directed through the maternal abdominal wall.

      (2) If the test is still nonreactive, then the **CST** or the **BPP** are performed.

D. **Contractions stress test (CST).** Any electronic fetal monitor strip with **both a FHR tracing and uterine contractions** can be evaluated for both NST and CST criteria.

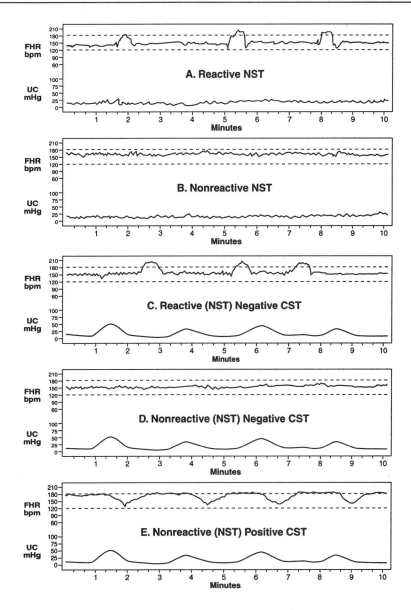

Figure 2-6. Antepartum electronic fetal monitor (EFM) tracings. All EFM stracings should be evaluated for two components: the nonstress test (NST) and the contraction stress test (CST). If a technically adequate fetal heart rate (FHR) tracing is present, the NST component can be assessed as reactive or nonreactive. If three or more uterine contractions (UCs) are present in 10 minutes, the CST components can be assessed as negative or positive. (*A*) The EFM tracing shows a normal baseline range, and no UCs are present. Thus, only the NST component can be assessed. Because three accelerations are present, the assessment is reactive NST. This is a reassuring tracing. (*B*) The EFM tracing shows a normal baseline range, and no UCs are present. Thus, only the NST component can be assessed. Because no accelerations are present, the assessment is nonreactive NST. Because this is not a reassuring tracing, the next step should be a vibroacoustic fetal stimulation. (*C*) The EFM tracing shows a normal baseline range, and four UCs are present in 10 minutes. Thus, both the NST and CST components can be assessed. Because three accelerations are present, and no late decelerations are present, the assessment is reactive NST, negative CST. This is a reassuring tracing. (*D*) The EFM tracing shows a normal baseline range, and four UCs are present in 10 minutes. Thus, both the NST and CST components can be assessed. Even though no accelerations can be seen, no late decelerations are present. The assessment is nonreactive NST, negative CST. This suggests fetal sleep, sedation, or central nervous system (CNS) abnormality. (*E*) The EFM tracing shows an elevated baseline range, and four UCs are present in 10 minutes. Thus, both the NST and CST components can be assessed. No accelerations can be seen, but repetitive late decelerations are present. The assessment is nonreactive NST, positive CST. This is highly suggestive of fetal compromise.

1. **Assumptions** are based on the presence or absence of FHR late decelerations.
   a. Uterine contractions diminish the flow of oxygenated **intervillous blood** to the fetus.
   b. A fetus with adequate **metabolic reserve** can cope satisfactorily with transient oxygen deprivation (i.e., **FHR remains at stable baseline through contractions**).
   c. A **compromised** fetus displays **late decelerations** (FHR decelerations persisting after a contraction).
2. **Method.** An external fetal cardiotocograph and contraction monitor is placed on the mother's abdomen, and the mother is positioned to avoid **supine hypotension.** Uterine contractions and FHR are recorded. If there are no spontaneous contractions, contractions may be induced by **nipple stimulation** (utilizing endogenous oxytocin) or intravenous (IV) **oxytocin infusion** (oxytocin challenge test). The goal is more than **three contractions in 10 minutes.** Baseline FHR, accelerations, and variability are noted, and reactive or nonreactive status is determined.
3. **Contraindications.** If the patient has a condition in which contractions may be hazardous, the CST should not be performed. These conditions include:
   a. Previous classic-incision uterine scar
   b. Previous myomectomy entering uterine cavity
   c. Premature rupture of membranes
   d. Incompetent cervix
   e. Placenta previa
4. **Interpretation**
   a. A **negative CST** (i.e., no late decelerations) is associated with a **fetal death rate** of 1 per 1000 within 1 week of the test.
      (1) If the test is **negative** and meets the criteria for a **reactive NST,** it is known as an **reactive-negative CST** and is highly predictive of fetal well-being, because both NST and CST components are reassuring (see Figure 2-6C).
      (2) If the test is **negative** but only meets the criteria for a **nonreactive NST,** it is known as a **nonreactive-negative CST** (see Figure 2-6D). The negative CST finding suggests adequate placental oxygenation, but the nonreactive-negative NST suggests fetal sleep, sedation, or CNS anomaly.
   b. An **equivocal CST** (nonrepetitive late decelerations) is worrisome.
      (1) If the test is **equivocal** but meets criteria for a **reactive NST,** fetal well-being may be present but cannot be assured.
      (2) If the test is **equivocal** and also meets the criteria for a **nonreactive NST,** it may indicate incipient fetal compromise.
   c. A **positive CST** (i.e., repetitive late decelerations with three consecutive contractions in 10 minutes) raises significant concerns regarding fetal jeopardy.
      (1) If the test is **positive** and meets the criteria for a **reactive NST,** it is known as a **reactive-positive CST** and may be falsely positive, but fetal well-being is not assured.

(2) If the test is both a **positive CST** and meets criteria for a **nonreactive NST,** it is known as a **nonreactive-positive CST** and is highly indicative of fetal compromise (see Figure 2-6E).

d. **Hyperstimulation** is diagnosed when late decelerations occur after coupled contractions (one contraction after another without relaxation time between) or when there are more than five contractions in 10 minutes, and each contraction lasts longer than 90 seconds. **Without uterine relaxation between contractions, intervillous blood flow ceases, and even a normal fetus shows late decelerations.**

5. **Recommendations**

   a. **If the CST is negative,** repeat it weekly or biweekly.

   b. **If the CST is either equivocal or positive-reactive:**

      (1) Labor should be induced if the fetus is mature ($\geq$ 36 weeks' gestation).

      (2) The CST should be repeated in 24 hours, or the BPP should be performed if the fetus is immature.

   c. **If the CST is positive-nonreactive,** the fetus should be delivered expeditiously. A vaginal delivery may be attempted if the cervix is favorable. A cesarean delivery should be performed if the cervix is unfavorable. A BPP should be performed if the fetus is markedly immature.

E. **Biophysical profile (BPP)**

1. **Assumptions**

   a. A healthy fetus moves, thereby accelerating its heart rate.

   b. Adequate fetoplacental blood flow results in normal amniotic fluid volume.

   c. Fetal compromise diminishes fetal movements, FHR accelerations, and amniotic fluid volume.

2. **Method**

   a. **Complete BPP involves five components.** An NST is performed (see II C), and then, **using ultrasound,** the following characteristics are assessed:

      (1) Size of **amniotic fluid** pockets

      (2) Presence of fetal **breathing** movements

      (3) Presence of gross **body** movement

      (4) Presence of **extremity extension,** flexion, and tone

   b. A **modified BPP** has only two components:

      (1) **NST,** which is most predictive for **immediate assessment** of placental function

      (2) **Amniotic fluid measurement,** which is most predictive for **long-term assessment** of placental function

3. **Interpretation of score** (Tables 2-3 and 2-4)

   a. **Negative test** is diagnosed when the BPP **score is 8 or 10.** Perinatal mortality rate is less than 1 per 1000 within 1 week.

   b. **Equivocal test** is diagnosed when the BPP **score is 4 or 6.** Perinatal mortality rate is 50–90 per 1000 within 1 week.

Table 2-3. Interpretation of the Biophysical Profile (BPP)

BPP Parameter	Score = 2 Points	Score = 0 Points
Amniotic fluid	≥ 1 × 1 cm pocket	Oligohydramnios
NST	Reactive	Nonreactive
Breathing	1 Episode of ≥ 30 sec	No breathing
Gross body motion	[≥ 3 Discrete movements]	[≤ 2 movements]
Extremity tone	[1 Extension/flexion]	[None]

NST = Nonstress test.

Table 2-4. Interpretation of the Biophysical Profile (BPP)

Total Score	Test Result	Perinatal Mortality/1000
0	Positive = fetal jeopardy	600
2	Positive = fetal jeopardy	120
4	Equivocal	90
6	Equivocal	50
8 or 10	Negative = fetal well-being	< 1

    c. Positive test is diagnosed when the BPP **score is 0 or 2.** Perinatal mortality rate is 120–600 per 1000 within 1 week. There is a 30% false-positive rate with a BPP, and most of these cases are associated with sedated fetuses (maternal use of alcohol or sedative–hypnotic drugs) or fetus with anomalies.

  4. Recommendations

    a. If the **score is 0 or 2,** delivery should be expeditious regardless of gestational age if no satisfactory nonhypoxic explanation is identified.

    b. If the **score is 4 or 6,** the fetus should be delivered if it is mature. If the fetus is immature, the BPP should be repeated in 24 hours.

    c. If the **score is 8 or 10,** the BPP should be repeated in 1 week.

III. PRENATAL DIAGNOSIS

  A. Indications for prenatal diagnosis

    1. Previous child with or family history of any of the following:

      a. Birth defects. Approximately 65% of newborn malformations are polygenic/multifactorial (see III B 3).

      b. Mental retardation

        (1) Fetal alcohol syndrome is the most commonly identified single cause.

        (2) Fragile X syndrome is the most common inherited cause.

    c. Chromosome disorder involving missing, extra, or rearranged chromosomes.

    d. Known genetic disorder passed from parents to children.

2. **Multiple fetal losses**

3. **Previous unexplained neonatal death** within the first 28 days of life.

4. **Maternal or paternal condition predisposing to congenital anomaly**

    a. Maternal factors include:

        (1) Age over 35 years, which predisposes to **nondisjunction trisomies** (e.g., trisomy 21, trisomy 18)

        (2) Overt diabetes, which predisposes to **CNS and cardiac anomalies** if hyperglycemia exists at embryogenesis

    b. Maternal or paternal factors include:

        (1) Balanced translocation, which is not affected by maternal age

        (2) Aneuploidy, in which the chromosome complement is more than or less than the normal 46

        (3) Mosaicism, in which one individual has two or more cell lines, each with differing chromosome complements

    c. Paternal factors include **autosomal dominant mutations,** which are associated with **advancing paternal age**

5. **Current pregnancy associated with** any of the following:

    a. History of teratogenic exposure (e.g., alcohol, drugs, radiation, chemicals, hyperthermia)

    b. Abnormal MSAFP

    c. Abnormal triple marker screen

    d. Abnormal fetus detected on ultrasound examination

B. Types of genetic problems for prenatal diagnosis (Figure 2-7)

1. **Chromosome or cytogenetic disorders**

    a. Small autosomal trisomy. Approximately 95% of trisomies 21, 13, and 18, which are caused by nondisjunction, are increased with advancing maternal age.

    b. Sex chromosome aneuploidy

        (1) Turner syndrome (45X) [see Chapter 3 I A 3]

        (2) Klinefelter syndrome (47XXY)

2. **Single gene disorders** (Table 2-5)

    a. Autosomal dominant disorders require only **one gene from either parent** for expression, although they may be first-time mutations. There is frequently a family history but no gender predominance, with a 50% chance of passage to offspring. **Examples,** which are often **gross anatomic lesions,** include:

        (1) Tuberous sclerosis

        (2) Neurofibromatosis

        (3) Achondroplasia

    b. Autosomal recessive disorders require **two genes, one from each parent,** for expression. Often there is no family history and no gender predominance, but there is a 25% chance of passage to offspring.

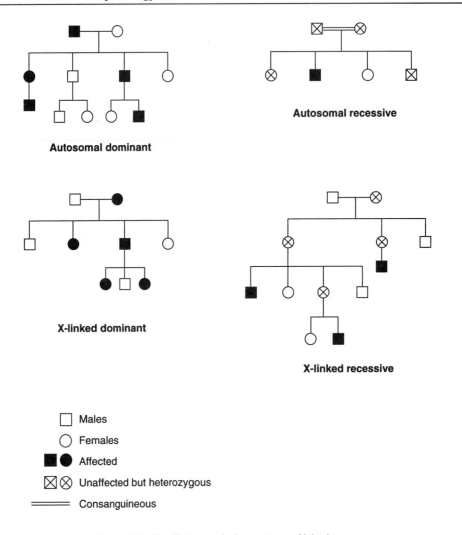

Figure 2-7. Familial transmission patterns of inheritance.

Examples, which are often **biochemical disorders,** include the following diseases and carrier frequencies:

(1) Cystic fibrosis (1 in 25 Caucasians)

(2) Tay-Sachs disease (1 in 30 Ashkenazi Jews)

(3) Thalassemia (1 in 20 Southeast Asians)

(4) Sickle cell disease (1 in 10 African-Americans)

c. **Sex-linked (X-linked)** disorders exist **only on the X chromosome.** These conditions, which may be either recessive or dominant in inheritance, may represent new mutations.

(1) **X-linked recessive disorders** are **more common than dominant ones.** Because males pass their X chromosome only to their daughters, affected males cannot pass the gene to their sons. **Only females can pass the gene.** On average, they give it to 50% of their sons, who are affected, and to 50% of their daughters, are carriers. Heterozygous females may manifest some aspects of the disease. **Examples** include:

Table 2-5.   Single-Gene (Mendelian) Disorders

	Autosomal Dominant	Autosomal Recessive	Sex (X) Linked) Dominant	Sex (X) Linked) Recessive
Genes needed for expression	1	2	1	1
% Passage to offspring	50%	25%	Fathers can pass only to females; mothers pass to both males and females	50% males affected 50% female carriers
% Carriers in unaffected offspring	None	50%	None	None in males 50% in females
Positive family history	Frequent	Seldom	Often	Often
Gender predominance	None	None	No	Yes
Examples	Achondroplasia Neurofibromatosis	Cystic fibrosis Tay-Sachs disease	Vitamin D– resistant rickets	Fragile X syndrome Hemophilia A

          (a) Duchenne muscular dystrophy

          (b) Fragile X syndrome

          (c) Hemophilia A (factor VIII deficiency)

      (2) Sex-linked dominant disorders are **uncommon** and tend to be **lethal in male offspring.** There are **no carrier** states. Any affected parent can transmit the gene. **Fathers can pass the gene only to their daughters.** Mothers can pass the gene to both their sons and daughters, who each have a 50% chance of being affected. **Examples** include:

          (a) Vitamin D–resistant rickets

          (b) Hyperammonemia

   3. Polygenic/multifactorial disorders

      a. These conditions **require both genetic and environmental influences and account for the majority of birth defects.** The recurrence rate is 2%.

      b. Examples include:

          (1) Cleft lip and palate

          (2) Neural tube defects (NTDs)

          (3) Congenital heart disease

          (4) Pyloric stenosis

  C. Timing and risk of teratogenesis (Table 2-6). Prior to **implantation,** before any germ layers have formed, exposure to any teratogen results in

Table 2-6. Timing and Risk of Teratogenesis

Timing from LMP	Developmental Event	Degree of Risk
0–2 weeks	Preconception	None*
2–3 weeks	Pre-implantation	None*
3–4 weeks	Gastrulation†	Least risk
4–8 weeks	Embryogenesis	Greatest risk

*Either normal development results or an embryonic death or pregnancy loss occurs.
†Formation of endo/meso/ectoderm.

either blastocyst death or intact survival. The greatest risk of teratogenesis exists 2–8 weeks' postconception (from development of the bilaminar and trilaminar germ discs to completion of organ system **development).**

1. **Substances that have documented teratogenic effects** (Table 2-7). Notice the predisposition for IUGR, microcephaly, and craniofacial anomalies.

2. **Substances that probably have no teratogenic effects** (Table 2-8).

D. **Prenatal diagnostic tests** (Table 2-9) are used to identify fetal abnormalities in utero.

1. **MSAFP**

a. **Timing.** Blood should be drawn from 15–20 weeks' gestation.

b. **Indication.** The MSAFP is used to detect **open NTDs.** This test has a sensitivity of 90% for fetuses with anencephaly and 85% for fetuses with spina bifida. However, the specificity is only 7%. Only 5% of NTDs occur in women who previously had a fetus affected with an NTD.

c. **Basis of test.** α-Fetoprotein (AFP) is synthesized by the fetal yolk sac, the GI tract, and the liver. It is the **major serum protein of the embryo** and the early fetus. Fetal urine is a major source of amniotic fluid AFP.

d. **Measurement.** Fetal serum AFP levels (measured in mg) are 100 times higher than amniotic fluid AFP levels (measured in μg) and 10,000 times higher than MSAFP (measured in ng). After 13 weeks, the amniotic fluid AFP level decreases, but the MSAFP level increases.

e. **Results** are reported as multiples of the median (MoMs).

(1) **High values** (> 2.5 MoM) are associated with the following:

(a) **Pregnancy dating errors (most frequent explanation)**

(b) Multiple fetuses

(c) Placental bleeding

(d) Open NTD (associated also with an increased level of amniotic fluid acetylcholinesterase)

(e) Ventral wall defects (e.g., gastroschisis, omphalocele)

(f) Renal anomalies (e.g., polycystic or absent kidneys, congenital nephrosis)

Table 2-7.   Substances With Documented Teratogenic Effects

Type of Substance	Teratogenic Effect
Abused substances	
Alcohol	**Midfacial hypoplasia,** IUGR, microcephaly
Cocaine	**Bowel atresias,** IUGR, microcephaly
Antibiotics	
Streptomycin	**VIII nerve** damage, hearing loss
Kanamycin	**VIII nerve** damage, hearing loss
Tetracycline	Deciduous **teeth discoloration,** tooth enamel hypoplasia
Anticonvulsants	
Carbamazepezine	**Fingernail hypoplasia,** IUGR, microcephaly, NTD
Phenytoin	**Nail hypoplasia,** IUGR, microcephaly, craniofacial dysmorphism
Trimethadione	**Facial dysmorphism,** IUGR, microcephaly, cleft lip or palate
Valproic acid	NTD **(spina bifida),** facial defects
Antivitamins	
Etretinate	Detectable levels may persist for more than 2 years after stopping use **(CNS malformations,** craniofacial dysmorphism, NTD/skeletal abnormalities)
Isotretinoin	**Microtia,** heart and **great vessel defects,** craniofacial dysmorphism
Methotrexate	**CNS malformations,** IUGR, craniofacial dysmorphism
Hormones	
Androgens	**Virilization** of female fetus
DES	**Müllerian duct anomalies,** clear cell carcinoma of vagina
Heavy metals	
Lead	Miscarriages, stillbirths
Mercury	Cerebral atrophy, microcephaly, blindness
Others	
ACE inhibitors	**Oligohydramnios,** renal tubular dysplasia, neonatal renal failure
Coumadin	**Strippled bone epiphyses,** IUGR, nasal hypoplasia
Lithium	**Ebstein's anomaly,** other cardiac disease
Thalidomide	**Phocomelia,** anotia

ACE = angiotension-converting enzyme; CNS = central nervous system; DES = diethylstilbestrol; IUGR = intrauterine growth restriction; NTD = neural tube defect.

       (g) Fetal demise

       (h) Sacrococcygeal teratoma

     (2) Low values are associated with the following:

       (a) Pregnancy dating error (most frequent explanation)

       (b) Trisomy 21. However, only 20% of cases are low MSAFP screen–positive.

  2. Triple marker screen. Three blood tests are performed on maternal serum **(MSAFP, estriol, and β-hCG)** and evaluated if in the normal range for gestational age. In **trisomy 18,** all levels are decreased. In **trisomy 21,** the MSAFP and estriol are decreased, but hCG is increased.

  a. Timing. Blood should be drawn from 15–20 weeks' gestation.

  b. Indication. The triple marker screen is used to detect abnormal fetal

Table 2-8. Substances That are Probably Nonteratogenic

Type of Substance(s)	Specific Agent
Abused substance	Marijuana
Antiacne agent	Tretinoin (topical)
Antiasthma agents	Beta agonists, prednisone, cromolyn, epinephrine, theophylline salts
Antibacterial agents	Penicillins, cephalosporins, clindamycin, erythromycin, metronidazole, nitrofurantoin, sulfa drugs (associated with neonatal jaundice at term)
Anticoagulant agents	Heparin, enoxaparin (low-molecular-weight heparin)
Antidepressant agents	Tricyclics, MAO inhibitors, SSRIs
Antiemetic agents	Cyclizine, emetrol, meclizine, chlorpromazine, promethazine
Antifungal agents	Clotrimazole, miconazole, nystatin, amphotericin B
Antihypertensive agents	Methyldopa, hydralazine, thiazides (associated with neonatal thrombocytopenia)
Antimalarial agent	Chloroquine
Antipsychotic agent	Chlorpromazine
Antituberculosis drugs	Isoniazid, PAS, rifampin, ethambutol
Antiviral agents	Zidovudine, acyclovir
Cardiovascular agents	Digoxin, quinidine, propranolol, nifedipine
Contraceptives	Depo-Provera, Norplant, oral contraceptives, spermicides
Minor analgesics	Acetaminophen, salicylates, ibuprofen (may cause oligohydramnios)
Narcotics	Codeine, propoxyphene, oxycodone, meperidine, morphine (all may result in neonatal withdrawal)
Others	Aspartame, caffeine, hair spray

MAO = monoamine oxidase; PAS = paraaminosalicylic acid; SSRI = selective serotonine reuptake inhibitor.

karyotypes. It identifies 60% of **trisomy 21** fetuses and also identifies **trisomy 18** fetuses.

    c. **Basis of test.** Aneuploid karotypes are associated with certain combinations of abnormally high or abnormally low levels of the three marker tests (Table 2-10).

3. **Amniocentesis**

    a. **Timing.** Amniocentesis is usually performed at 15 weeks' gestation.

    b. **Indication.** Amniocentesis is used to detect cytogenetic abnormalities and to measure amniotic fluid AFP.

    c. **Basis of test.** A needle is inserted transabdominally into the amni-

Table 2-9. Prenatal Diagnostic Tests

Test	Timing	Test Basis	Target	Limitations	Fetal Risk
Maternal serum α-fetoprotein (MSAFP)	15–19 weeks	Fetal AFP in maternal serum	• NTD • VWD • Trisomy 21	• True positive rate only 7% for NTD • Detects only 20% trisomy 21	None
Triple marker screen	15–19 weeks	• Serum AFP • Serum estriol • Serum β-hCG	• NTD • VWD • Trisomy 21	• Detects 60% of trisomy 21	None
Amniocentesis	≥ 15 weeks	Desquamated fetal cells in amniotic fluid AF-AFP	• Cytogenetic disorders • Enzyme disorders	• Amniotic fluid not obtainable • Amniocytes do not grow	0.5% loss rate
Chorionic villus sampling (CVS)	9–12 weeks	Transvaginal or transabdominal aspiration of chorionic villus tissue	• Cytogenetic disorders • Enzyme disorders	• Villus tissue not obtainable • Placental mosaicism though fetus is normal • Maternal cell contamination	0.7% loss rate Possible limb reduction defects if done at < 10 weeks
Percutaneous umbilical blood sampling (PUBS)	> 20 weeks	Fetal blood from umbilical cord	Any blood test	• Isoimmunization (diagnosis & treatment) • Karyotyping • Fetal infection	1%–2% loss rate
Sonography	18–20 weeks (optimal)	Assessment of fetal anatomy	Identification of gross structural anomalies	• Maternal obesity • Sonologist expertise	None
Fetoscopy	15–20 weeks	Transabdominal placement of fiber-optic scope into amniotic sac	• Visualize fetal anatomy • Biopsy fetal skin	• Technical problems	2%–5% loss rate

NTD = neural tube defect; VWD = ventral wall defect.

otic sac to obtain **amniocytes** (i.e., desquamated fetal cells suspended in amniotic fluid), which are then cultured and subjected to karyotyping. Approximately 20–30 ml of amniotic fluid is aspirated using continuous ultrasound localization.

    d. Risk and limitation

        (1) Risk of spontaneous abortion. The pregnancy loss rate is 0.5% (over background loss rate of 2%–3%). Loss may result from needle insertion, causing fetal trauma; infection; ruptured membranes; or stimulation of uterine contractions, leading to premature delivery.

        (2) Limitation. Amniocentesis for fetal karyotype cannot detect

Table 2-10. Test Values for Triple Marker Screen

Test	Trisomy 18	Trisomy 21
MSAFP	↓	↓
Estriol	↓	↓
hCG	↓	↑

hCG = human chorionic gonadotropin; MSAFP = maternal serum α-fetoprotein.

mendelian (single gene) disorders or polygenic/multifactorial disorders (e.g., CNS and cardiac anomalies). However, fetal amniocytes can be analyzed by the polymerase chain reaction method and other techniques to identify genetic abnormalities.

4. **Chorionic villus sampling (CVS)**
   a. **Timing.** CVS may be performed from 9–12 weeks' gestation.
   b. **Basis of test.** Because both the fetus and the placenta originate from the same zygote, it should be possible to infer the fetal karyotype from the placental karyotype. The chorionic villus is the precursor to the placenta. Under ultrasound guidance, samples of the chorionic villus are aspirated through a transcervical catheter or transabdominal needle.
   c. **Advantages.** CVS results can be obtained at an early gestational age, and biochemical and molecular diagnoses can be made.
   d. **Disadvantages**
      (1) In approximately 1%–2% of cases in which mosaicism is found in the placenta, the fetus has a normal karyotype.
      (2) Occasionally, the chorionic villus can be contaminated with maternal cells.
      (3) If the test is performed at less than 10 weeks' gestation, there may be a risk of fetal limb reduction defects.
      (4) The **fetal loss rate** may be higher **with CVS** than with amniocentesis.

5. **Percutaneous umbilical blood sampling (PUBS; cordocentesis)**
   a. **Timing.** PUBS is performed in the second and third trimester when the umbilical cord vessels are large enough to puncture safely.
   b. **Indications**
      (1) Isoimmunization (fetal transfusion)
      (2) Fetal karyotyping (anomalies, severe IUGR)
      (3) Fetal infection [e.g., cytomegalovirus (CMV), toxoplasmosis, rubella]
      (4) Genetic diseases (e.g., hemophilia A and B, sickle cell disease, thalassemia)
      (5) Evaluation of fetal acid–base condition
   c. **Disadvantages.** PUBS has a **1%–2% fetal loss rate.**
   d. **Basis of test and results.** Fetal blood is obtained transabdominally using a sterile needle under ultrasound guidance. The blood can be analyzed for chromosome anomalies, evidence of intrauterine infection, or genetic–metabolic abnormalities.

6. **Targeted sonography.** Specific gross structural anomalies may be identified using targeted sonography.

   a. **Scheduling.** Optimally, sonography is performed between 18–20 weeks' gestation when fetal anatomical structures are large enough to assess visually.

   b. **Safety.** Ultrasound appears biologically safe. No fetal risks have been independently confirmed in over 25 years of use in the low-intensity range of medical ultrasound.

   c. **Accuracy.** The precision of ultrasound diagnosis may be limited by the following variables:

      (1) Fetal position within the uterus

      (2) Anterior placental implantation

      (3) Thickness of maternal abdominal wall

      (4) Abdominal wall scar tissue

      (5) Expertise of the sonologist

7. **Fetoscopy** utilizes a thin-caliber fiberoptic scope that is placed transabdominally into the amniotic cavity.

   a. The **purpose** is to visualize external fetal anomalies and to biopsy fetal skin in utero.

   b. The **main indication** is fetal skin biopsy in suspected congenital icthyosis.

   c. The **disadvantages include** a 1%–2% fetal loss rate.

E. **Prevention of neural tube defects (NTDs). Maternal folate supplementation** has been shown to **decrease the risk** of NTDs.

   1. For **all women of reproductive age,** the dose is **0.4 mg daily** preconceptionally.

   2. For **high-risk women** (i.e., those with overt diabetes, seizure disorders or previous history of an infant with an NTD), the dose is **4 mg daily** starting 3 months prior to planned pregnancies.

IV. DISCREPANT FUNDAL SIZE means the uterine fundus measures 3 cm (or more) larger or smaller than expected for the supposed week of gestation.

A. **False positives.** The uterine size initially appears discrepant, but actually it is appropriate for gestational age.

   1. **Measurement errors** may be caused by different examiners, inexperienced examiners, or difficult examinations caused by a woman's exogenous obesity.

   2. **Gestational age calculation errors** can occur with any of the following: unsure LMP, unplanned pregnancy, and unusual or irregular LMP. Recent steroid contraceptive use, abortion, or lactation are associated with anovulation, which may mask the true date of conception.

B. **True positives.** Uterine size is truly **too small** for dates.

   1. **IUGR** (Table 2-11) is the failure of one or more of the following standard sonographic fetal growth parameters to follow a normal growth curve: **biparietal diameter (BPD), head circumference (HC), abdominal circumference (AC), femur length (FL).**

Table 2-11. Intrauterine Growth Restriction (IUGR)

	Symmetric	Asymmetric
Ultrasonic parameters		
Biparietal diameter (BPD)	↓	Normal
Head circumference (HC)	↓	Normal
Abdominal circumference (AC)	↓	↓ Decreased
Femur length (FL)	↓	Normal
Time of insult	Early pregnancy	Late pregnancy
Etiology	Fetal problem	Placenta mediated
	• Cytogenetic	• Hypertension
	• Infection	• Poor nutrition
	• Anomalies	• Maternal smoking
Amniotic fluid volume	Normal levels	Often decreased

   a. **Symmetric IUGR** occurs when the **BPD,** the **HC,** the **AC,** and the **FL** are **all decreased.**
       (1) It tends to develop from an insult **early** in the pregnancy (i.e., first or early second trimester).
       (2) It usually is attributed to **fetal causes** such as cytogenetic disorders, intrauterine infection (e.g., toxoplasmosis, rubella, CMV, herpes, syphilis), or gross structural anomalies.
       (3) The **amniotic fluid** volume usually is **normal.**
   b. **Asymmetric IUGR** occurs when the **AC** is **decreased,** but the **BPD, HC,** and **FL** are **normal.**
       (1) It tends to develop from an insult **late** in the pregnancy (i.e., in the late second or the third trimester).
       (2) It usually is attributed to **placental causes** such as hypertension (chronic, pregnancy-induced), poor maternal nutrition, and maternal smoking.
       (3) The **amniotic fluid** volume usually is **decreased.**
 2. **Oligohydramnios** is defined as an inadequate volume of amniotic fluid.
   a. **Amniotic fluid index (AFI)** is the sum of ultrasound measurements of amniotic fluid in the four abdominal quadrants: right upper quadrant, left upper quadrant, right lower quadrant, and left lower quadrant.
       (1) The **greatest** amniotic fluid **vertical** pocket in each of the four quadrants is measured.
       (2) The AFI should normally be between 5 and 25 cm.
       (3) Oligohydramnios is diagnosed if the **AFI is less than 5 cm.**
   b. **Fetal significance.** Reduced amniotic fluid volume limits the normal freedom of fetal extremity and chest wall movement.
       (1) Thus, fetuses affected by oligohydramnios may have musculoskeletal deformations (e.g., clubfoot), pulmonary hypoplasia, or umbilical cord compression.
       (2) IUGR is found in 60% of fetuses in pregnancies with oligohydramnios.

      c. Causes of oligohydramnios include:

        (1) Premature rupture of membranes

        (2) Fetal urinary tract anomaly (e.g., renal agenesis, obstructive lesions)

        (3) Maternal medications [e.g., angiotensin-converting enzyme (ACE) inhibitors, indomethacin]

        (4) Placental insufficiency (can be caused by preeclampsia and is often associated with IUGR)

  3. Fetal demise (see Chapter 3 IV). Fetal death from any cause results in the uterus being smaller than expected for dates.

C. True positives. Uterine size is truly **too large** for dates.

  1. Molar pregnancy most commonly presents as a uterus larger than dates (see Chapter 3 VII)

  2. Leiomyomas are benign smooth muscle tumors that may cause external enlargement of the uterine wall (see Chapter 13 III B). Their anatomic location is usually **intramural, subserosal,** or **pedunculated subserous.**

  3. Multiple gestation (see Chapter 3 V) can result from either **assisted reproduction** or **spontaneous ovulation.**

  4. Fetal macrosomia is defined as a fetus who has a birth weight greater than 4000–4500 g (8.75–9.84 lb) and whose weight is above the 90th to 95th percentile.

    a. Diagnosis. Fetal macrosomia can be suggested clinically by fundal palpation or by ultrasound examination. Both methods have significant error rates.

    b. Hazards of macrosomia

      (1) Maternal risks

        (a) Traumatic delivery

        (b) Shoulder dystocia

        (c) Increased rate of operative vaginal or cesarean delivery

        (d) Postpartum hemorrhage

      (2) Fetal risks

        (a) Shoulder dystocia

        (b) Hypoglycemia

    c. Causes of macrosomia

      (1) Postdates pregnancy (see V)

      (2) Glucose intolerance (see Chapter 4 VIII)

      (3) Constitutional (i.e., large parents)

      (4) Beckwith-Wiedemann syndrome (rare)

  5. Polyhydramnios is defined as either **excessive amniotic fluid** (> 2000 ml), a single amniotic fluid vertical pocket greater than 15 cm, or a **four-quadrant AFI greater than 25 cm.**

    a. Classification (Table 2-12)

      (1) Acute polyhydramnios usually has an onset **before 24 weeks'** gestation. Amniotic fluid accumulated **rapidly** with a high incidence of identifiable **fetal anomalies.** Acute polyhydramnios is frequently associated with **perinatal loss.**

Table 2-12. Types of Polyhydramnios

	Acute	Chronic
Onset	< 24 weeks	> 30 weeks
Amniotic fluid level	Increases rapidly	Increases gradually
Etiology	Often identified: • Decreased fetal swallowing • Fetal gastrointestinal obstruction • Twin-twin transfusion	Seldom found
Perinatal outcome	Frequent mortality	Often normal

> **(2) Chronic** polyhydramnios usually has an onset **after 30 weeks'** gestation. Amniotic fluid accumulates **gradually,** and often there is **no identifiable etiology.** Frequently, the **perinatal outcome is good.**

   b. **Known mechanisms** include either **increased production** and/or **decreased removal** of amniotic fluid

   (1) Decreased fetal swallowing. A fetus normally swallows up to 1500 ml/day. Fetal anomalies include anencephaly, spina bifida, and arthrogryposis.

   (2) Fetal GI tract obstruction (most severe with proximal lesions). Conditions include duodenal atresia (double-bubble sign: stomach plus dilated duodenum) and tracheoesophageal fistula.

   (3) Twin–twin transfusion syndrome (see Chapter 3 V C 2 a). The recipient twin has enhanced renal blood flow resulting in excessive urine production, leading to polyhydramnios.

   c. **Unknown mechanisms** are functioning for fetal pulmonary anomalies (e.g., cystic adenomatoid malformation), maternal diabetes, and fetal hydrops (immune, nonimmune).

V. POSTDATES PREGNANCY

   A. **Definition.** Postdates pregnancy is diagnosed when a pregnancy persists after:

   1. **42 weeks of amenorrhea,** assuming ovulation occurred on day 14

   2. **294 days of amenorrhea,** assuming ovulation occurred on day 14

   3. **280 days' postconception,** assuming conception date is known

   B. **Incidence.** Approximately 8% of all pregnancies are diagnosed as postdates pregnancies based on LMP. The actual rate of pregnancies that truly go longer than 280 days' postconception is 4% when based on a known ovulation date. The majority of women completing 42 postmenstrual weeks have less advanced gestations based on their ovulation date occurring after day 14 of their cycle..

   C. **Etiology.** Most postdates pregnancies are **idiopathic** (no explanation found). However, the following conditions or factors may be associated:

1. Lack of normally high estrogen levels
2. Anencephaly
3. Fetal adrenal hypoplasia
4. Absence of fetal pituitary gland
5. Placental sulfatase deficiency (X-linked trait)

D. **Abdominal pregnancy.** In this rare condition where the fetus is not contained within the uterus, uterine contractions obviously do not lead to labor and delivery.

E. **Hazards of postdates pregnancies** (Table 2-13). Perinatal morbidity and mortality rates are increased two to three times. Postdates fetuses usually manifest one of the two following outcomes:

1. **Fetal macrosomia** occurs in **70%–80%** of postdates pregnancies and is characterized by:
   a. **Maintenance of placental oxygenation and nutrition,** leading to:
      (1) Normal oxygenation and absence of fetal hypoxia
      (2) Excessive fetal growth and deposition of subcutaneous tissue resulting in a fetus with a birth weight of more than 4000–4500 g
   b. **Intrapartum complications** resulting from fetal macrosomia that include:
      (1) Failure of normal labor progression leading to increased cesarean delivery
      (2) Delivery shoulder dystocia leading to birth trauma, brachial plexus injury, or even death

Table 2-13.   Hazards of Postdates Pregnancies

Characteristic	Dysmaturity Syndrome	Macrosomia
Incidence	20%–30%	70%–80%
Placental function	Deteriorating (from infarction and aging)	Maintained
Amniotic fluid	Decreased	Normal
Neonatal appearance	Scawny (decreased subcutaneous tissue)	Large (increased subcutaneous tissue)
Causes of cesarean section	Cord compression Placental insufficiency	Fetopelvic disproportion
Causes of meconium passage	GI tract maturity Anal sphincter hypotonia from acidosis	GI tract maturity
Causes of neonatal morbidity	Acidosis Meconium aspiration Hypoglycemia	Birth trauma

GI = gastrointestinal.

    c. Passage of meconium in utero from normal peristalsis from fetal GI tract maturity

  2. Postmaturity/dysmaturity syndrome occurs in **20%–30%** of post-dates pregnancies and is characterized by:

    a. Aging or infarction of the placenta that can lead to uteroplacental insufficiency, which results in:

      (1) Decreased oxygenation leading to fetal hypoxia

      (2) Decreased nutrition resulting in decreased fetal subcutaneous tissue and a scrawny neonate

    b. "Dehydration" of the fetoplacental unit, which can lead to:

      (1) Oligohydramios resulting in umbilical cord compression

      (2) Decreased Wharton's jelly (which supports umbilical vessels on the cord), resulting in umbilical cord compression

      (3) Dry, peeling fetal skin

    c. Passage of meconium in utero, which can result from two different mechanisms:

      (1) Normal peristalsis from fetal GI tract maturity

      (2) Anal sphincter hypotonia from fetal acidosis

F. Clinical management

  1. Determine confidence of the gestational age using the following parameters:

    a. Menstrual history. This tends to be reliable if:

      (1) Patient is **sure** of her last menstrual period.

      (2) Pregnancy was **planned.**

      (3) Menstrual cycle was **not irregular.**

      (4) Menstrual cycle **duration was usual** for patient

      (5) No recent history of **factors** associated with **anovulation** such as oral contraceptive use, abortion, pregnancy, or lactation

    b. Clinical parameters. These are pregnancy landmarks associated with certain gestational ages.

      (1) Uterine size estimated by early pelvic examination ($<$ 12 weeks)

      (2) Fetal heart tones detected early by Doppler stethoscope ($<$ 12 weeks)

      (3) Fundal size estimated by abdominal palpation

        (a) At the symphysis pubis at 12 weeks

        (b) At the umbilicus at 20 weeks

      (4) Maternal first report of fetal movement (quickening)

        (a) Occurs in a multigravida at 16–18 weeks' gestation

        (b) Occurs in a primigravida at 18–20 weeks' gestation

      (5) Fetal heart tones heard with fetoscope at 18–20 weeks' gestation

    c. Ultrasound parameters. The earlier the ultrasound is performed in the pregnancy, the higher the confidence and accuracy that can be placed in the gestational age (Table 2-14).

      (1) Crown–rump length (CRL) is accurate $\pm$ 5 days between 8–12 weeks.

      (2) BPD is accurate $\pm$ 7 days between 12–18 weeks.

Table 2-14.   Comparison of Ultrasound Dating with Gestational Age

Gestational Age	Parameter	Accuracy
<12 weeks	CRL	±5 days
12–18 weeks	BPD HC AC FL	±1.0 week
18–24 weeks	BPD HC AC FL	±1.5 weeks
24–30 weeks	BPD HC AC FL	±2.0 weeks
30–36 weeks	BPD HC AC FL	±2.5 weeks
36–40 weeks	BPD HC AC FL	±3.0 weeks
> 40 weeks	BPD HC AC FL	±3.5 weeks

AC = abdominal circumference; BPD = biparietal diameter; CRL = crown-rump length; FL = fetal length; HC = head circumference.

2. **If dates are firm, and the cervix is favorable (i.e., dilated, effaced soft), the goal is delivery.**
   a. Labor should be induced via artificial rupture of membranes or IV oxytocin.
   b. Continuous intrapartum fetal monitoring should be performed watching for:
      (1) **Variable decelerations** from umbilical cord compression
      (2) **Late decelerations** from fetal hypoxia
3. **If dates are firm, but the cervix is unfavorable (i.e., closed, uneffaced, firm), two options are appropriate.**
   a. **Cervical ripening** can be induced using intracervical or intravaginal **prostaglandin** E_2 (PGE$_2$).
      (1) The induction-to-delivery interval may be shortened, but the rate of cesarean delivery is unchanged.
      (2) The patient should be monitored for uterine hyperstimulation.
      (3) IV oxytocin is started after cervical ripening is achieved.
   b. Both **NSTs and AFIs** can be performed **twice weekly.**
      (1) Fetal surveillance should be continued until spontaneous labor occurs.
      (2) Induction of labor should be performed if the NST becomes nonreactive or the AFI is less than 5 cm.
4. **If dates are questionable or uncertain, conservative management is appropriate.**
   a. Both **NSTs and AFIs** should be performed twice weekly.
   b. Fetal surveillance should be continued until spontaneous labor occurs.
   c. Induction of labor should be performed if the NST becomes nonreactive or the AFI is less than 5 cm.
5. **Meconium aspiration syndrome (MAS)**
   a. **Pathophysiology.** Thick meconium is four times more common in

postdates pregnancies and is often associated with decreased amniotic fluid. Gasping in utero, occurring in the hypoxic fetus, can lead to MAS in the neonate.

b. **Mechanisms.** Meconium passage in utero may result from mature bowel function and peristalsis (usually no problem) or fetal acidosis with decreased anal sphincter tone (worrisome).

c. **Prevention**

(1) **Amnioinfusion therapy** involves infusion of normal saline through an intrauterine catheter to provide pseudoamniotic fluid, which dilutes the meconium and prevents umbilical cord compression

(2) **Suctioning fetal nares and pharynx** on the perineum (after the head is delivered but before delivery of the body) removes meconium that could be aspirated on the first breath.

(3) **Neonatal tracheal aspiration** after delivery, using a laryngoscope, is performed to remove meconium found below the vocal cords.

Review Test

Directions: Each of the numbered items or incomplete statements in this section is followed by answers or by completions of the statement. Select the ONE lettered answer or completion that is BEST in each case.

1. Which one of the following conditions is the most common cause of maternal mortality in the United States?

(A) Infection
(B) Hemorrhage
(C) Hypertension
(D) Trauma
(E) Thromboembolism

2. Which one of the following conditions is the most common cause of perinatal morbidity and mortality in the United States?

(A) Congenital malformation
(B) Preterm delivery
(C) Intrauterine growth restriction (IUGR)
(D) Infection
(E) Abnormal karyotype

3. Which one of the following statements regarding Naegele's rule and estimated due date (EDD) is true?

(A) EDD = date of last menstrual period (LMP) minus 3 months plus 3 days
(B) EDD is falsely prolonged when the menstrual cycle exceeds 28 days
(C) EDD must be adjusted to the duration of the proliferative phase of cycle
(D) EDD calculation assumes a variable follicular phase
(E) If LMP is July 4, then EDD is February 7

4. A 23-year-old primigravida presents for a routine prenatal visit. She is currently 16 weeks pregnant. Which of the following gestational age–specific prenatal laboratory tests should now be performed?

(A) Hepatitis B surface antigen
(B) Syphilis serology
(C) Complete blood count
(D) Maternal serum α-fetoprotein (MSAFP)
(E) Urine culture

5. A presumptive sign of pregnancy is

(A) Hegar's sign
(B) palpation of fetal parts
(C) uterine enlargement
(D) amenorrhea
(E) auscultation of fetal heart tones

6. A pregnant woman who is 5′0″ tall weighs 160 pounds before conception. Which one of the following is closest to her recommended total pregnancy weight gain?

(A) 10 pounds
(B) 15 pounds
(C) 25 pounds
(D) 30 pounds
(E) 35 pounds

7. Which one of the following conditions causes the majority of birth defects?

(A) Polygenic/multifactorial disorders
(B) Cytogenetic disorders
(C) Teratogenic exposure
(D) Single gene disorders
(E) Sporadic disorders

8. A 35-year-old multigravida undergoes maternal serum α-fetoprotein (MSAFP) screening during her pregnancy. Analysis shows a positive high/elevated level. Which of the following is the most likely explanation for this finding?

(A) Open neural tube defect (NTD)
(B) Ventral wall defect
(C) Gestational-age dating error
(D) Placental bleeding
(E) Fetal demise

9. A 28-year-old woman with a family history of birth defects comes to the office requesting preconception counseling regarding prevention of congenital anomalies. Which one of the following birth defects can be prevented by administering this woman preconceptional folate supplementation?

(A) Ventral wall defects
(B) Neural tube defects (NTDs)
(C) Trisomy 21
(D) Turner syndrome
(E) Fetal alcohol syndrome

10. A 20-year-old pregnant woman undergoes a 28-week obstetric ultrasound examination. Decreased amniotic fluid is evident. Which one of the following fetal anomalies is most likely associated with this finding?

(A) Anencephaly
(B) Obstructive renal lesions
(C) Obstructive gastrointestinal (GI) lesions
(D) Neuromuscular disorders
(E) Tracheoesophageal fistula

11. A 26-year-old woman presents to the maternity unit with preterm contractions. To determine gestational age you review the prenatal chart and find a number of prenatal ultrasound reports. Which one of the following measurements is the most accurate sonographic dating parameter?

(A) Crown–rump length (CRL) at 10 weeks
(B) Biparietal diameter (BPD) at 15 weeks
(C) Abdominal circumference (AC) at 25 weeks
(D) Head circumference (HC) at 30 weeks
(E) Femur length (FL) at 35 weeks

12. Which one of the following clinical parameters is the most helpful in confirming accurate gestational dating?

(A) Fetal heart tones by Doppler stethoscope at 16 weeks
(B) Multigravida report of quickening at 20 weeks
(C) Primigravida report of quickening at 18 weeks
(D) Fetal heart tones by fetoscope at 24 weeks
(E) Uterine fundal height at 26 weeks

13. A 20-year-old primigravida is seen in the outpatient prenatal clinic. According to her last menstrual period (LMP), her estimated due date was two weeks ago. Fundal height is 42 cm, and the fetus is in longitudinal lie and cephalic presentation. In the management of this patient, it is most crucial to answer which one of the following clinical questions?

(A) What is the estimated fetal weight?
(B) How dilated is the cervix?
(C) What is the station of the presenting fetal part?
(D) How accurate is the estimated due date (EDD)?
(E) What has been the maternal weight gain?

Directions: Each of the numbered items or incomplete statements in this section is negatively phrased, as indicated by a capitalized word such as NOT, LEAST, or EXCEPT. Select the ONE lettered answer or completion that is BEST in each case.

14. All of the following perinatal rates are calculated per 1000 events EXCEPT

(A) infant mortality rate
(B) neonatal mortality rate
(C) fetal mortality rate
(D) maternal mortality rate
(E) perinatal mortality rate

15. A 17-year-old (gravida 2, para 1) woman presents to the maternity unit with irregular uterine contractions. According to her last menstrual period (LMP), she is 32 weeks pregnant. You perform the four Leopold maneuvers. In making these assessments, you have answered all of the following questions EXCEPT

(A) how dilated is the cervix?
(B) to what extent has the presenting part descended into the pelvis?
(C) on which side of the uterus is the cephalic prominence?
(D) on which side of the uterus are the fetal small parts?
(E) what fetal part is in the uterine fundus?

16. All of the following are standard sonographic fetal growth parameters EXCEPT

(A) biparietal diameter (BPD)
(B) head circumference (HC)
(C) abdominal circumference (AC)
(D) transcerebellar diameter
(E) femur length (FL)

Directions: The group of items in this section consists of lettered options followed by a set of numbered items. For each item, select the ONE lettered option that is most closely associated with it. To avoid spending too much time on matching sets with large numbers of options, it is generally advisable to begin each set by reading the list of options. Then, for each item in the set, try to generate the correct answer and locate it in the option list, rather than evaluating each option individually. Each lettered option may be selected once, more than once, or not at all.

Questions 17–24

For each of the following characteristics, select the most appropriate antepartum fetal assessment method.
(A) Fetal kick count
(B) Nonstress test (NST)
(C) Contraction stress test (CST)
(D) Biophysical profile (BPP)

17. Does not involve fetal movements

18. Is based on the presence or absence of late decelerations

19. Has the lowest rate of false-positive tests

20. Requires no costly technology

21. Is based only on the presence or absence of fetal heart accelerations

22. Is contraindicated in those with placenta previa

23. Is inadequate for primary screening in high-risk patients

24. Uses primarily real-time ultrasound assessment of fetus

Answers and Explanations

1. The answer is E [I B 3; Figure 2-1].

Maternal mortality in the United States is approximately 8 per 100,000 live births. Cesarean delivery increases this risk twofold to threefold. Although infection, hemorrhage, hypertension, and trauma are factors contributing to maternal deaths, thromboembolisms are the largest single contributor to maternal deaths in the United States. Most thromboembolic disease in pregnancy occurs in the immediate postpartum period.

2. The answer is B [I B 7; Figure 2-2].

The perinatal mortality rate in the United States is approximately 10 per 1000 live births. This rate is one third of what it was 30 years ago. Although the other conditions mentioned do result in perinatal complications, preterm delivery contributes more to perinatal morbidity and mortality than does any other single cause in the United States.

3. The answer is C [I C 1 b].

Naegele's rule is a handy and simple method of arriving at an estimated due date (EDD) if the date of the last menstrual period (LMP) is known. It is based on a number of assumptions that may not always be present. Adjustments must be made if the proliferative phase of the cycle is other than 14 days. Naegele's rule is based on subtracting 3 months and adding 7 days to the LMP. The EDD for an LMP of July 4 is April 11.

4. The answer is D [I C 2; Table 2-1].

Prenatal laboratory tests are performed to identify either whether a patient is at risk for a particular problem or to make an early diagnosis of a problem that is already present. Some of these tests depend on gestational age, when the interpretation of test results varies with changing weeks of pregnancy, and results must be compared with known normal values. This is the case with maternal serum α-fetoprotein (MSAFP) and the triple marker screen [i.e., AFP, human chorionic gonadotropin (hCG), estriol]. Other tests do not depend on gestational age. Tests for perinatal infectious diseases are usually in this category. The MSAFP test must be performed between 15 and 19 weeks. The other tests (i.e., hepatitis B surface antigen, syphilis serology, complete blood count, and urine culture) do not depend on gestational age; therefore, they may be performed in the first trimester.

5. The answer is D [I C 5].

Evidence that suggests a diagnosis of pregnancy both to the patient and an external observer can be divided into three categories: presumptive, probable, and positive. The presumptive signs of pregnancy are generic changes that are not specific to pregnancy. The probable signs are related to physical changes in the uterus. The positive signs are related to specific changes related to the fetus. Of the five options—Hegar's sign, palpation of fetal parts, uterine enlargement, amenorrhea, and auscultation of fetal heart tones—only amenorrhea is a presumptive sign of pregnancy.

6. The answer is B [I C 6 a].

Overall, weight gain in pregnancy is a minor factor in pregnancy outcome in the United States. The major effect of lack of maternal weight gain is observed among underweight patients. Therefore, dietary recommendations for pregnant women should be individualized. Recommended weight gain for women with a low prepregnancy weight (PPW) [i.e., < 90% of ideal body weight (IBW)] is 30–40 pounds. For women with an average PPW (i.e., 90%–135% IBW), the recommendation is 25–30 pounds. For women with a high PPW (i.e., > 135% IBW), the recommendation is 15–20 pounds.

7. The answer is A [III A 1 a, B 3].

Polygenic/multifactorial disorders are responsible for 65% of all newborn malformations. Examples include neural tube defects (NTDs), congenital heart disease, and cleft lip or palate.

8. The answer is C [III D 1 d].

Gestational age–dating errors are the most common cause of an elevated maternal serum α-fetoprotein (MSAFP) level. The major concern with an elevated level of MSAFP is an open neural tube defect (NTD). Ventral wall defects, placental bleeding, and fetal demise can also elevate the level of MSAFP. However, statistically the most common problem is gestational dating error. If the pregnancy is more advanced than the date of the last menstrual period (LMP) indicates, the maternal blood specimen may show an elevated AFP value, which although normal for the actual gestational age, artifactually appears high for the calculated gestational age. When the sonographic dating correctly identifies the true gestational age, the AFP value is seen to be within normal limits.

9. The answer is B [III E].

Only neural tube defects (NTDs) can statistically be prevented by maternal supplementation of 4 mg of folate at the time of early embryogenesis. None of the other disease entities listed (i.e., ventral wall defects, trisomy 21, Turner syndrome, fetal alcohol syndrome) can currently be prevented through nutritional supplementation.

10. The answer is B [IV B 2].

Low amniotic fluid, or oligohydramnios, is a finding that merits concern and requires a thorough investigation to identify the cause. Because normal amniotic fluid dynamics are dependent on fetal urine output, obstructive renal lesions decrease amniotic fluid and lead to oligohydramnios. Anencephaly, obstructive gastrointestinal (GI) lesions, neuromuscular disorders, and tracheoesophageal fistula are associated with increased, not decreased, amniotic fluid. The nervous system anomaly or GI obstruction prevents normal fetal swallowing and ingestion of amniotic fluid. Thus, in these cases, the amniotic fluid builds up because the normal mechanism for removing it from the uterus is not operative.

11. The answer is A [V F].

The earlier in pregnancy a sonographic growth parameter can be identified, the better. This is predicated on the finding that when a value can be placed on a growth curve when the slope is the maximum, the more accurate it is in dating the pregnancy. The crown–rump length (CRL) at 10 weeks should be accurate to within 5 days. The rate of growth of the first-trimester CRL is so rapid that it provides a very accurate dating parameter.

12. The answer is C [V F 1 b (4)].

Confirming a clinical dating parameter at the earliest gestational age possible is the most helpful. Eighteen weeks is generally the earliest that a primigravida woman reports quickening. Fetal heart tones by Doppler stethoscope at 16 weeks are not very helpful, because 6 weeks have passed since the fetal heart tones could first have been heard with a Doppler stethoscope. The reporting of quickening by a multigravida woman at 20 weeks is not very helpful, because 4 weeks have passed from when a multigravida woman should first detect quickening (at 16 weeks). Fetal heart tones by fetoscope at 24 weeks are not helpful, because 4 weeks have passed from when fetal heart tones could first have been detected via fetoscope (at 20 weeks). Measuring uterine fundal height at 26 weeks is not helpful, because the fundal height is most accurately measured during the first trimester.

13. The answer is D [V B].

Unless the gestational age is firmly established, a diagnosis of postdates pregnancy cannot be made. Therefore, the confidence in the due date is the most important question to answer.

14. The answer is D [I B 4].

Maternal mortality rate is calculated on the basis of 100,000 events. Infant mortality rate, neonatal mortality rate, fetal mortality rate, and perinatal mortality rate are calculated on the basis of 1000 events.

15. The answer is A [I C 3].

The purpose of Leopold maneuvers is to identify (before delivery) the physical relationships between the fetus and the uterine cavity. These include the lie, presentation, station, and degree of flexion of the head. Leopold maneuvers are performed by careful abdominal palpation. Cervical dilation cannot be assessed by abdominal palpation, which is the essential activity in the Leopold maneuvers.

16. The answer is D [IV B 1].

Many fetal anatomic structures have been measured sequentially throughout pregnancy, and the measurements have been used to form reference tables so that the normal limits of antenatal growth can be identified. However, only four measurements are currently used as the standard parameters: biparietal diameter (BPD), head circumference (HC), abdominal circumference (AC), and femur length (FL). Whereas transcerebellar diameter in mm does approximate the gestational age in weeks, it is not used as a standard measurement of fetal growth.

17–24. The answers are: 17-C [II D], 18-C [II D 1], 19-D [II E 3], 20-A [II B], 21-B [II C 1], 22-C [II D 3], 23-A [II B 4], 24-D [II E 2 a].

The contraction stress test (CST) does not assess the degree of fetal movement. The CST focuses only on the presence or absence of late decelerations in response to uterine contractions. The biophysical profile (BPP) is the most specific of the four testing modalities presented as options. Maternal perception of fetal kick counts requires no specialized technology. The BPP includes the nonstress test (NST), but the NST used alone measures accelerations of fetal heart rate (FHR). Inducing contractions with placenta previa could cause bleeding, which contraindicates the CST in those with placenta previa. Only counting fetal kicks may not be sensitive enough to pick up early fetal compromise, so it should not be used for primary surveillance of high-risk pregnancies. Of all the tests presented in this question set, only the BPP uses real-time ultrasound technology.

3

Pregnancy: Obstetric Complications

I. FIRST-TRIMESTER LOSS. Overall, 15% of clinically recognized pregnancies undergo first-trimester loss.

    A. Cytogenetic abnormalities are found with increasing frequency as the gestational age of pregnancy loss decreases (Figure 3-1).

        1. Almost 50% of abortuses show autosomal **trisomies.** Trisomies of all chromosomes except chromosome 1 have been found.

        2. Nearly 20% of abortuses show **polyploidy** (i.e., more than two **haploid** chromosome complements), 75% of which are **triploid** (69,XXX), and 25% of which are **tetraploid** (92,XXXX).

        3. Monosomy X (Turner's syndrome) is the **single most common aneuploidy.** This condition usually occurs from paternal sex chromosome loss. The classic sonographic fetal finding is a **cystic hygroma.** Approximately 2% survive to term, and they usually lack germ cells. Characteristic physical findings include sexual infantilism, ovarian streak gonads, and short stature.

        4. Ultrasound findings suggestive of aneuploidy include choroid plexus cysts, thickened nuchal skin fold, hyperechogenic bowel, echogenic intracardiac foci, dilated renal pelves, omphalocele, and cardiac anomalies.

    B. Noncytogenetic abnormalities may be responsible for the loss of cytogenetically "normal" first-trimester abortuses. Examples include the following:

        1. Mendelian genetic problems involving lethal genes of a dominant, recessive, or X-linked nature

        2. Polygenic/multifactorial genetic problems

        3. Gross structural anomalies

    C. The **clinical approach** to a woman suspected of having or confirmed as having a first-trimester loss consists of gathering the following information.

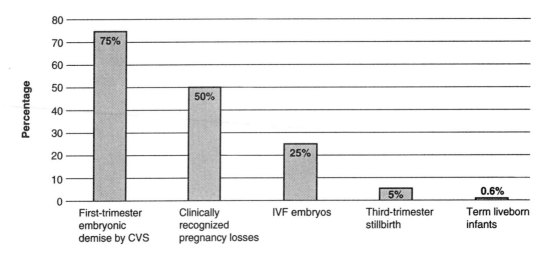

Chromosome anomalies

Figure 3-1. Frequency of chromosome anomalies among categories of pregnancy outcomes. Note that the earlier the loss occurs, the higher the percentage of aneuploidy. *CVS* = chorionic villus sampling; *IVF* = in vitro fertilization.

1. **Are the patient's vital signs stable?** If the patient's vital signs are not stable, the following must be determined.
   a. **Is there evidence of hypovolemia?**
      (1) **Postural pulse and blood pressure** (BP) [lying, sitting, standing] should be obtained.
      (2) Does the patient appear to be in **shock?**
   b. **Is there evidence of infection?**
      (1) The patient's **temperature** should be assessed.
      (2) A **pelvic examination** should be performed to check for tenderness or purulent cervical discharge.
   c. **Is there adequate intravenous (IV) access?**
      (1) An **IV** line with a large-bore needle (e.g., 16- or 18-gauge) should be started.
      (2) An **isotonic IV solution** (e.g., Ringer's lactate, normal saline) should be infused at the maximum rate if the patient is unstable.
   d. **Is there adequate urine output?** An indwelling **urinary catheter** should be placed and **hourly urine production** should be monitored if there is evidence of hypovolemia.
2. **Is the patient pregnant?**
   a. **Qualitative assessment.** A **urine or serum human chorionic gonadotropin (hCG) test** is reported as either positive or negative for pregnancy.
   b. **Quantitative assessment.** This **serum β-hCG test** estimates gestational age and is expressed as milli-international units (mIU). Sensitivity as low as 5 mIU/ml is possible with radioimmunoassay methods. The international reference preparation (IRP) criteria are used in the United States.

3. Is the pregnancy viable? Transvaginal sonographic parameters are sought in assessing pregnancy viability.

   a. A normal gestational sac can be seen at **five menstrual weeks.**

   (1) Shape. The sac is round or oval.

   (2) Position. The sac is in the fundal or middle portion of the uterus.

   (3) Contour. The sac is smooth and rounded.

   (4) Trophoblastic reaction. The sac is surrounded by an echogenic reaction of at least 3 mm in thickness.

   (5) Growth. The diameter of a normal sac increases approximately 1 mm/day in early pregnancy.

   b. Normal internal landmarks that should be seen within the gestational sac are:

   (1) A yolk sac, measuring 3–5 mm in diameter, should be seen when the gestational sac is greater than 10 mm. The yolk sac disappears at 10–12 weeks' gestation.

   (2) An embryo should be seen when the gestational sac is greater than 20 mm. Cardiac activity can be observed in an embryo that is at least 3 mm in length.

   c. The **discriminatory threshold** is the critical β-hCG value above which a normal intrauterine gestational sac can be seen (Figure 3-2).

   (1) Transabdominal sonography uses the β-hCG value of **6500 mIU/ml** (42 postmenstrual days' gestation) as the discriminatory threshold.

   (2) Transvaginal sonography uses the value of **1500 mIU/ml** (38 postmenstrual days' gestation) as the discriminatory threshold.

   d. Normal sonographic appearance is highly reassuring. Pregnancy loss rates with normal sonographic findings are 2% at 8 weeks' gestation and 1% at 16 weeks' gestation.

D. Types of spontaneous abortions (Table 3-1) consist of the following:

   1. A missed abortion (or embryonic demise) can be diagnosed if there is **sonographic evidence of a nonviable pregnancy without bleeding or cramping.**

   a. Abnormal sonographic findings

   (1) Gestational sac that is collapsing or irregularly shaped

   (2) Trophoblastic reaction that is irregular and thin

   (3) Yolk sac that is not seen

   (4) Embryo that is absent or amorphous

   (5) Cardiac activity that is absent

   b. Management is a scheduled suction dilation and curettage (D&C). Expectant observation may be followed awaiting spontaneous expulsion of products of conception. However, there is a risk of acute and unpredictable onset of hemorrhage, requiring an emergency D&C.

   2. Threatened abortion occurs in approximately **25% of pregnancies. Minimal bleeding** is the key element for the diagnosis of threatened abortion. Frequently benign bleeding can occur from irritation of columnar epithelium in the endocervical canal.

   a. Diagnostic criteria include **all** of the following: minimal bleeding

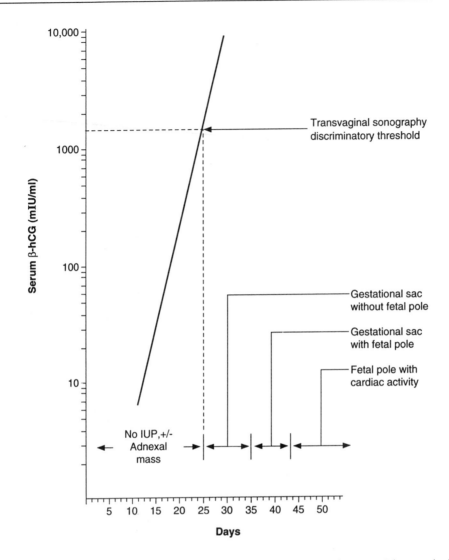

Figure 3-2. The discriminatory threshold for transvaginal sonography indicates the serum β-human chorionic gonadotropin (β-hCG) titer above which an intrauterine gestational sac should be seen. *IUP* = intrauterine pregnancy. (Reprinted with permission from Beckmann CR, Ling FW, Barzansky BM, et al (eds): *Obstetrics and Gynecology*, 1st ed. Williams & Wilkins, 1992, p 290.)

with or without mild cramping, a closed internal cervical os, and normal sonographic findings.

   b. **Management** is **expectant observation.** Use of pharmacologic agents such as progesterone does not change the outcome. There is no evidence of benefit from bed rest, although it is often advised.

3. **Inevitable abortion** indicates the pregnancy is doomed to end shortly. **Progressive cervical dilation without the passage of tissue** is the key element for the diagnosis of inevitable abortion.

   a. **Diagnostic criteria,** regardless of sonographic findings, include heavy, **profuse bleeding** and/or **severe cramping,** and a **dilated** internal cervical os.

Table 3-1. First-Trimester Bleeding: Differential Diagnoses*

Type of Abortion	Is the Embryo Viable?	Is the Patient Bleeding?	Is the Patient Cramping?	Is the Internal Cervical Os Open?	Was Tissue Passed?	Is the Patient Febrile?
Missed abortion	None seen	No	No	No	No	No
Threatened abortion	Yes	Yes	Mild	No	No	No
Inevitable abortion	Variable	Yes	Yes	Yes	Variable	No
Incomplete abortion	NA	Yes	Yes	Yes	Yes	No
Completed abortion	NA	Minimal	Minimal	Yes	Yes	No
Septic abortion	NA	Variable	Variable	Yes	Yes	Yes

NA = not applicable.
*Always consider the possibility of a molar or ectopic pregnancy.

> (1) **Assessment of blood loss** should be done objectively by estimating the number of soaked sanitary pads. Subjective assessment is often unreliable and exaggerated.
> (2) **Assessment of internal cervical os.** The internal cervical os is considered dilated if no resistance is encountered as a **ring forceps is passed** through the os. Passing a cotton swab through the os is inaccurate because a cotton swab may normally pass through the patient's os.

> b. **Management** is **emergency suction D&C.**

4. **Incomplete abortion** is the diagnosis if the **internal cervical os is open** and the **patient has passed some tissue.**

   a. **Diagnostic criteria** include the ability to pass ring forceps through the internal cervical os and the passing of tissue. However, the passing of tissue can be subjective (patient history). Objective determination can be made if the patient brings the specimen or tissue is found on speculum examination.

   b. **Management** is **emergency suction D&C.**

5. **Completed abortion** can be diagnosed if the patient **has passed tissue** but now is only **minimally cramping and bleeding.**

   a. **Diagnostic criteria** include **all** of the following:
      (1) Historical finding of bleeding, cramping, and passage of tissue
      (2) Examination finding of a dilated internal cervical os
      (3) Minimal current bleeding
      (4) Transvaginal sonogram shows empty uterus with normal "endometrial stripe"

   b. **Management** includes **ruling out of ectopic pregnancy** via transvaginal sonography followed by cautious observation. **Following the serial quantitative serum β-hCG titers** until they are negative ensures that no trophoblastic villi remain in the uterus.

E. Additional concerns

1. **Rh blood typing status.** If the patient is **Rh$_o$ (D) negative** [and her partner is Rh$_o$ (D) positive], an atypical antibody screen (AAS) must be obtained to ensure that the patient is not isoimmunized. If the AAS is negative, Rh$_o$ (D) immune globulin (e.g., RhoGAM) should be administered within 72 hours to prevent sensitization.

2. **Infectious complications.** If the patient is **febrile, infected, or septic,** an unsterile, lay abortion procedure may have been performed.
   a. **Physical examination.** The patient should be evaluated for cervical purulence and pelvic or uterine tenderness.
   b. **Management.** Cervical cultures should be obtained, and IV antibiotics with broad-spectrum coverage for gram-positive and gram-negative aerobic organisms as well as anaerobic organisms should be initiated. A gentle suction D&C should then be performed.

3. **Emotional reaction to the pregnancy loss**
   a. **Establish** whether the pregnancy was wanted or unwanted.
   b. **Reassure** the patient and her partner that grief and guilt are part of the normal response.
   c. **Inform** the patient and her partner that the normal sequence of recovery from a perinatal loss includes trouble sleeping and eating, crying, and thinking of the lost infant.

4. **Likelihood of having another first-trimester pregnancy loss**
   a. **Risks for the next pregnancy** include the following:
      (1) If this pregnancy was the patient's first, the risk of losing the next pregnancy is **15%.**
      (2) If the patient's first pregnancy was a normal fetus, and this loss was her second pregnancy, the risk of losing a third pregnancy is **15%.**
      (3) If the patient's first pregnancy was a first-trimester loss, and this pregnancy was another loss, the risk of losing the third pregnancy is **40%.**
      (4) If the first pregnancy was a normal fetus, the second pregnancy was a first-trimester loss, and this pregnancy was another loss, the risk of losing her fourth pregnancy is **25%.**
   b. **Medical workup** for **recurrent first-trimester losses** should include the following:
      (1) Thyroid studies to rule out a hypothyroid state
      (2) Parental karyotype to rule out aneuploidy
      (3) Hysterosalpingography to rule out a uterine anomaly
      (4) *Mycoplasma* **culture** to rule out infectious etiology
      (5) Anticardiolipin antibody test to rule out antiphospholipid syndrome (see IV C 3 a).

5. **Preconception counseling.** Loss of a pregnancy presents an opportunity to implement changes that could improve the next pregnancy outcome.

   a. **Behavior changes** can improve some pregnancy outcomes.

      (1) If the patient has **overt diabetes,** normoglycemia should be attempted to prevent fetal anomalies.

      (2) If the patient is at increased risk for **neural tube defects (NTDs),** daily folic acid (4 mg/day) should be initiated.

      (3) If the patient has **phenylketonuria,** she should begin a phenylalanine-restricted diet.

      (4) The patient's medications should be reviewed. She should be switched to alternative medications if she takes any of the following **teratogenic medications:**

         (a) Hydantoin/phenytoin

         (b) Warfarin (Coumadin)

         (c) Isotretinoin

         (d) Valproic acid

         (e) Folic acid antagonists (e.g., methotrexate)

      (5) The use of **recreational and addictive drugs** should be strongly discouraged, and the use of harmful substances, including alcohol and tobacco, should be discontinued.

   b. **Active maternal immunizations** that may protect the fetus during the next pregnancy include:

      (1) Attenuated live-virus **rubella** vaccine (pregnancy should be avoided for 3 months; see Chapter 5 III)

      (2) Three-injection series against **hepatitis B** (see Chapter 5 VII)

   5. Ectopic pregnancy should always be considered in the differential diagnosis of first-trimester bleeding (see Chapter 13 V).

   6. Molar pregnancy should always be considered in the differential diagnosis of first-trimester bleeding (see VII).

II. SECOND-TRIMESTER LOSS.

Whereas first-trimester losses are most often caused by cytogenetic abnormalities, second-trimester losses are caused by **uterine anatomic defects, incompetent cervix, or fetal death.**

   A. **Maternal causes**

      1. **Uterine anatomic defects**

         a. **Müllerian duct fusion anomalies,** including uterine septum and uterine duplication, can contribute to pregnancy losses (Figure 3-3). Müllerian system anomalies are associated with an increase in the risk of urinary tract anomalies. An IV pyelogram (IVP) should be performed.

            (1) **Diagnostic methods** for müllerian duct anomalies include the following:

               (a) **Hysterosalpingography:** instilling radio-opaque dye transcervically into the uterine cavity and taking radiographs

               (b) **Hysteroscopy:** inspecting the uterine cavity through a transcervical fiberoptic scope

               (c) **Laparoscopy:** inspecting the external uterine contour through a transabdominal fiberoptic scope

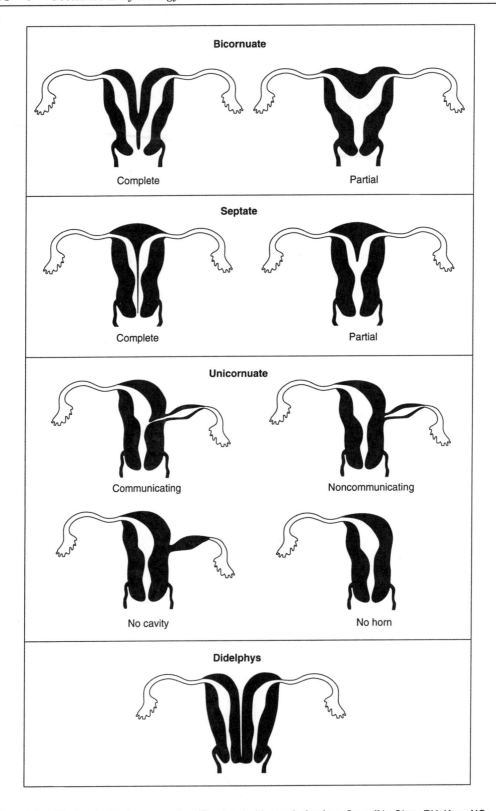

Figure 3-3. Müllerian duct fusion anomalies. (Reprinted with permission from Speroff L, Glass RH, Kase NG: *Clinical Endocrinology and Infertility,* 5th ed. Williams & Wilkins, Baltimore, 1994, p 370.)

(2) A **uterine septum** may receive an inadequate vascular supply for placentation if implantation occurs on the septum. A thin septum is more worrisome than a thick septum, because the blood supply is more attenuated.

(a) Treatment for a **thin** uterine septum is **hysteroscopic resection.**

(b) Treatment for a **thick** uterine septum may involve **exploratory laparotomy** to bivalve the uterus, removal of the septum, and repair of the uterus (Strassman procedure). Labor is unsafe in patients who have been repaired with bivalving of the uterus because of the risk of uterine rupture.

(3) Uterine duplication with the fetus growing in one of the two uterine horns limits the space available for expansion that is necessary to reach term gestation. Half of these patients undergo preterm delivery, some prior to fetal viability.

b. A submucous **uterine leiomyoma** limits the vascular supply for placentation and contributes to atypical hormone responsiveness of the overlying endometrium. If the supply of oxygen and nutrition to the fetus is inadequate, fetal demise can occur.

(1) Diagnosis involves **hysterosalpingography** or **hysteroscopy.**

(2) Treatment involves **hysteroscopic resection.**

2. Incompetent cervix

a. Definitions

(1) Functional. Passive, painless midtrimester cervical dilation results in membrane prolapse and rupture leading to expulsion of an immature, nonviable fetus.

(2) Anatomic. A cervical structural weakness results in the patient being unable to carry a fetus to viability.

b. Etiology

(1) Congenital

(a) In utero **diethylstilbestrol (DES) exposure.** A nonsteroidal estrogen, DES was used to treat threatened abortions up to 1970. Females exposed in utero to DES have an increased risk of müllerian duct anomalies, including uterine and cervical malformations.

(b) Spontaneous occurrence

(2) Traumatic

(a) Mechanical cervical dilation

(b) Second-trimester abortion

(c) Cervical amputation, conization, or laceration

c. Diagnosis

(1) History. The **most accurate diagnosis is a retrospective one** based on a history of painless midtrimester cervical dilation resulting in expulsion of a nonviable fetus. History of any of the congenital or traumatic causes of an incompetent cervix contributes strongly to the diagnosis (see II A 2 b).

(2) Pelvic examination. An examination for vaginal septae, cervical anomalies, and abnormal uterine configuration should be performed. Cervical length, thickness, and dilation should be assessed.

(3) **Vaginal ultrasound.** If the history is suggestive but not confirmatory, start serial weekly sonographic examinations during the next pregnancy. Parameters assessed include shortening of cervical length and widening of the endocervical canal starting at the internal os. Such widening is known as funneling or beaking.

(4) **Nonpregnant workup.** A number of methods for assessing cervical incompetence before pregnancy have been suggested. There should be no internal os resistance to an 8-mm Hegar dilator. A traction test with an inflated Foley balloon or balloon hysterography has been proposed. None of these nonpregnant diagnostic methods are reliable.

d. **Management.** The primary approach to a patient with an incompetent cervix is **cervical cerclage,** which involves the placement of a circumferential cervical suture that externally supports the internal os (Figure 3-4).

(1) **Methods.** Cervical cerclage is scheduled for placement between 10–12 weeks' gestation, after a sonogram shows a normal viable fetus. This allows the suture to be placed before cervical dilation, effacement, and prolapse of membranes through a dilated cervical os.

(a) The **Shirodkar method** is performed vaginally, leaving a merseline tape suture buried submucosally. The cerclage usually is not removed. Rather, a scheduled cesarean delivery is performed.

(b) The **McDonald method** is performed vaginally, leaving the suture easily accessible. The cerclage is removed at 36 weeks to allow labor and vaginal delivery.

(c) The **transabdominal method** is performed by laparotomy if the cervix is too short to allow a vaginally placed cerclage.

A. McDonald **B.** Shirodkar **C.** Transabdominal

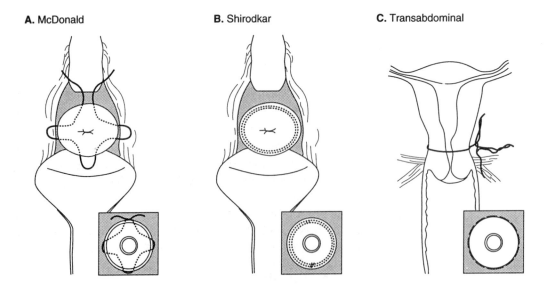

Figure 3-4. Management of a patient with an incompetent cervix: McDonald, Shirodkar, and transabdominal methods. (Reprinted with permission from Scott JR, DiSaia PJ, Hammond CB, et al (eds): *Danforth's Obstetrics and Gynecology,* 6th ed. J.B. Lippincott, Philadelphia, 1990, p 219.)

The cerclage is left in place, and cesarean delivery is performed.

(2) **Complications of cerclage** may include premature rupture of membranes, infection, bleeding, and subsequent preterm delivery.

B. **Fetal causes.** Any disease process that can lead to fetal death can lead to a second-trimester loss (see IV). Two etiologic categories with examples include:

1. **Diseases intrinsic to the fetus** such as:

   a. **Chromosome anomalies** (e.g., monosomy X, trisomy 21)

   b. **Anatomic anomalies** (e.g., cardiac, osteochondrodysplasias)

   c. **Nonimmune hydrops** (e.g., tumor, α-thalassemia, tachyarrhythmias)

2. **Diseases mediated through the placenta,** such as:

   a. **Immune hydrops,** which is the most severe form of isoimmunization (e.g., from maternal anti-D or anti-Kell antibodies)

   b. **Nonimmune hydrops** (from fetomaternal hemorrhage)

   c. **Maternal infections** (e.g., syphilis, parvovirus B19)

   d. **Maternal systemic conditions** [e.g., type I diabetes mellitus (DM), anticardiolipin antibody]

III. THIRD-TRIMESTER BLEEDING (Table 3-2)

A. **Causes**

1. **Abruptio placentae** (Figure 3-5) is the premature separation of a **normally implanted placenta** (not in lower uterine segment), which causes **painful bleeding.**

   a. **Incidence.** Abruptio placentae affects approximately 1 in 100 deliveries at term. It is the **most common obstetric cause of disseminated intravascular coagulation (DIC).**

Table 3-2. Third-Trimester Bleeding

	Abruptio Placenta	Placenta Previa	Vasa Previa	Uterine Rupture
Painful bleeding?	Yes	No	No	Yes
Incidence	1%	0.5% (at 40 weeks)	Rare	Rare
Mechanism of bleeding	Separation of normally implanted placenta	Separation of placenta implanted in lower uterine segment	Ruptured fetal vessels traversing membranes over cervix	Ruptured myometrial vessels
Types	• External or overt • Internal or concealed	• Complete • Partial • Marginal • Low-lying	NA	NA

NA = not applicable.
SPROM = spontaneous premature rupture of membranes.

A. Partial separation

B. Marginal separation

C. Complete separation with concealed hemorrhage

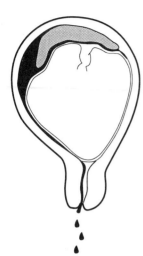 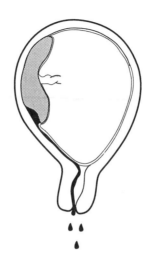 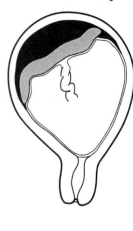

Figure 3-5. Diagnostic classification of types of placental abruptio: partial, marginal, and complete separation with concealed hemorrhage. (Reprinted with permission from Scott JR, DiSaia PJ, Hammond CB, et al (eds): *Danforth's Obstetrics and Gynecology,* 6th ed. J.B. Lippincott, Philadelphia, 1990, p 560.)

    b. Pathophysiology

        (1) Hemorrhage occurs into the decidua basalis, separating part of the placenta from the uterus.

        (2) Blood from the forming hematoma may remain retroplacental (concealed) or may progress to the edge of the placenta, where it may break through the membranes and enter the amniotic cavity or may flow between the chorion and decidua to the cervix and vagina (overt).

        (3) Couvelaire uterus (uteroplacental apoplexy) is caused by extensive extravasation of blood into the myometrium.

    c. Diagnosis of abruptio placentae is **best made clinically.** Ultrasound often fails to detect retroplacental bleeding, causing false-negative diagnoses. Bleeding may be either overt or concealed.

        (1) External (overt) abruption

            (a) Blood may be bright red or dark and clotted.

            (b) The patient has only mild pain, unless she is in labor.

            (c) The degree of anemia and shock is equivalent to apparent blood loss.

        (2) Internal (concealed) abruption

            (a) There is little vaginal bleeding because the blood is trapped in the uterus.

            (b) Pain is severe; the uterus is hard and tender.

            (c) Fetal heart tones may be absent because of fetal demise.

            (d) The degree of shock is more than expected for the amount of visible blood.

2. **Placenta previa** (Figure 3-6) is the premature separation of an **abnormally implanted placenta** (in the lower uterine segment) that causes **painless bleeding.**

  a. **Incidence**

    (1) **Sonographic diagnosis of placenta previa** decreases with gestational age.

      (a) At 16 weeks' gestation, as many as 25% of pregnancies demonstrate asymptomatic placenta previa.

      (b) By 40 weeks' gestation, only 0.5% of pregnancies show lower segment placental implantation.

    (2) The **mechanism** of this phenomenon is "apparent" **placental migration.** The inferior aspect of the placenta, implanted lower in the uterus with poor blood supply, undergoes **atrophy.** The superior aspect of the placenta, implanted higher in the uterus with richer blood supply, undergoes **hypertrophy.**

  b. **Pathophysiology**

    (1) With **advancing pregnancy,** the passive lower **uterine segment stretches and thins,** which alters the lower segment implantation site of the placenta.

    (2) The **venous sinuses are exposed** as the placental anchoring villi are avulsed from the decidua.

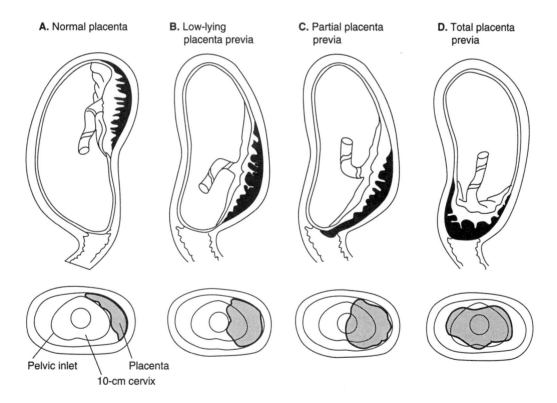

A. Normal placenta   **B.** Low-lying placenta previa   **C.** Partial placenta previa   **D.** Total placenta previa

Pelvic inlet   Placenta   10-cm cervix

Figure 3-6. Diagnostic classification of placenta previa: (*A*) Normal, (*B*) Low-lying, (*C*) Partial, and (*D*) Total. (Reprinted with permission from DeCherney AH, Pernoll ML (eds): *Current Obstetrics and Gynecologic Diagnosis & Treatment,* 8th ed. Appleton & Lange, East Norwalk, Conn., 1994, p 404.)

      (3) Timing of the first bleed is determined by how early in pregnancy the lower segment begins to form and by how low the placenta is implanted.

      (4) The **extent** of the first bleed is variable, and each successive bleed tends to be heavier.

    c. Diagnostic classification is based on the relationship of the placenta to the cervical os as visualized by ultrasound.

      (1) Total placenta previa. The internal os is completely covered by the placenta, and the placenta is unlikely to "move" away to allow vaginal delivery.

      (2) Partial placenta previa. The internal os is partially covered by the placenta, and the placenta may "move" away from the os. Vaginal delivery may be possible.

      (3) Low-lying placenta previa. The placenta is implanted in the lower uterine segment. Vaginal delivery is likely.

3. Vasa previa is bleeding arising from **ruptured fetal vessels** crossing the placental membranes overlying the cervix. Bleeding results most commonly from vessels from a **velamentous insertion** of the umbilical cord but can also occur from vessels joining an **accessory placental lobe** to the main placental disk. The classic **diagnostic triad** of vasa previa is **membrane rupture** leading to **vaginal bleeding** followed by **fetal bradycardia**.

    a. Incidence. Vasa previa is rare.

    b. Pathophysiology of bleeding from a velamentous insertion

      (1) Umbilical cord takes its origin removed from placental disk.

      (2) The fetal vessels traverse the membranes for a variable distance before joining together.

      (3) The vessels cross membranes overlying the internal cervical os.

      (4) The rupture of membranes causes tearing of fetal vessels.

      (5) If the fetus is not immediately delivered, it may undergo rapid exsanguination.

4. Uterine rupture is a full-thickness laceration of the myometrial wall. This can occur at the site of a previous uterine incision, or it can arise spontaneously without predisposition. The diagnosis should be considered with heavy vaginal bleeding in the presence of a well-contracted uterus. **Classification and pathophysiology** are described as follows:

    a. Incomplete. The peritoneal cavity remains separated from the uterine cavity by visceral peritoneum.

    b. Complete. The laceration communicates directly with the peritoneal cavity.

    c. Rupture of cesarean scar. Traumatic rupture of an old uterine incision throughout most of its length with extrusion of part or all of the fetus into the peritoneal cavity usually results in massive bleeding, with a 50% risk of fetal death and a 5% risk of maternal death.

    d. Dehiscence. Separation of a scar is usually gradual and asymptomatic, involving only part of the old incision without bleeding and leaving the peritoneum intact This is not a true rupture.

B. Risk factors (Table 3-3). Note that a previous history of third-trimester bleeding increases the risk of recurrence. Although multiple risk factors have been identified for the various kinds of bleeding, no risk factors are identifiable in most cases.

C. Clinical approach

1. **Vital signs.** The patient's heart rate and BP should be monitored, and intravascular volume should be assessed.

2. **Clinical characteristics** (Table 3-4). Distinguishing between placenta previa and abruptio placentae can be refined by comparing bleeding characteristics, fetal status, and uterine characteristics.

3. **Origin of bleeding.** The **Apt test** is a rapid but crude bedside method for assessing if bleeding is maternal or fetal. It is based on the resistance of fetal hemoglobin F to alkali. Sodium hydroxide is mixed with the blood. If the resulting color is **pink** it indicates **fetal blood,** whereas a **brown** color indicates **maternal blood.**

   a. **Maternal** bleeding can be found with abruptio placentae, placenta previa, or uterine rupture.

   b. **Fetal blood is found only with vasa previa.**

4. **Maternal complications**

   a. **Hemorrhagic shock** can be caused by both apparent as well as concealed blood loss.

   b. **DIC** can be caused when thromboplastin enters the maternal circulation, which leads to hypofibrinogenemia.

   c. **Postpartum hemorrhage** can be caused by failure of the uterus to contract properly or by coagulopathy.

   d. **Renal failure** may occur as a consequence of ischemic necrosis of the kidneys, acute tubular necrosis, or bilateral cortical necrosis.

   e. **Sheehan syndrome** is caused by ischemic necrosis of the anterior pituitary gland due to shock.

Table 3-3. Risk Factors for Third-Trimester Bleeding

Abruptio Placentae	Placenta Previa	Vasa Previa	Uterine Rupture
Previous abruption	Previous placenta previa	Velamentous cord insertion	Previous classic uterine incision
Hypertension			
Maternal-fetal trauma	Multiparity	Multiple gestation	Injudicious use of oxytocin
	Advanced maternal age		
Polyhydramnios with rapid decompression			Grandmultiparity
	Multiple gestation		Marked uterine distention
Maternal use of cocaine or tobacco			
Spontaneous premature rupture of membranes (SPROM)			External/internal version
Short umbilical cord			

Table 3-4. Clinical Characteristics of Third-Trimester Bleeding

Clinical Finding	Suggestive of Placenta Previa	Suggestive of Abruptio Placentae
Bleeding characteristics		
Onset	May be gradual, progressive	Often abrupt, unexpected
How evident	Always external	May be either external or concealed
Color	Bright red	Dark
Fetal status		
Fetal heart tones	Usually present	May be absent (if fetal demise)
Engagement	Absent (placenta obstructs)	May be present
Presentation	Often malpresentation	Unaffected by bleeding
Uterine characteristics		
Pain	Painless unless labor	Intense and steady
Tenderness	Absent	Present
Tone	Soft and relaxed	Firm to stony hard
Shape	Normal	May enlarge and change shape

5. **Management of third-trimester bleeding**
    a. **Initial evaluation and stabilization** should be obtained.
        (1) **Avoid digital cervical examination or speculum examination until ultrasound has been obtained to rule out placenta previa.**
        (2) **Obtain patient's history** rapidly, and perform a quick physical examination.
        (3) **Obtain the following laboratory test results** promptly:
            (a) Complete blood cell count and peripheral smear
            (b) Platelets, prothrombin time (PT), fibrinogen, and fibrin split products
            (c) Typing and cross-matching of 4 U of blood
        (4) **Establish an IV line** with an 18-gauge needle.
        (5) **Transfuse** selected blood products when indicated.
    b. **Treatment of bleeding** includes:
        (1) **Packed red blood cells** (RBCs) should be transfused to maintain adequate oxygen carrying capacity.
        (2) **Fresh-frozen plasma and platelets** should be administered if DIC is present. Fibrinogen is seldom used today.
        (3) **Hysterectomy** should be performed if bleeding from a noncontracting uterus cannot be controlled.
    c. **Timing and route of delivery** are summarized in Table 3-5. Note

Table 3-5. Management Criteria for Third-Trimester Bleeding

	Allow Vaginal Delivery	Emergency Cesarean Delivery	Scheduled Cesarean Delivery	Conservative Management*
Abruptio placentae	**All criteria needed** at any gestational age if: • bleeding controlled • mother and fetus stable • rapid vaginal delivery expected	**Perform if any criteria present** at any gestational age if: • bleeding or DIC uncontrolled • mother and fetus unstable • vaginal delivery unlikely	**Never appropriate**	**All criteria needed:** • fetus is immature • bleeding stopped • mother and fetus stable • no evidence of DIC
Placenta previa	**Never appropriate**	**Perform if any criteria present** at any gestational age: • bleeding uncontrolled • mother and fetus unstable • vaginal delivery unlikely	**All criteria needed:** • fetal lung maturity confirmed by amniotic fluid surfactant studies • mother and fetus stable	**All criteria needed:** • fetus is immature • bleeding controlled • mother and fetus stable
Vasa previa	**Never appropriate**	**Crucial to perform as soon as diagnosis is made**	**Never appropriate**	**Never appropriate**
Uterine rupture	**Never appropriate**	**Crucial to perform as soon as diagnosis is made**	**Never appropriate**	**Never appropriate**

*Consists of admission to hospital at bed rest using maternal corticosteroids, tocolytics, and blood component transfusions as indicated.
DIC = disseminated intravascular coagulation.

that vasa previa and uterine rupture are managed by emergency cesarean section as soon as the diagnosis is made. Abruptio placentae and placenta previa management vary according to gestational age as well as maternal and fetal status.

IV. FETAL DEMISE

    A. Confirming fetal death

        1. Initial indicators of fetal death

            a. Early pregnancy: absence of uterine growth

            b. Late pregnancy: absence of fetal movement

        2. Confirmatory findings by physician

            a. Absence of fetal cardiac activity

      (1) Auscultation with a fetoscope or Doppler stethoscope does not detect fetal heart tones.

      (2) Electronic fetal monitoring (EFM) using an external sonocardiogram or an internal scalp electrode does not detect fetal cardiac activity.

      (3) Ultrasound visualization of the fetus reveals no cardiac or great vessel vascular motion. This is 100% accurate and is **the method of choice in confirming fetal demise.**

    b. **Radiographic findings** are seldom used today.

      (1) Robert's sign (gas in the great vessels) is caused by postmortem blood degeneration.

      (2) Spalding's sign (overlapping skull bones) is caused by collapse of the fetal brain.

      (3) Angulation of the spine (exaggeration of fetal spinal curvature) is caused by loss of tone of paraspinal muscles and ligaments.

    c. Absence of fetal motion by ultrasound (i.e., lack of gross body movements, lack of extremity flexion and extension)

  3. Pseudocyesis. **"False pregnancy"** is diagnosed when a nonpregnant woman believes she is pregnant and develops signs and symptoms suggestive of pregnancy, yet her uterus is nonpregnant on sonogram, and a β-hCG level is negative. This is a **conversion reaction** in which psychic conflict is expressed in physical terms.

B. Determining how long the fetus has been dead is important to assess the risk of DIC.

  1. Changes noted immediately include ultrasound findings of absent cardiac activity and absent fetal movement.

  2. Changes noted after a few days

    a. Radiographic findings include Spalding's sign and Robert's sign.

    b. Amniocentesis reveals port wine–colored amniotic fluid.

    c. Ultrasound findings include Spalding's sign and generalized fetal edema.

C. Causes of fetal demise

  1. Idiopathic deaths, accounting for half of the fetuses that die, show no obvious cause of death even after extensive testing.

  2. Placenta or cord problems include abruptio placentae with fetomaternal hemorrhage (i.e., fetus becomes hypovolemic by bleeding into maternal circulation).

  3. Maternal systemic diseases

    a. Anticardiolipin antibody–lupus anticoagulant–antiphospholipid syndrome. This refers to a group of autoimmune conditions in which maternal antibodies attack the lipid membranes of a pregnant woman's vascular system and the fetoplacental unit.

      (1) A **history** of cerebrovascular accident, venous thrombosis, or repeated pregnancy losses is associated with this syndrome.

      (2) The **diagnosis** is confirmed by a consistent history; a prolonged activated partial thromboplastin time (PTT); and an elevated level of anticardiolipin antibodies, lupus anticoagulant, or antiphospholipid antibodies.

(3) The **treatment** is controversial and consists of one or more of the following agents: low-dose aspirin, heparin, and prednisone.

b. **Type I DM** (see Chapter 4 VIII)

(1) Fetal death occurs mostly in diabetics with vascular disease, poor glycemic control, polyhydramnios, and fetal macrosomia.

(2) The precise cause is unknown but probably involves fetal hyperinsulinemia, chronic intrauterine hypoxia, and reduced placental blood flow. The macrosomic fetus outgrows the ability of the placenta to supply it with adequate oxygen.

5. **Maternal trauma** can cause hemorrhage with resulting hypotension leading to peripheral vasoconstriction, which diminishes uteroplacental blood flow and thus placental gas exchange. The result is fetal death.

a. **Penetrating trauma** to the uterus (e.g., gunshots, stab wounds) often leads to fetal death by direct fetal injury.

b. **Blunt trauma** to the uterus (e.g., falls, motor vehicle accidents, domestic violence) is less likely to lead to direct fetal injury because of the force-absorbing uterine wall and amniotic fluid.

6. **Maternal isoimmunization** (see VI) results in hemolysis of fetal RBCs by maternal immunoglobulin G antibodies that have crossed transplacentally into the fetus from the maternal circulation. If the fetal anemia is sufficiently severe, fetal hydrops and subsequent demise can occur.

7. **Fetal causes**

a. **Abnormal karyotype.** Aneuploidy of the large autosomes leads to first-trimester embryonic demise. Later fetal deaths largely involve either the sex chromosomes (e.g., monosomy X) or the smaller autosomes (e.g., trisomy 13, 18, 21).

b. **Anatomic anomalies.** Examples include cardiac defects and osteochondrodysplasias (e.g., osteogenesis imperfecta).

c. **Infections.** Severe first-trimester infections lead to embryonic demise or cause teratogenesis. Second-trimester infections primarily involving the fetus seldom lead to fetal death. The following are exceptions.

(1) **Parvovirus B19.** Fetal **erythroid progenitor cell destruction** leads to severe anemia and hydrops.

(2) **Syphilis,** *Listeria, Mycoplasma,* and **cytomegalovirus (CMV).** Severe **inflammation and edema of placental villi** leads to fetal hypoxia from decreased oxygen transport.

d. **Nonimmune hydrops**

(1) This is caused by a **wide variety of fetal causes,** including aneuploidy, gross anomalies, or infections, as well as fetomaternal hemorrhage, α-thalassemia, and fetal tachyarrhythmias.

(2) The **fetal mortality rate** for fetuses with nonimmune hydrops is as high as **90%.**

D. **Determining the cause of fetal demise** (Table 3-6). To assess the possibility of recurrence of a fetal death, it is important to ask, **"Why did it happen?"** The optimal time to gather any data that could shed light on this question is at the time of diagnosis and delivery.

Table 3-6. Determining the Cause of Fetal Demise

Test	Clinical Condition
TORCHES studies	Fetal infection
Listeria **culture**	Fetoplacental infection
Anticardiolipin antibodies/ lupus anticoagulant	Antiphospholipid syndrome
Fetal autopsy	Abnormal gross anomalies suggesting a syndrome
Karyotype	Abnormal fetal chromosomes
Total body fetal radiograph	Osteochondrodystrophic disorders
Maternal Kleihauer-Betke test	Fetomaternal bleed
Atypical antibody titer	Maternal isoimmunization

TORCHES = toxoplasmosis, rubella, cytomegalovirus, herpes simplex virus (syphilis).

    E. Appropriate management. This generally includes expeditious termination of the pregnancy.

      1. Cervical examination should be performed to assess whether the cervix is favorable (i.e., dilated, effaced, soft) for labor and delivery.

        a. If favorable, labor can be induced, anticipating vaginal delivery. Artificial rupture of membranes and IV oxytocin infusion are used to induce labor. There is no benefit to delivering a dead fetus via cesarean section.

        b. If unfavorable, use of the following should be considered.

          (1) Cervical ripening agents such as cervical laminaria/dilateria or prostaglandin E_2 (PGE$_2$) medications (i.e., vaginal suppositories, intracervical jelly) shorten the induction-to-delivery interval but do not decrease the cesarean delivery rate.

          (2) Dilation and evacuation (D&E) [see Chapter 10 III F 1] can be performed if:

            (a) Gestational age is less than 20 weeks.

            (b) Autopsy on an intact fetus is not necessary.

      2. Maternal psychologic issues are important.

        a. Grief response. Time should be allowed for an appropriate grief response to begin. The grief response includes denial, anger, bargaining, and acceptance. Crying, difficulty sleeping, and loss of appetite are commonly experienced.

        b. Support. Time should be allowed for the rallying of family and social support.

        c. Delaying intervention. Delaying induction of labor or D&E temporarily for these reasons may be appropriate.

        d. Disposition of fetal remains. Parents should not be discouraged from seeing and holding the fetus or obtaining mementos (e.g., pictures, handprints, or footprints). Autopsies and funerals may help in the grieving process. Parental participation in decision making can help them achieve more control in coping with their loss.

3. The length of time that the fetus has been dead is important.

    a. DIC is a serious complication of prolonged retention of a dead fetus, which can be triggered by the release of **tissue thromboplastin** from the deteriorating fetus and placenta into the maternal circulation.

    b. Baseline coagulation studies should be obtained if the mother refuses immediate intervention, with repeat testing weekly. **DIC is rare until 4 weeks after fetal demise.**

    c. Delivery should be attempted in the following instances:

       (1) Four weeks have passed since fetal demise.

       (2) Serum fibrinogen level is less than 200 mg/ml.

       (3) Platelet count is decreasing ($< 100,000$/ml).

V. MULTIPLE GESTATION

A. Incidence

1. Clinically recognized

    a. Twins: 1 in 90 births at term. (**Vanishing twin syndrome** is noted often in early pregnancy when one twin undergoes developmental arrest and resorption, resulting in a singleton birth.)

    b. Triplets: 1 in about 8000 births (90^2)

    c. Quadruplets: 1 in about 730,000 births (90^3)

2. According to mode of ovulation

    a. 1%: spontaneous ovulation

    b. 10%: clomiphene ovulation induction

    c. 30%: gonadotropin ovulation induction

B. Classification of twins (Table 3-7) may be based on identifying the number of eggs, placentas, or amniotic sacs.

1. By zygosity (number of **eggs** from which the multiple fetuses arose). Sonographic clues to zygosity are given in Table 3-8.

    a. Monozygotic or **identical** twins arise from **one egg** and represent **one-third** of all twins.

    b. Dizygotic or **fraternal** twins arise from **two eggs** and represent **two-thirds** of all twins.

2. By chorionicity [number of **placentas** within the uterus (Figure 3-7)]

    a. Monochorionic (one shared placenta) twins can only be monozygotic. One twin (i.e., recipient) may take disproportionately more placental blood flow than the other (i.e., donor), resulting in **twin–twin transfusion syndrome** (see V C 2). The septum dividing the two sacs has **two layers** only—an amnion from each fetus.

    b. Dichorionic (two placentas) twins can be monozygotic or dizygotic. The placentas may be **separate** (two different locations on the uterine wall) or **fused** (immediately adjacent to each other). The septum dividing the two sacs has **four layers**—a chorion and an amnion from each fetus.

Table 3-7. Twin Gestation Types

	DiDi (Dichorionic-Diamnionic)		MonoDi (Monochorionic-Diamnionic)	MonoMono (Monochorionic-Monoamnionic)	Conjoined (Monochorionic-Monoamnionic
	Different Gender	Same Gender			
Placenta number	2	2	1	1	1
Amnion number	2	2	2	1	1
Incidence of occurrence	1 in 300	1 in 300	1 in 400	1 in 3,000	1 in 50,000
Time of cleavage	NA	NA or 0–72 hrs	4–8 days	9–12 days	> 12 days
Zygosity of twins	Di	Di or Mono	Mono	Mono	Mono
Related to fertility treatment	Yes	Yes or No	No	No	No
Risk of twin-twin transfusion	None	None	Present	Present	NA
Risk of cord entangle	None	None	None	Present	NA
Risk of malformation	Low	Low-Med	Medium	High	NA
Risk of vasa previa	Low	Low	Higher	Higher	NA
Risk of placenta previa	High	High	High	High	High
Risk of preterm delivery	High	High	High	High	High

NA = not applicable.

Table 3-8. Sonographic Clues to Zygosity

Findings	Zygosity	Frequency
Different genders	Dizygotic	30%
Two placentas, same gender, different blood groups	Dizygotic	27%
One placenta	Monozygotic	23%
Two placentas, same gender, same blood group	Monozygotic	20%

    3. By amnionicity (number of **amniotic sacs** within the uterus)
        a. Monoamnionic (one sac) twins can be only monozygotic. There is a **high risk of cord entanglement,** because there is no septum between the two fetuses. **Conjoined twins** must always be monoamnionic.
        b. Diamnionic (two sacs) twins can be either monochorionic or dichorionic. If they are dichorionic, they may be either monozygotic or dizygotic.

  C. Clinical approach
    1. Multiple gestation
      a. Suggestive signs of multiple gestation include:

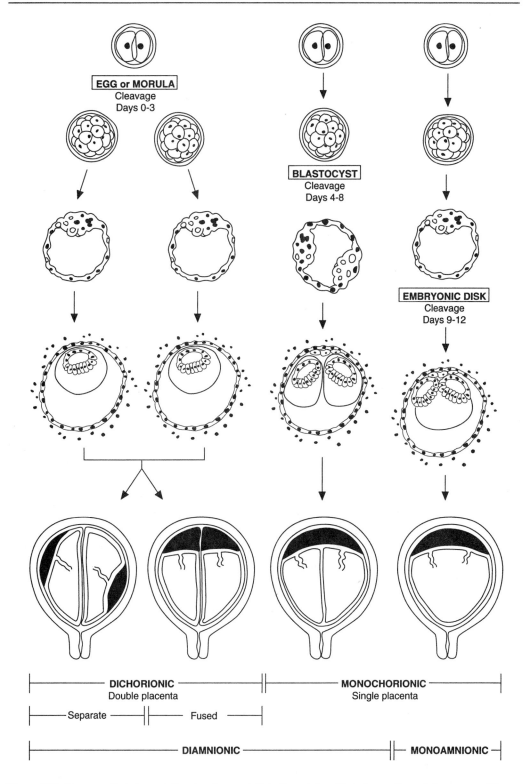

Figure 3-7. Monozygotic twin gestation development. Note the relationship between time of cleavage and the embryonic tissue that divides on the number of chorions and amnions. (After DeCherney AH, Pernoll ML (eds): *Current Obstetric and Gynecologic Diagnosis & Treatment,* 8th ed. Appleton & Lange, East Norwalk, Conn., 1994, p 359.)

       (1) Large-for-dates uterus (> 4 cm larger than expected)

       (2) Excessive weight gain for singleton pregnancy

       (3) Abnormally high levels of maternal serum β-hCG and α-feto-protein

   b. Definitive diagnosis of multiple gestation is via **ultrasound visualization** of two or more embryos or fetuses. Confirmation is possible at less than 7 weeks' gestation.

   c. Other causes of uterus large-for-dates (e.g., hydramnios, hydatidiform mole, tumors) should be ruled out (see Chapter 2 IV C).

  2. Fetal risks

   a. Twin–twin transfusion (Table 3-9)

     (1) Diagnosis is by a significant **size discordance** (> 25% difference in sonographic-estimated fetal weight) between the twins. Discordance is often associated with the finding of **polyhydramnios** in one amniotic sac and **oligohydramnios** in the other.

     (2) Mechanism of twin–twin transfusion is the **unequal distribution** of placental blood flow between twins.

       (a) The **donor twin** tends to be **smaller** and **anemic** with decreased renal blood flow, resulting in **oligohydramnios.**

       (b) The **recipient twin** is **larger** and **polycythemic** with enhanced renal blood flow, resulting in **polyhydramnios.**

       (c) Monochorionic placentation is required. Vascular anastomosis is required and may be arteriovenous, artery–artery, or venous–venous.

     (3) Risk is only present when the twins are of the **same gender** and there is only **one placenta.** There is almost no risk with different fetal genders and two placentas.

   b. Fetal malformations. These are diagnosed by ultrasound examination. The rate of occurrence is **three times higher** in multiple pregnancies than in singleton fetuses.

     (1) The risk of malformation is **highest** with **monozygotic** twins who, by definition, are of the same fetal gender and who share one placenta. **The later the cleavage occurs, the higher the risk.**

     (2) The risk is **lowest** with **dizygotic** twins having two placentas.

Table 3-9. Twin–Twin Transfusion

	Donor Twin	Recipient Twin
Fetal size	Smaller	Larger
Amniotic fluid	Oligohydramnios	Polyhydramnios
Neonatal appearance	Pale	Plethoric
Neonatal outcome	Good	Poor
Hematocrit	Anemic	Polycythemic

c. Umbilical cord abnormalities

(1) Types of umbilical cord abnormalities include a two-vessel cord, marginal or velamentous insertion (5% of monochorionic twins), and vasa previa.

(2) Risk is **highest** with **monozygotic twins** who, by definition, are of the same gender and who share one placenta. The risk of umbilical cord abnormalities is lowest with dizygotic twins of different genders having two placentas.

(3) Umbilical cord entanglement risk is present only with mono-amniotic twins who must be monozygotic and monochorionic.

3. Maternal risks

a. Nutritional anemias (e.g., iron deficiency, folate deficiency) occur **twice as often** in multiple pregnancies as in singleton pregnancies because of the demands on the mother's iron and folate stores to expand the RBC mass (see Chapter 4 IX).

b. Pregnancy-induced hypertension occurs **three times** more often in multiple pregnancies than in singleton pregnancies (see Chapter 4 I).

c. Preterm labor occurs in **50%** of twin pregnancies. The use of tocolytic agents exposes the mother to risks from side effects and other hazards (see Chapter 6 V).

d. Postpartum uterine atony with hemorrhage results from the inability of the overdistended uterus to contract well and remain contracted after delivery (see Chapter 7 II). **Uterine atony is the most common cause of postpartum hemorrhage.**

e. Cesarean delivery is performed in **50%** of twin pregnancies. It requires an incision through the abdominal and uterine walls for delivery of the fetuses.

4. Late pregnancy, labor, and delivery risks

a. Placenta previa is more common, because a wider uterine surface area is covered by the placenta(s).

b. Velamentous insertion of the cord occurs in **7%** of twins but in only 1% of singleton pregnancies.

c. Spontaneous premature rupture of membranes occurs in **25%** of twin pregnancies, which is more than double the percentage that occurs in singleton pregnancies.

d. Preterm labor and delivery occur in **50%** of twins, resulting in a perinatal mortality rate that is sevenfold higher than singleton pregnancies.

e. Intrauterine growth restriction (IUGR) is found in **25%** of twins, with twin–twin transfusion being a common cause.

f. Malpresentation occurs 10 times more often than in singleton pregnancies, leading to a **50%** cesarean delivery rate. The various types of twin presentation and their relative frequencies are:

(1) 50%: cephalic-cephalic

(2) 30%: breech-cephalic (30%)

(3) 10%: breech-cephalic (10%)

(4) 10%: single or double transverse lie

5. Management of the patient with a multiple pregnancy

a. Antepartum care

(1) Counsel on increased nutritional needs. The two fetuses and the even higher expanded blood volume of a twin pregnancy (compared with a singleton fetus) increase the need for calories, iron, and folate.

(2) Monitor for preterm labor and delivery. The mother should be instructed to **decrease** her physical activity and work. She should undergo **serial cervical examinations** assessing for change in cervical dilation and effacement. She should also be educated about the **symptoms and signs of labor:**

(a) Menstrual-like cramps

(b) Onset of new low-back pain

(c) Pelvic pressure

(d) Change in vaginal discharge

(3) Monitor for pregnancy-induced hypertension. Serial BP determinations and urine protein measurements should be made. The mother should be educated about the signs and symptoms of hypertension (i.e., headaches, visual changes, epigastric pain).

(4) Monitor for appropriate fetal growth. Sonograms measuring biparietal diameter (BPD), head circumference (HC), abdominal circumference (AC), and femur length (FL) should be performed every 3–4 weeks for growth parameters. Calculations can then be performed to assess concordance of the fetal weight and determine if twin–twin transfusion is present.

(5) Monitor for fetal well-being. Serial biophysical profiles (BPPs) should be performed when the sonograms are performed. Serial nonstress tests (NSTs) are performed if there is more than 25% discordance. The contraction stress test (CST) is not performed because stimulation of uterine contractions is contraindicated.

b. Intrapartum care

(1) Route of delivery is based on fetal presentation.

(a) If both twins are cephalic presentations, **vaginal delivery** can be safely attempted.

(b) If both twins are estimated to weigh 2000 g or more, and if the first twin is cephalic, vaginal delivery can be attempted regardless of the presentation of the second twin. The second twin can undergo an **external version,** or a **vaginal breech** delivery can take place.

(c) If the presentation of the first twin is not cephalic, and the twins are at a viable gestation, then **cesarean delivery** should be performed.

(2) EFM of heart rates of both fetuses should be performed during labor. Formerly, two EFM machines were necessary. New technology allows one EFM machine to monitor both fetuses simultaneously.

(3) Have access to full perinatal services.

(a) Obstetric/perinatology services are needed for such a high-risk delivery.

       (b) Obstetric anesthesia services are required in case an emergency cesarean delivery is necessary.

       (c) Pediatric/neonatology services are needed, with separate teams for each neonate.

   c. Postpartum care. Oxytocin should be administered intravenously as soon as the placenta(s) is (are) delivered. Additional oxytocin, methylergonovine maleate, and dinoprost (e.g., Hemabate) should be ready for administration in case uterine atony and postpartum hemorrhage occur.

VI. ISOIMMUNIZATION. This condition occurs when a woman produces **antibodies** directed against **foreign RBC surface antigens,** often those of her fetus. The most common antigens involved are those of the rhesus blood group system, but any RBC antigens may be involved.

  A. Nomenclature and genetics

    1. Blood group antigens. Five major rhesus blood group antigens have been identified with specific antisera: C, c, D, E, e. Antiserum specific for a "d" antigen has not been found.

      a. D antigen is the main rhesus blood group antigen in isoimmunization.

      b. Du+ designation is given when a partial D antigen immunologically responds as a regular D antigen (i.e., Du+ acts as a "weak D" antigen).

    2. Genetics

      a. The **locus** is on the short arm of chromosome 1.

      b. The **zygosity** of D antigen–positive men is as follows:

        (1) 60% are heterozygous (Dd).

        (2) 40% are homozygous (DD).

      c. Incidence of Rh negativity varies according to race (Table 3-10).

  B. Pathophysiology

    1. Sensitizing pregnancy

      a. A significant number of fetal RBCs, most often at time of delivery, cross the placenta into the mother's circulation.

      b. Her lymphocytes become activated to produce antibodies against the foreign fetal RBC antigens.

      c. The level of antibodies produced is usually low.

    2. Subsequent pregnancy

      a. A minimal number of fetal RBCs, often prenatally, cross the placenta into the mother's circulation, stimulating an **amnestic response** from her **lymphocytes.**

      b. A high number of **antibodies** are produced crossing the placenta into the fetal circulation adsorbing to the antigen-positive RBCs, **causing** their **hemolysis.**

      c. If the rate of hemolysis is faster than rate of hematopoiesis, **fetal anemia** develops.

Table 3-10. Racial Variations in Incidence of Rh Negativity

Race	Incidence
Basques of France and Spain	30%
Caucasian Americans	15%
Hispanic Americans	10%
African Americans	6%

    d. Extramedullary hematopoiesis can cause hypoproteinemia and ascites leading to heart failure, circulatory collapse, and fetal death.

C. Requirements for maternal RBC isoimmunization

    1. The **fetus** must have **antigen-positive** RBCs.

    2. The **mother** must have **antigen-negative** RBCs.

    3. **Sufficient fetal RBCs** must gain access to the maternal circulation.

    4. The **mother** must have the **immunogenic capacity** to produce antibodies against the fetal RBC antigen.

D. Factors that reduce the risk of isoimmunization with fetomaternal hemorrhage

    1. The **mother is an immunologic nonresponder.** Therefore, she is not sensitized, although she has received large volumes of antigen-positive blood from the fetus.

    2. **ABO incompatibility is present.** The protective effect is most pronounced when the mother has an O blood type and the father has an A, B, or AB blood type.

        a. Naturally occurring maternal anti-A or anti-B antibodies lyse the fetal RBCs before maternal lymphocyte activation occurs and causes isoimmunization.

        b. ABO-incompatible cells are cleared more rapidly by the maternal spleen.

    3. **Rh_o (D) immune prophylaxis** reduces the risk of isoimmunization if the mother is Rh-negative and the fetus is Rh-positive (Box 3-1).

E. Fetomaternal hemorrhage of some degree can occur.

    1. **Spontaneously** (without obvious antecedent event)

        a. 5% of pregnancies in the first trimester

        b. 15% of pregnancies in the second trimester

        c. 30% of pregnancies in the third trimester

    2. **In 20%** of pregnancies **after second- or third-trimester amniocentesis**

    3. **In 15%** of pregnancies **after spontaneous or induced abortion**

F. Clinical approach

    1. **Evaluate if the fetus is at risk for isoimmunization.**

Box 3-1. Risk of Isoimmunization With and Without
Rh_0 (D) Immune Prophylaxis

If Rh_0 (D) Immune Globulin Is Administered Prophylactically:	Risk is:
• At 28 weeks and after delivery	0.2%
• After delivery (but not given at 28 weeks)	2.0%

If Rh_0 (D) Immune Globulin is not given at 28 weeks or after delivery:

• and it is the mother's first pregnancy	15.0%
• and the number has had several pregnancies	50.0%

---

a. **What is parental blood type and Rh status?**

(1) Blood type and Rh status (anti-D) of the mother and father should be determined.

(2) **There is no fetal risk if both the mother and father are negative for the antigen.**

b. **Are atypical antibodies present?**

(1) Antibodies against fetal RBC antigens should be screened for by the indirect Coombs test or by the atypical antibody test (AAT).

(2) **There is no fetal risk if the indirect Coombs test or AAT is negative.**

c. **What is the identity of atypical antibodies present?**

(1) If present, the atypical antibody should be typed to determine whether it is associated with hemolytic disease of the newborn (HDN). This condition can result from anti-Kell, anti-Kidd, or anti-Duffy antibodies and does not result from anti-Lewis antibodies.

(2) **There is no fetal risk if the atypical antibodies are not associated with HDN.**

d. **What is the atypical antibody titer?** If the atypical antibody is associated with HDN, the titer of the antibody should be determined. Enough antibodies must exist in the maternal circulation to cross the placenta into the fetal circulation and cause a sufficient degree of fetal RBC hemolysis to cause anemia in the fetus. If the concentration of antibodies is high enough to cause concern regarding fetal anemia, it is considered a **significant titer.**

(1) An **insignificant titer is less than 1:8,** because the risk of HDN is negligible. The titer should be repeated monthly as long as the titer remains less than 1:8.

(2) A **significant titer** for HDN is **greater than 1:8** dilution. Further fetal evaluation must be pursued to assess if there is evidence for fetal anemia.

2. **Evaluate the fetus for hemolysis (fetal anemia) if the titer is greater than 1:8.**

a. **The fetal hematocrit can be assessed indirectly through amniotic fluid bilirubin.**

(1) **Amniotic bilirubin** correlates inversely with cord blood hemoglobin at delivery. The higher the rate of fetal RBC hemolysis, the higher the amniotic bilirubin and the lower the fetal hemoglobin.

(2) When the gestational age is advanced enough for intervention to be feasible, ultrasound-guided amniocentesis can be performed. Unconjugated amniotic bilirubin can be assessed by amniotic fluid spectrophotometry focusing on the bilirubin absorption wavelength, which is 450 nm. The optical density (OD) reading is measured at 450 nm (ΔOD_{450} value) and plotted on a Liley graph, which gives normal ranges for each gestational age greater than 20 weeks (Figure 3-8). Three zones, I, II, and III, are designated.

(a) **Zone I** is the normal range for amniotic fluid bilirubin, suggesting that the rate of RBC hemolysis can be cleared by the fetal liver. Either the fetus is unaffected or only mildly affected, with a low risk of fetal anemia.

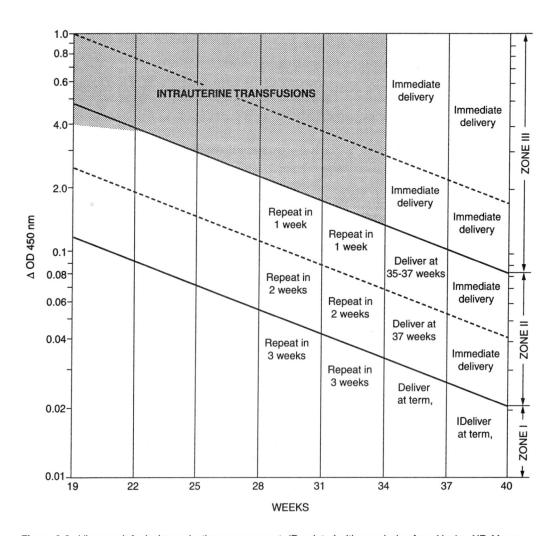

Figure 3-8. Liley graph for isoimmunization management. (Reprinted with permission from Hacker NF, Moore JG (eds): *Essentials of Obstetrics and Gynecology,* 2nd ed. W.B. Saunders, Philadelphia, 1992, p 303.)

        (i) Conservative management has a lower risk than intervention.

        (ii) Management. Repeat amniocentesis in 3 weeks. If the gestational age is greater than 37 weeks, deliver the fetus.

    (b) Zone II is a range higher than expected for amniotic fluid bilirubin, suggesting that the rate of RBC hemolysis can be cleared by the fetal liver. The fetus is probably affected, with a moderate, but not severe, risk of fetal anemia.

        (i) Conservative management has a lower risk than intervention.

        (ii) Management. Repeat amniocentesis in 1–2 weeks. If the gestational age is 37 weeks or more, deliver the fetus.

    (c) Zone III is markedly higher than expected for amniotic fluid bilirubin. The fetus is most probably anemic and is at high risk for development of hydropic changes.

        (i) At this point, doing nothing is more hazardous than intervention.

        (ii) Management. Either deliver the fetus or perform an intrauterine transfusion, depending on the gestational age (see VI F 3 b).

  b. Fetal hematocrit can be assessed directly.

    (1) Percutaneous umbilical blood sampling (PUBS) is performed under sonographic guidance, when technically feasible, usually after 25 weeks' gestation.

    (2) Optimal PUBS needle placement is where the umbilical cord inserts into the placenta. The needle site can be confirmed by vessel flow turbulence when saline is injected or by identification of fetal mean corpuscular volume.

    (3) Critical fetal hematocrit is less than 25%.

  c. Fetal status can be evaluated by ultrasound.

    (1) Evidence of **hydropic changes** (e.g., ascites, skin edema, pleural or pericardial effusions) should be sought.

    (2) Evidence of **heart failure** [e.g., increasing biventricular outer end-diastolic (BVOD) diameter of the fetal heart] should be sought.

3. Evaluate whether the risk of fetal anemia is high enough to warrant intervention.

  a. Indications for fetal intervention

    (1) ΔOD_{450} value in zone III

    (2) Hematocrit < 25%

    (3) Presence of hydropic changes

    (4) BVOD diameter greater than 95th percentile

  b. Intervention options

    (1) Delivery should be performed if the gestational age is **at least 34 weeks** and the fetal lung maturity is confirmed.

    (2) Intrauterine transfusion should be performed if the gestational age is **less than 34 weeks.**

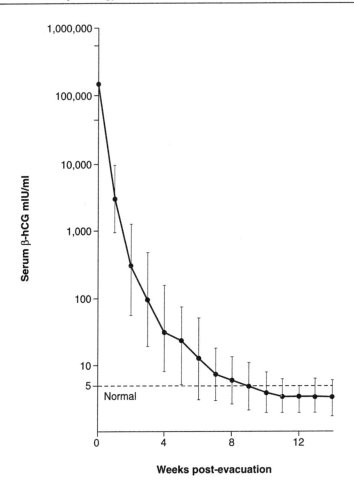

Figure 3-9. Normal regression curve of β-human chorionic gonadotropin (β-hCG) after molar evacuation. (Reprinted with permission from Beckmann CR, Ling FW, Barzansky BM, et al (eds): *Obstetrics and Gynecology,* 1st ed. Williams & Wilkins, Baltimore, 1992, p 290. Data from Morrow CP, et al: Clinical and laboratory correlates of molar pregnancy and trophoblastic disease. *Am J Obstet Gynecol* 128:428, 1977.)

        (a) Intraperitoneal transfusion. RBCs infused into the peritoneal cavity pass into fetal subdiaphragmatic lymphatics and are absorbed within 7 days if the fetus is not hydropic. Absorption is slower if hydrops is present. Ascitic fluid should be withdrawn first. Fetal bradycardia may occur.

        (b) Intravascular transfusion. RBCs are infused directly into the fetal umbilical vessels. This method is preferred if ascites or hydrops are present. Fetal bradycardia may occur.

    4. Prevent Rh isoimmunization in an Rh-negative gravida by use of Rh$_o$ (D) immune globulin

        a. RBC antigen sites on fetal blood cells in the maternal circulation are bound using **passive immunization.**

        b. Immunize within 72 hours of the bleeding event to prevent the activation of maternal lymphocyte production of unwanted antibodies.

   c. **Intramuscular injection** of Rh_o (D) immune globulin is performed if the AAT is negative.

   (1) A **dosage of 300 μg** neutralizes either 15 ml of fetal RBCs or 30 ml of fetal whole blood (assuming the hematocrit is 50%). More than one vial of Rh immune globulin may be needed depending on the volume of the fetomaternal bleed.

   (2) **With routine administration,** Rh_o (D) immune globulin should be given at **28 weeks' gestation** and **after delivery** (if the neonate is Rh-positive). The half-life of Rh_o (D) immune globulin is 21 days.

   (3) **Special circumstances** exist after D&C, amniocentesis, and antepartum hemorrhage, when there is a risk of the mixing of fetal and maternal blood. If there is excess fetomaternal hemorrhage, the **Kleihauer-Betke test** should be performed on the mother's blood to estimate the fetal blood volume in the maternal circulation.

   (a) **Acid** is used to extract hemoglobin through RBC membranes. Adult hemoglobin is readily extracted, and fetal hemoglobin is eluted slowly.

   (b) **Differential staining** of the slide yields an estimate of the volume of fetal RBCs in the maternal circulation.

VII. GESTATIONAL TROPHOBLASTIC NEOPLASIA (GTN). This disease is composed of a **spectrum of neoplasms** having in common a proliferative trophoblastic abnormality of pregnancy. It can range from **benign** (hydatidiform mole) to gestational trophoblastic tumor (GTT) with **malignant** potential. They arise from fetal tissues at the inner cell mass stage prior to formation of the germ layers, and they are composed of both syncytiotrophoblast and cytotrophoblast cells. The highest incidence occurs in Taiwan and the Philippines (1 in 125 deliveries). The incidence in the United States is 1 in 1500 deliveries.

   A. **Clinical classification** (Table 3-11)

   1. **Hydatidiform moles** account for most cases of gestational trophoblastic neoplasia. Two types exist:

   a. **Complete,** or classic, hydatidiform moles (20% progress to GTT)

   b. **Incomplete,** or partial hydatidiform moles (5% progress to GTT)

   2. **GTT** has neoplastic malignant potential and can be nonmetastatic or metastatic. Low-risk metastatic GTT has a good prognosis for the mother, whereas high-risk metastatic GTT has a poor prognosis.

   B. **Risk factors for GTN**

   1. **Nonmetastatic risks** include:

   a. **Maternal age extremes** (i.e., < 20 years, > 40 years)

   b. **Diet** (i.e., low in beta-carotene, folate deficiency)

   c. **Blood group.** Type A women impregnated by type O men (AO) have 10 times the risk of choriocarcinoma compared with AA coupling.

   2. **Metastatic risks** include:

   a. Large uterus

Table 3-11. Types of Molar Pregnancies

	Complete (Common)	Incomplete (Partial)
Karyotype	Paternally derived euploidy 46, XX > 46, XY	Triploidy 69, XXY (80%) 69, XXX (20%)
Fetus present	No	Yes
Vessels in villii	Absent	Normal
Edema of villii	Yes	Some
Trophoblastic cells	Proliferative	Atrophic

        b. High β-hCG titer

        c. Low gestational age

        d. Presence of theca lutein cysts

  C. Characteristic features of hydatidiform moles

     1. Gross features. Most hydatidiform moles have multiple grape-like vesicles filling the uterus. Some are not detectable on gross examination, and thus appear as normal tissue. A histologic diagnosis is imperative to rule out molar pregnancy. A **coexistent fetus** may be found with **incomplete moles.**

     2. Histologic features. There is a poor correlation of hydatidiform mole histology with the malignant course of GTT.

        a. Complete moles. These feature edema of the villus stroma, absence of fetal vessels, and trophoblastic hyperplasia.

        b. Incomplete moles. Some villi are edematous, and others are normal. Fetal vessels are seen, and there is minimal trophoblastic hyperplasia.

     3. Cytogenetic features

        a. Complete moles are 46,XX but chromosomes are **paternally derived.** The ovum nucleus was absent or became inactivated. Two sperm penetrated the egg, or a single sperm duplicated its chromosomes.

        b. Incomplete moles show triploidy. There is an 80% incidence of 69,XXY and a 20% incidence of 69,XXX or 69,XYY.

  D. Clinical approach

     1. Clinical findings are suggestive of GTN (Table 3-12). These include both historical as well as physical examination details.

     2. Test results that help **confirm the diagnosis** and **assess the extent of disease** include:

        a. Sonogram, which shows multiple echoes without a gestational sac or fetal parts ("snowstorm" pattern)

        b. Chest radiograph, which may show lung metastasis, the most common metastatic site

Table 3-12. Clinical Findings Suggestive of Gestational Trophoblastic Neoplasia

Findings in History	Rate	Findings on Examination
Bleeding during first half of pregnancy (usually prior to 16 weeks gestation)	90%	Expulsion of vesicles via vagina
Passage of vesicles	80%	No fetal heart tones
Preeclampsia <24 weeks	10%	Uterine fundus is larger than dates
Severe hyperemesis	10%	Theca lutein ovarian cysts
Hyperthyroidism (from placental thyrotropin production)	10%	

      c. Serum β-hCG titer, which is markedly elevated (Figure 3-9) [e.g., values > 100,000 mIU/ml].

  3. Appropriate management of patients with benign GTN

    a. Surgical management

      (1) A suction D&C is the method of choice.

        (a) Oxytocin is administered intravenously to contract the uterus and close the large venous sinuses providing blood supply to the molar tissue. Gentle, sharp curettage is performed to rule out invasion of the mole into the myometrium. Decidua basalis tissue is obtained for histology.

        (b) Complications include massive hemorrhage and uterine perforation. A laparotomy setup should be available to perform a hysterectomy if necessary.

      (2) Hysterectomy is an option in women who have completed childbearing or who are older (and have a higher risk of malignant sequelae).

      (3) Inappropriate treatments include hysterotomy and induction of labor.

    b. Medical management. Prophylactic single-agent chemotherapy may be used in women with a large uterus or in women who are poor follow-up candidates. **Chemotherapeutic agents** used include methotrexate or actinomycin D.

    c. Follow-up protocol. Obtain weekly β-hCG titers until they are negative for 3 weeks, then monthly titers until they are negative for 12 months. Effective contraception should be used in the follow-up period to prevent confusion of recurrent disease with rising titers from pregnancy.

  4. Prognostic indicators in patients with malignant GTN include the following:

    a. Low risk/good prognosis factors are:

      (1) Serum β-hCG titer < 40,000 mIU/ml at the onset of therapy (not at diagnosis)

      (2) Therapy started within 4 months of antecedent pregnancy

      (3) Metastasis only to lungs or pelvis

b. **High risk/poor prognosis** factors are:

   (1) Serum β-hCG titer > 40,000 mIU/ml at the onset of therapy (not at diagnosis)

   (2) Therapy initiated > 4 months after antecedent pregnancy

   (3) Metastasis to brain or liver

   (4) Failed response to a single chemotherapeutic agent

   (5) Choriocarcinoma after full-term delivery

5. **Management of patients with malignant GTN** differs based on prognosis.

   a. **Patients with a good prognosis GTN**

      (1) **Single-agent therapy** is almost uniformly successful, with 100% of patients having complete remission, 90% of patients having preserved reproductive function, and only 10% of patients having the risk of recurrence. **Methotrexate** is the drug of choice, and actinomycin D is also used.

      (2) **Follow-up protocol** includes a 5-day treatment cycle every other week until β-hCG titers are negative. Weekly titers are performed until three are negative, and then monthly titers are performed until 12 are negative.

   b. **Patients with poor prognosis GTN**

      (1) **Prolonged hospitalization and aggressive therapy** are required with multiple courses of combined-agent chemotherapy (e.g., methotrexate, actinomycin D, chlorambucil/cyclophosphamide). Whole-brain or whole-liver irradiation may be necessary to prevent a fatal cerebral or liver hemorrhage.

      (2) **Follow-up protocol** involves weekly serum β-hCG titers until three are negative and then monthly titers for 2 years. Thereafter, titers should be obtained every 3 months up to 5 years.

Review Test

Directions: Each of the numbered items or incomplete statements in this section is followed by answers or by completions of the statement. Select the **ONE** lettered answer or completion that is **BEST** in each case.

1. Most first-trimester spontaneous abortuses fall into which one of the following types of cytogenetic abnormalities?

(A) Monosomies
(B) Disomies
(C) Trisomies
(D) Triploidies
(E) Tetraploidies

2. A 25-year-old woman experiences unexplained vaginal bleeding and cramping. Her last menstrual period (LMP) is uncertain. She has a qualitative serum β-human chorionic gonadotropin (β-hCG) test, which is positive, and a transvaginal pelvic sonogram, which reveals an intrauterine gestational sac. Which one of the following quantitative serum β-hCG values represents the lowest level at which these sonographic findings could be found?

(A) 1000 mIU/ml
(B) 1500 mIU/ml
(C) 2500 mIU/ml
(D) 4500 mIU/ml
(E) 6500 mIU/ml

3. A 34-year-old woman (gravida 2, para 1) experiences fetal demise at 22 weeks' gestation. Labor is induced, and she undergoes a vaginal delivery of a grossly normal-appearing fetus. Pelvic ultrasound shows uterine leiomyomas. Which one of the following uterine leiomyoma locations within this woman's uterus is the most likely cause of this second-trimester pregnancy loss?

(A) Intramural
(B) Subserosal
(C) Submucosal
(D) Pedunculated
(E) Intraligamentous

4. A 20-year-old woman (gravida 3, para 0, abortus 2) has experienced two second-trimester losses characterized by painless cervical dilation and rupture of the membranes followed by expulsion of grossly immature, nonviable fetuses. Which one of the following is the primary management intervention in this pregnancy?

(A) Progestational agents
(B) Bed rest
(C) Tocolytic agents
(D) Cervical cerclage
(E) Myomectomy

5. A 39-year-old multigravida at 30 weeks' gestation presents to the maternity unit complaining of not feeling fetal movement for the past 24 hours. Obstetrical ultrasound reveals a singleton fetus in complete breech presentation. No cardiac or great vessel motion can be identified. Which one of the following questions is the most crucial in determining the urgency to induce labor in this patient?

(A) What does the cervical examination show?
(B) How long has the fetus been dead?
(C) Why did the fetus die?
(D) What is the mother's mental status?
(E) What is the gestational age?

6. What is the frequency of spontaneous twin gestation in the United States?

(A) 1 in 50
(B) 1 in 90
(C) 1 in 200
(D) 1 in 300
(E) 1 in 500

109

7. A 29-year-old multigravida presents for her first prenatal visit at 10 weeks' gestation. Specimens for a routine prenatal laboratory panel are obtained. The indirect Coombs test [or atypical antibody test (AAT)] is positive, but no antibody identification is provided. Which one of the following is the most common major Rh blood-group antigen that may be responsible for these findings?

(A) C
(B) c
(C) D
(D) E
(E) e

8. Which one of the following statements about Rh_o (D) immune globulin (RhoGAM) is true?

(A) It binds red blood cell (RBC) antigen sites through active immunization.
(B) It should be given within 72 hours of the fetomaternal bleed.
(C) It has a half-life of 30 days.
(D) An amount of 300 μg neutralizes 30 ml of fetal RBCs.
(E) It is not indicated if the fetomaternal bleed occurs before 15 weeks.

Directions: Each of the numbered items or incomplete statements in this section is negatively phrased, as indicated by a capitalized word such as NOT, LEAST, or EXCEPT. Select the ONE lettered answer or completion that is BEST in each case.

9. A 37-year-old (gravida 2, para 1, abortus 1) reports she lost two pregnancies at 19 and 21 weeks' gestation. She denies any systemic diseases and states she is in good health. Which one of the following is LEAST likely to be the cause of her pregnancy losses?

(A) Incompetent cervix
(B) Uterine anomalies
(C) Fetal infections
(D) Fetal hydrops
(E) Fetal cytogenetic abnormalities

10. All the following are characteristics of complete moles EXCEPT

(A) the chromosome complement is paternally derived
(B) a coexistent fetus is never seen
(C) the risk of progression to invasive disease is higher than in incomplete moles
(D) the tissue karyotype is usually triploidy
(E) the villus stroma shows marked edema

Directions: The set of matching questions in this section consists of a list of four to twenty-six lettered options (some of which may be in figures) followed by several numbered items. For each numbered item, select the ONE lettered option that is most closely associated with it. To avoid spending too much time on matching sets with large numbers of options, it is generally advisable to begin each set by reading the list of options. Then, for each item in the set, try to generate the correct answer and locate it in the option list, rather than evaluating each option individually. Each lettered option may be selected once, more than once, or not at all.

Questions 11–15

For each of the characteristics identified, select the associated cause of third-trimester bleeding.
(A) Abruptio placentae
(B) Placenta previa
(C) Vasa previa
(D) Uterine rupture

11. Bleeding is of fetal origin

12. It is associated with transverse lie at term

13. It is the most common cause of bleeding at term

14. Diagnosis is best made by sonography

15. It is the most common obstetric cause of disseminated intravascular coagulation (DIC).

Answers and Explanations

1. The answer is C [I A 1].

The incidence of early pregnancy losses is approximately 15% in known pregnancies. Up to 50% of clinically recognized first-trimester pregnancy losses are the result of autosomal trisomies. Monosomies, disomies, triploidies, and tetraploidies represent a smaller fraction of losses. The most common single trisomy found in all spontaneous abortions is trisomy 16, whereas the most common trisomy of liveborns is trisomy 21. The single most common aneuploidy is monosomy X or Turner's syndrome.

2. The answer is B [I C 3 c].

The discriminatory threshold is the β-human chorionic gonadotropin (β-hCG) value below which a gestational sac could not be expected to be seen by sonography. Because transvaginal sonography has a higher resolution than transabdominal sonography, one would expect transvaginal sonography to identify a gestational sac at an earlier gestational age. The critical level is 1500 mIU/ml for transvaginal sonography. The critical level is 6500 mIU/ml for transabdominal sonography.

3. The answer is C [II A 1 b].

Uterine leiomyomas are the most common neoplasm of the female genital tract; 25%–50% of women are affected. The great majority of these are asymptomatic. In second-trimester pregnancy loss, however, a submucosal location is correct. The mechanism by which submucosal leiomyomas cause second-trimester pregnancy losses is that implantation occurs over the myoma with inadequate vascular supply for satisfactory placentation. Intramural, subserosal, pedunculated, and intraligamentous uterine leiomyomas are not usual causes of second-trimester losses.

4. The answer is D [II A 2 d].

Many patients have undergone cerclage placement without an adequate workup to exclude other causes of pregnancy loss. Once the diagnosis has been carefully made, however, cervical cerclage is the primary management. The pathophysiology of an incompetent cervix is believed to be inability to retain an intrauterine pregnancy to viability because of cervical structural weakness. The cornerstone of treatment is mechanical strengthening of the cervix by placement of a cervical cerclage. Progestational agents and tocolytic agents may relax the myometrium but do not address cervical weakness. Bed rest is a useful adjunct in management but is not the primary therapy. Myomectomy is a spurious distractor.

5. The answer is B [IV E 3].

If the fetus has been dead for a significant period, tissue thromboplastin could have been released from the fetus, causing disseminated intravascular coagulation (DIC) in the mother. This is a potentially life-threatening problem that would significantly affect all other decisions regarding management. Questions regarding the cervical examination, the cause of fetal demise, the mother's mental status, and the gestational age are important questions that need to be addressed for other reasons, but they are not the most critical in deciding the urgency of pregnancy termination.

6. The answer is B [V A 1].

Most twins occur spontaneously and are not the consequence of ovulation induction. Approximately 1% of pregnancies in the United States are found to be twin gestation at delivery. The multiple gestation rates when clomiphene citrate and menotropins are used for ovulation induction are 10% and 30%, respectively. Twinning rates also vary geographically; the highest rates in the world are found in Nigeria.

7. The answer is C [VI A 1 a].

Half of maternal isoimmunization cases in the United States are caused by the D antigen. Isoimmunization in pregnancy involves maternal production of antibodies directed at red blood cell (RBC) antigens foreign to the mother. Because only immunoglobulin G (IgG) antibodies cross the placenta, IgM antibodies are not of concern. Not all antibodies are associated with hemolytic disease of the newborn (HDN). Of the antibodies that do cause HDN, some cause only mild cases. The remainder of isoimmunization cases are caused by a variety of less common antigens such as C, c, E, e, or others such as Kidd, Kell, and Duffy.

8. The answer is B [VI F 4].

Rh_0 (D) immune globulin (RhoGAM) should be given within 72 hours of the fetomaternal bleed because failure to do so would allow the binding of red blood cells (RBC) to receptors that initiate irreversible lymphocyte activations. The statement about the binding of RhoGAM to RBC antigen sites through active immunization is incorrect because RhoGAM works through passive immunization to bind the antigen sites on the foreign RBC. RhoGAM has a half-life of 21 days. If the fetomaternal bleed occurs before 15 weeks, 300 μg of RhoGAM neutralizes binding sites on 15 ml of fetal RBC and should be given earlier than 15 weeks if fetomaternal bleeding is suspected.

9. The answer is E [II A–B].

Second-trimester losses are much less frequent than first-trimester losses. Fetal cytogenetic abnormalities are more frequent in first-trimester losses than in second-trimester losses. The majority of second-trimester losses involve incompetent cervix, uterine anomalies, fetal infections, and fetal hydrops.

10. The answer is D [VII A 1 a, C 2 a, 3 a].

Complete, or hydatidiform, moles are far more common than incomplete moles. The highest rates of molar pregnancies in the world are found in Taiwan and the Philippines, where rates are 10 times higher than in the United States. The correct answer (but incorrect statement) is that the tissue karyotype is usually triploid. Complete moles usually have a paternally derived 46,XX chromosome complement. This can occur by either two separate sperm fertilizing an egg with either an inactivated or absent nucleus, or a single sperm that duplicates its chromosomes after penetrating the same non-nucleated egg. Other characteristics of complete moles include the absence of a coexistent fetus, a risk of progression to invasive disease that is higher than in incomplete moles, and marked edema in the villus stroma.

11–15. The answers are: 11-C [III A 3], 12-B [III A 2], 13-A [III A 1], 14-B [III A 2], 15-A [III A 1].

Bleeding in vasa previa originates from fetal vessels that are removed from the placental disk, which crosses the fetal membranes that overlie the cervical os. Placenta previa, which has a lower uterine segment implantation site, may obstruct the pelvic inlet and lead to abnormal fetal lies. Abruptio placentae, which is a premature separation of a normally implanted placenta, is the most common cause of bleeding at term with an incidence of 1% of pregnancies. The definitive diagnosis of placenta previa is made by sonography. Abruptio placentae is the most common obstetric cause of disseminated intravascular coagulation (DIC).

4

Pregnancy: Medical Complications

I. HYPERTENSIVE DISORDERS

A. **Criteria for diagnosis**

1. **Blood pressure (BP) elevation** must be sustained, and **one** of the following conditions must be present:

   a. Absolute BP of $\geq$ 140/90 mm Hg, **or**

   b. An increase in baseline diastolic BP of $\geq$ 15 mm Hg, **or**

   c. An increase in baseline systolic BP of $\geq$ 30 mm Hg

2. **BP elevation** must be **confirmed** on at least **two occasions** at least 6 hours apart and at bed rest.

B. **Classification** (Table 4-1)

1. **Mild preeclampsia.** Criteria for diagnosis include:

   a. **BP of $\geq$ 140/90 mm Hg** or increase in diastolic BP of $\geq$ 15 mm Hg or increase in systolic BP of $\geq$ 30 mm Hg

   b. **Proteinuria of 1–2+** on dipstick or $\geq$ 300 mg on 24-hour urine collection

   c. **Edema** of the face or upper extremities

2. **Severe preeclampsia.** Criteria for diagnosis include:

   a. **BP of $\geq$ 160/110 mm Hg**

   b. **Proteinuria of $\geq$ 3–4+** on dipstick or $\geq$ 5 g on 24-hour urine collection

   c. **Symptoms**

      (1) **Headaches** resulting from cerebral edema

      (2) **Visual disturbances** resulting from decreased cerebral perfusion of the occipital cortex

      (3) **Epigastric pain** resulting from hepatocellular necrosis, edema, and ischemia stretching Glisson's capsule

   d. **Laboratory findings**

Table 4-1. Hypertensive Disorders of Pregnancy

	Mild Preeclampsia	Severe Preeclampsia	Eclampsia	Chronic HTN	Chronic HTN with Superimposed Preeclampsia	Transient HTN
Blood pressure	Relative increased dias 15 mm Hg, or increased syst 30 mm Hg, or absolute 140/90	≥160/110 mm Hg	At least mild preeclampsia criteria	Preexisting HTN or HTN <20 weeks	Increased over baseline	At least mild pre eclampsia criteria
Proteinuria	1–2+ on dipstick, or ≥300 mg/24 hr	3- 4+ on dipstick or ≥5 g/24 hr	At least mild preeclampsia criteria	Variable (may be none)	At least mild preeclampsia criteria or increased over baseline	None
Edema of face, hands	Variable	Variable	Variable	None	Variable (may be none)	None
Convulsions	None	None	Present	None	None	None
Symptoms*	None	Possible	Possible	None	Possible	None
DIC findings†	None	Possible	Possible	None	Possible	None
Hemoconcentration	Mild	Marked	Marked	None	Variable	None
Cyanosis, oliguria, pulmonary edema	None	Possible	Possible	None	Variable	None

DIC = disseminated intravascular coagulation; *HTN* = hypertension; *PIH* = pregnancy-induced hypertension.
*Symptoms include headache, epigastric pain, and visual disturbances.
†DIC findings include decreased platelets and decreased fibrinogen as well as increased PTT and increased PT.

   (1) Thrombocytopenia (< 100,000/ml) resulting from vasospasm-induced macroangiopathic hemolysis

   (2) Elevated liver enzymes resulting from hepatocellular necrosis

  e. Clinical findings

   (1) Pulmonary edema resulting from increased capillary membrane permeability

   (2) Oliguria resulting from intrarenal vasospasm

   (3) Cyanosis resulting from right heart failure

 3. Eclampsia is diagnosed in the presence of unexplained convulsions with other criteria for preeclampsia.

  a. Approximately 25% occur **antepartum** (before labor).

  b. Approximately 50% occur **intrapartum** (during labor).

  c. Approximately 25% occur **postpartum** (most within first 24 hours).

 4. Chronic hypertension is diagnosed with a history of preexisting hypertension either before the onset of pregnancy or before 20 weeks' gestation (without coexisting molar pregnancy) and persisting past 6 weeks postpartum.

 5. Chronic hypertension with superimposed preeclampsia has a worse outcome than either chronic or pregnancy-induced hypertension alone. Diagnosis requires **all** of the following criteria:

  a. Presence of chronic hypertension

  b. Increase in diastolic BP of $\geq$ 15 mm Hg or systolic BP of $\geq$ 30 mm Hg

  c. Increase in proteinuria

 6. Transient hypertension, which is diagnosed with the development of hypertension without other findings of preeclampsia, is largely a **retrospective diagnosis** that is made after the pregnancy is over.

 7. HELLP syndrome is a subtype of preeclampsia. The five letters make up a mnemonic device representing the unique disease findings: *H*emolysis, *E*levated *L*iver enzymes, and *L*ow *P*latelets.

C. Preeclampsia–eclampsia spectrum

 1. Epidemiology of preeclampsia. Preeclampsia occurs only in humans and only in pregnant women beyond 20 weeks' gestation.

  a. Incidence. Approximately 8% of the general obstetric population develop preeclampsia.

  b. Risk factors

   (1) Nulliparity (most common risk factor; eight times greater than in multiparas)

   (2) Age extremes (i.e., < 20 years, > 34 years)

   (3) Multiple gestation

   (4) Hydatidiform mole

   (5) Diabetes mellitus (DM)

   (6) Nonimmune fetal hydrops

   (7) Chronic hypertension

   (8) Preexisting renal disease

   (9) Small vessel disease (e.g., systemic lupus erythematosus, longstanding type 1 DM)

2. **Characteristic pathology** involves **renal glomerular endotheliosis,** which refers to swelling of the endothelial cells of the capillary loops in the glomerular tuft.

3. **Pathogenesis** involves **diffuse vasospasm** and **capillary wall endothelial injury.**

   a. **Diffuse vasospasm** produces:

     (1) **Altered refractory state of pregnancy** against the pressor effect of renin, angiotensin II, and aldosterone

     (2) **Systolic and diastolic hypertension**

     (3) **Increased capillary permeability,** which results in:

       (a) **Hemoconcentration** from decreased intravascular volume, which leads to increased blood urea nitrogen (BUN), creatinine, uric acid, hemoglobin, and hematocrit. Diuretics should be avoided, because they may exacerbate hemoconcentration by further reducing intravascular volume.

       (b) **Edema** from loss of protein into extravascular space

       (c) **Excessive weight gain** from fluid retention

     (4) **Reduced systemic perfusion** of the following organ systems:

       (a) **Kidneys,** resulting in increased BUN, creatinine, and uric acid

       (b) **Uteroplacental unit,** resulting in placental insufficiency, which may decrease placental **nutritional function** and lead to intrauterine growth restriction (IUGR) as well as decrease placental **respiratory function** that leads to fetal hypoxia

     (5) **Vasoactive prostaglandins imbalance,** with levels of vasoconstricting **thromboxane** exceeding the vasodilating effect of **prostacyclin**

   b. **Capillary wall endothelial injury** results in:

     (1) Fibrin deposition in the capillary beds (microangiopathic hemolytic anemia)

     (2) Platelet destruction

     (3) Disseminated intravascular coagulation (DIC)

     (4) Consumptive coagulopathy

D. Evaluation of maternal-fetal status. Management is based on type and severity of hypertensive disease as well as gestational age.

1. **Indicators of a decline in maternal well-being**

   a. **Increasing BP** (systolic and/or diastolic)

   b. **Worsening symptoms** (i.e., headache, visual disturbances, epigastric pain)

   c. **Increasing hemoconcentration** (i.e., BUN, creatinine, uric acid, hemoglobin, hematocrit)

   d. **Increasing proteinuria** on 24-hour urine collection

   e. **Worsening DIC** laboratory tests [e.g., decreasing platelet count, lengthening prothrombin/partial thromboplastin times (PT/PTTs), decreasing fibrinogen)

2. **Indicators of a decline in fetal well-being**

   a. **Nonreactive nonstress test (NST)**

    b. Positive contraction stress test (CST)

    c. Declining biophysical profile (BPP)

    d. Serial sonographic growth parameters showing slowing or arrest of growth.

    e. Decreasing fetal movements

E. Clinical approach. Management is based on the type and severity of hypertensive disease as well as gestational age. Options include aggressive inpatient, conservative inpatient, and conservative outpatient.

    1. Aggressive inpatient management includes:

      a. Diagnostic criteria

        (1) Mild or severe preeclampsia; ≥ 37 weeks' gestation

        (2) Severe preeclampsia; < 26 weeks' gestation

        (3) Severe preeclampsia; 26–34 weeks' gestation, when associated with **maternal jeopardy:**

          (a) Severe persistent headache

          (b) Persistent visual changes

          (c) Hepatocellular injury

          (d) Thrombocytopenia or other evidence of DIC

          (e) Pulmonary edema

          (f) Abruptio placentae

        (4) Severe preeclampsia; 26–34 weeks' gestation, when associated with **fetal jeopardy:**

          (a) Repetitive severe variable decelerations

          (b) Repetitive late decelerations

          (c) Repetitive BPP ≤ 4

          (d) Oligohydramnios [amniotic fluid index (AFI) ≤ 4 cm]

          (e) IUGR (estimated fetal weight ≤ fifth percentile)

        (5) Chronic hypertension with superimposed preeclampsia at any gestational age

        (6) Eclampsia or HELLP syndrome at any gestational age

      b. Guidelines

        (1) Maintenance of diastolic BP between 90 and 100 mm Hg. Further reduction of BP jeopardizes placental blood flow. Appropriate antihypertensive medications include:

          (a) Hydralazine (direct arteriolar vasodilator), which causes baroreceptor sympathetic stimulation [increasing heart rate (HR) and cardiac output (CO)], thus preserving placental blood flow

          (b) Labetalol (nonselective β-blocker), which preserves uteroplacental blood flow

        (2) Prevention of convulsions with intravenous (IV) magnesium sulfate

          (a) Administration of loading dose of 5 g IV over 20 minutes, and maintenance infusion at 2 g/hr. The maintenance IV infusion should be given for 24 hours after delivery.

          (b) Watching for clinical evidence of magnesium toxicity (Box 4-1)

          (c) Absence of toxicity is ensured as long as deep tendon reflexes are obtainable.

Box 4-1. Clinical Findings for Parenteral Magnesium Sulfate

Dose	Effect
5–8 mg/dl	Therapeutic level
10 mg/dl	Loss of deep tendon reflexes
15 mg/dl	Respiratory paralysis
25 mg/dl	Cardiac arrest

         (d) **IV calcium gluconate** is the **antidote** for magnesium toxicity.

      (3) **Initiation of delivery.** Labor can be induced anticipating vaginal delivery if the patient is stable and there are no contraindications. Otherwise, cesarean delivery is indicated.

  2. **Conservative inpatient management** is appropriate in the following cases:

    a. **Mild preeclampsia that is remote from term (< 37 weeks). Guidelines include:**

      (1) Monitoring BP every 4 hours

      (2) Performing a daily urine dipstick for protein

      (3) Performing twice-weekly 24-hour urine protein measurements

      (4) Performing weekly liver function tests and electrolyte levels

      (5) Initiating delivery if criteria for severe preeclampsia are met

    b. **Severe preeclampsia in carefully selected cases**

      (1) **All of the following criteria must be met.**

        (a) Gestational age > 26 weeks but < 34 weeks

        (b) BP persistently ≥ 160/110 mm Hg

        (c) Absence of fetal jeopardy

        (d) Absence of maternal jeopardy

      (2) **Guidelines include:**

        (a) Intensive maternal and fetal monitoring in a tertiary perinatal center

        (b) Cautious volume expansion

        (c) Aggressive antihypertensive therapy (e.g., hydralazine, labetalol)

        (d) Anticonvulsant therapy (e.g., magnesium sulfate)

        (e) Corticosteroids to enhance fetal lung maturity

      (3) **Initiation of delivery** if maternal or fetal deterioration occurs

  3. **Conservative outpatient management**

    a. **Patient selection criteria** include:

      (1) **Transient hypertension** (i.e., BP in the mildly elevated range, no proteinuria)

      (2) **Uncomplicated chronic hypertension** (without superimposed preeclampsia)

    b. **Guidelines include:**

      (1) Bed rest in the left lateral position

      (2) Home BP monitoring

(3) Twice-weekly outpatient visits

c. **Initiation of delivery** if maternal or fetal deterioration occurs

F. **Prevention.** Large, prospective, randomized studies have shown that no prophylactic intervention for preeclampsia improves pregnancy outcome. This includes use of **aspirin** and supplemental **calcium.**

II. CARDIAC DISEASE

A. **Effect of normal physiologic changes of pregnancy on heart disease:**

1. **Stenotic lesions** are **tolerated poorly**

   a. The augmented blood volume and CO **raise** left ventricular preload, **increasing** the rate of blood flow that must cross the stenotic valve.

   b. The increased HR of pregnancy **shortens** the diastolic filling time, which is the only time blood can flow across the stenotic valve.

   c. If the pregnancy-induced increase in preload and the shortened diastolic filling time exceed the ability of the stenotic valve to allow forward blood flow to the left ventricle, **pulmonary vascular pressure** rises and **pulmonary edema** develops.

2. **Insufficiency lesions** are **tolerated better** for the following reasons:

   a. The augmented blood volume and CO raise left ventricular preload, thus increasing the rate of blood flow that flows across the insufficient valve.

   b. The increased HR reduces the time that regurgitation may occur within the cardiac cycle.

   c. The decreased peripheral vascular resistance (PVR) reduces the backward pressure of blood returning into the cardiac chamber, thus less blood flows backward through the insufficient valve.

B. **Types of heart disease in pregnancy**

1. **Functional classification** (Box 4-2) is based on the nature of **cardiac symptoms** along with the **degree of maternal disability** regardless of the underlying cardiac lesion.

   a. The **value of this approach** is in:

      (1) Comparing status of patients within a given diagnosis

---

Box 4-2. New York Functional Classification of Heart Disease

Lower risk

Class I	No signs or symptoms of cardiac decompensation
Class II	No symptoms at rest; minor limitations with activity

Higher risk

Class III	No symptoms at rest; marked limitations with activity
Class IV	Symptoms at rest

(2) **Reassessing** patients who change functional categories during pregnancy

b. **Symptoms of cardiac disease** to ask the patient about include:

(1) Severe or progressive dyspnea

(2) Paroxysmal nocturnal dyspnea

(3) Progressive orthopnea

(4) Hemoptysis

(5) Syncope with exertion

(6) Chest pain related to effort or emotion

c. **Signs of cardiac disease** to look for include:

(1) Loud systolic murmur or click

(2) Diastolic murmur

(3) Cardiomegaly, including parasternal heave

(4) Cyanosis or clubbing

(5) Persistent jugular venous distention (JVD)

(6) Features of **Marfan syndrome**

2. **Structural classification** is based on the cardiac anatomic lesion involved. It can be subdivided into acquired and congenital heart disease.

a. **Acquired heart disease** (mostly rheumatic in origin)

(1) **Mitral stenosis** is the **most common** type (90%). Problems occur as a result of:

(a) **Left atrial enlargement,** which can lead to atrial fibrillation, subacute bacterial endocarditis, and emboli

(b) **Slow diastolic filling,** which can lead to pulmonary congestion, congestive heart failure, and pulmonary edema

(2) **Mitral insufficiency** is usually well tolerated by pregnant women.

b. **Congenital heart disease**

(1) **Atrial septal defect (ASD)** and **ventricular septal defect (VSD). ASD is the most common congenital heart lesion in the adult population.**

(a) **If surgically corrected,** ASD and VSD pose no problems during pregnancy.

(b) **If uncorrected,** the septal defects are usually well tolerated during pregnancy.

(2) **Tetralogy of Fallot** consists of right ventricular outflow obstruction, right ventricular hypertrophy, large VSD, and overriding aorta. It is the **most commonly encountered cyanotic heart lesion in pregnancy.**

(a) **If surgically corrected,** without major residual defects, pregnancy is tolerated well.

(b) **If uncorrected,** with persistent cyanotic heart disease, there is a **10% mortality rate.**

(3) **Eisenmenger's syndrome** has the **highest morality rate (50%)** of any heart disease in pregnancy.

(a) **Criteria for diagnosis** include **pulmonary hypertension** that is greater than or equal to the systemic resistance and a **biventricular shunt** between right and left ventricles.

(b) Pathophysiology. Systemic hypotension is tolerated poorly because a right-to-left shunt develops, which bypasses the pulmonary circulation, sending unoxygenated blood into the peripheral circulation. This leads to rapid circulatory collapse.

(4) Mitral valve prolapse occurs in 5% of normal young women, most of whom are asymptomatic.

c. Peripartum cardiomyopathy is rare, idiopathic heart failure that develops during the latter part of pregnancy or within the first 6 months postpartum. It is often associated with pulmonary embolus (PE).

(1) Risk factors include age over 30 years, multiparity, racial background (black), multiple gestation, and hypertension.

(2) Symptoms are those of congestive heart failure: dyspnea, chest pain, fatigue, orthopnea, palpitations, and syncope.

(3) Signs include jugular venous distention, rales, edema, cardiomegaly, third heart sound, and arrhythmias.

(4) Laboratory findings. A chest radiograph demonstrates cardiomegaly and pulmonary edema, and an echocardiogram shows decreased ejection fraction.

(5) Treatment includes bed rest, sodium restriction, diuresis, digitalis, and anticoagulation.

(6) Prognosis is 75% mortality within 5 years if cardiomegaly does not resolve within 6 months from onset.

C. Maternal mortality risk (Table 4-2)

D. Principles of prenatal management

1. Fluid retention should be avoided. The patient should be placed on a 2-g sodium diet. Left lateral decubitus rest for 1 hour three times a day should be encouraged. Digitalis and diuretics should be used if necessary.

Table 4-2. Maternal Mortality Risk

Low Mortality ($< 1\%$)	Moderate Mortality (5%–15%)	High Mortality (25%–50+%)
Uncomplicated ASD, VSD, or PDA	Artificial heart valve	Pulmonary hypertension
Pulmonic or tricuspid valve disease	Mitral stenosis with atrial fibrillation	Complicated coarctation of the aorta
Uncomplicated bioprosthetic heart valve	Aortic stenosis	Marfan syndrome with dilated aortic root (diameter > 40 mm)
Mitral stenosis; functional class I or II disease (see Box 4-2)	Uncomplicated coarctation of the aorta	Peripartum cardiomyopathy
Corrected tetraology of Fallot	Marfan syndrome with normal aortic root (diameter < 40 mm)	
	Uncorrected tetralogy of Fallot	
	Previous myocardial infarction	

ASD = atrial septal defect; PDA = patent ductus arteriosus; VSD = ventral septal defect.

2. **Strenuous activity,** which tends to shunt blood away from uteroplacental circulation, should be avoided.

3. **Anemia** should be avoided so that the compensatory tachycardia that follows anemia is prevented.

4. **Each prenatal visit** should include close observation for evidence of worsening disease.

E. **Principles of intrapartum management**

1. **Reassurance and sedation** decreases epinephrine response and tachycardia.

2. **Use of epidural analgesia** decreases pain leading to tachycardia.

3. **Placement in the left lateral position** enhances uteroplacental/intervillous blood flow.

4. **Invasive monitoring** such as an arterial line and a Swan-Ganz catheter if the patient is class III or class IV in the New York functional classification system should be used (see Box 4-2).

5. **Forceps delivery should be used,** and second-stage valsalva should be avoided.

6. **Use of subacute bacterial endocarditis (SBE) antibiotic prophylaxis guidelines [American Heart Association (1997)]**

   a. SBE prophylaxis is **not recommended** in the following circumstances:
      (1) **Any cesarean deliveries,** regardless of cardiac lesion or history
      (2) Vaginal delivery in low-to-moderate risk individuals

   b. SBE prophylaxis is **optional** in only the following **high-risk patients** undergoing a **vaginal delivery** with the following conditions:
      (1) Previous SBE
      (2) Prosthetic heart valve
      (3) Complex cyanotic congenital heart disease
      (4) Surgically constructed shunts

   c. **Recommended antibiotics**
      (1) Ampicillin 2 g IV plus gentamicin IV or
      (2) Vancomycin 1 g IV

F. **Principles of postpartum management**

1. Close observation for volume overload is essential immediately after the placenta is expelled.

2. CO increases 15% immediately after delivery of the placenta as a result of the autotransfusion of uteroplacental blood rapidly being infused into the peripheral circulation.

3. PVR increases resulting from the sudden loss of the placental low-resistance arteriovenous shunt.

III. **THROMBOEMBOLIC DISEASE,** which affects 1% of pregnant women, varies in prognosis from benign to lethal. Thromboembolic phenomena are the predominant cause of maternal mortality.

A. **Pathophysiology**

1. **Endothelial injury** from traumatic vaginal delivery or abdominal delivery increases the relative risk fivefold postpartum.

2. **Vascular stasis,** the strongest single predisposing factor, is augmented by decreased pelvic and lower extremity blood flow and vessel wall tone.

3. **Enhanced blood coagulability** involves pregnancy-induced increases in factors II, VII, VIII, IX, X and fibrinogen.

4. **Coagulation protein deficiencies** (antithrombin III, protein C, protein S, plasminogen) markedly increase the risk of thrombosis.

B. **Superficial thrombophlebitis** does **not** predispose patients to embolic disease.

1. **Symptoms** include pain and sensitivity in the affected lower extremity.

2. **Signs** include erythema, tenderness, and swelling at the involved site.

3. **Diagnosis** is one of exclusion after deep venous thrombosis (DVT) is ruled out.

4. **Treatment** is conservative and includes bed rest, local heat, and nonsteroidal anti-inflammatory agents (NSAIDs).

C. **Deep venous thrombosis (DVT)** does predispose patients to embolic disease. In 50% of cases, the site of thrombosis is the pelvic veins, and in the remaining 50%, it is the lower extremities.

1. **Symptoms** may include pain and sensitivity in the affected lower extremity. However, the condition may also be asymptomatic.

2. **Signs** may include tenderness and edema with calf pain with ankle dorsiflexion (Homans' sign).

3. **Diagnosis** is by duplex Doppler studies or impedance plethysmography (above the knee) or venography (below the knee).

4. **Treatment** is full anticoagulation initially by IV or subcutaneous (SQ) heparin in sufficiently high doses to prolong the partial thromboplastin time to 1.5 to 2.5 times the laboratory control value.

   a. **Heparin** does not cross the placenta because of its high molecular weight.

   b. **Oral warfarin** may be used in puerperal cases (after thrombus stabilization with heparin), but it is not used antenatally because it crosses the placenta, exposing the fetus.

   c. **Protamine sulfate** reverses life-threatening heparin overdose.

D. **Pulmonary embolus (PE)** is the potentially fatal consequence of DVT.

1. **Symptoms** include **chest pain** and **dyspnea** (> 80% of patients). No single symptom or combination of symptoms is specific, because the location and size of thrombi in the lung varies.

2. **Findings** include **tachypnea** (> 90% of patients). The chest radiograph is commonly normal. Although arterial blood gas (ABG) measurements may show low PO_2, they are usually normal. The electrocardiogram (EKG) may show tachycardia and right axis deviation, but it is also generally normal.

3. **Diagnosis** is dependent on pulmonary imaging modalities.

    a. **Ventilation–perfusion (V̇/Q̇) scan** is the most accurate noninvasive method. Technically satisfactory V̇/Q̇ scans are reported as normal or low probability, intermediate probability, or high probability of PE. Technically suboptimal V̇/Q̇ scans may be reported as indeterminate or suspicious.

    b. **Pulmonary angiography,** which involves involving injection of contrast media into the lobar or segmental branches of the pulmonary artery, is the most definitive diagnostic method. It is indicated when the V̇/Q̇ scan is of intermediate probability or indeterminate for technical reasons.

  4. **Treatment** is full anticoagulation with IV or SQ heparin as described for DVT (see III C 4).

IV. OBSTETRIC SHOCK.

Shock can be defined as a state of **inadequate tissue perfusion.** This condition can arise from a variety of causes in pregnant women, including hypovolemia and sepsis.

  A. Hypovolemic shock

    1. **Etiology**

      a. **Antepartum** causes include ruptured ectopic pregnancy, abruptio placentae, placenta previa, and uterine rupture (see Chapter 3 III A).

      b. **Intrapartum** causes include surgical procedures such as cesarean delivery (see Chapter 6 VI).

      c. **Postpartum** causes include placenta accreta/increta/percreta, uterine atony, uterine inversion, lacerations, and retained placenta. (see chapter 7 II)

    2. **Pathophysiology**

      a. **Hypotension is initially corrected** by hemodynamic autoregulation, which maintains arterial perfusion until 25% of the intravascular volume is lost.

        (1) The **sympathetic nervous system** causes peripheral vasoconstriction and blood flow redistribution to vital organs.

        (2) **Volume shifts** occur as fluid from the extravascular space moves into the intravascular space.

        (3) **Adrenal gland epinephrine** secretion exerts inotropic and chronotropic effects on cardiac function.

      b. **If hypotension is uncorrected,** a series of downward spiraling events begins.

        (1) **Fetal hypoxemia** as a result of declining uteroplacental perfusion (resulting from limited uterine artery autoregulation), producing metabolic acidosis and ultimately fetal death.

        (2) **Maternal hypoxemia** leads to anaerobic metabolism, also producing metabolic acidosis and ultimately maternal death.

    3. **Clinical findings** include:

      a. **Initial findings** are orthostatic changes, noted when patient is moved from lying to sitting to standing position.

        (1) **Rise in HR** ($\geq$ 20 beats/min)

        (2) **Fall in BP** ($\geq$ 15 mm Hg)

(3) Fall in pulse pressure ($\leq$ 30 mm Hg)

b. **Subsequent changes,** which occur as the patient's condition worsens, reflect loss of target tissue perfusion and oxygenation.

(1) Symptoms include altered mentation and dizziness.

(2) Signs include diaphoresis, cold extremities, supine tachycardia, and hypotension.

(3) Maternal monitoring indicates central venous pressure less than 5 cm H_2O, a pulmonary capillary wedge pressure (PCWP) less than 5 mm Hg, and a urine output less than 30 ml/hr.

(4) Fetal monitoring reveals bradycardia or repetitive late decelerations.

4. **Treatment**

a. **Control of the bleeding source** by uterine massage, administration of uterotonic agents (oxytocin, methylergonovine, dinoprostone), and ligation of vessels

b. **Replacement of functional blood volume** using military antishock trousers (MAST) garment and intravenous crystalloid, colloid, or red blood cells (RBCs) as needed

c. **Correction of coagulation disorders** using platelets or fresh frozen plasma as needed. Abnormal hemostasis is likely if at least 15 units of whole blood are lost or if at least 10 units of RBCs are given.

d. **Vessel embolization** may be effective in unresponsive conditions.

B. **Septic shock**

1. **Epidemiology**

a. **Antepartum** causes include septic abortion and pyelonephritis.

b. **Postpartum** causes include puerperal sepsis (see Chapter 7 III).

2. **Pathophysiology.** Lysis of bacterial cell walls release **endotoxin,** which leads to:

a. **Consumptive coagulopathy** and fibrinolysis activation

b. **DIC** from complement activation, producing leukocyte-mediated endothelial injury and platelet aggregation

c. **Capillary permeability,** third spacing, vasodilation, and hypotension from mast cell degranulation, resulting in histamine release

3. **Phases of septic shock**

a. **Early or** *warm phase* **shock has a better prognosis** and is characterized by warm extremities due to increased CO. Clinical findings are warm extremities, hyperthermia, confusion, tachypnea, respiratory alkalosis, and only minimal hypotension. Without aggressive intervention, deterioration occurs, leading to severe hypotension and late phase shock.

b. **Late or** *cold phase* **shock has a poorer prognosis** and is characterized by cold extremities resulting from decreasing CO and increasing PVR. Clinical findings are cold and clammy skin; obtundation; and **multiple organ failure,** including systemic cardiac (myocardial depression), renal (oliguria, acute tubular necrosis), pulmonary (adult respiratory distress syndrome), and hematologic (hemoconcentration, DIC) conditions.

4. **Treatment**
   a. **Fever reduction using** antipyretic agents and cooling blankets
   b. **Aggressive stabilization of vital signs by:**
      (1) Expanding IV volume with 2 L crystalloid wide open and blood products as needed
      (2) Placing pulmonary artery catheter if systolic BP is < 80 mm Hg
      (3) Continuing volume expansion until PCWP is > 15 mm Hg
      (4) Providing inotropic therapy (digoxin and dopamine) if left ventricular function is depressed
      (5) Initiating peripheral vasoconstrictors (phenylephrine) if no response
   c. **Removal of underlying causes** of sepsis such as products of conception
   d. **Initiation of triple-agent antibiotics** with broad-spectrum coverage:
      (1) Ampicillin 2 g IV q6hr
      (2) Gentamicin 1.5 mg/kg IV q8hr
      (3) Clindamycin 900 mg IV q8hr

V. PULMONARY DISORDERS

A. **Amniotic fluid embolism**

1. **Epidemiology**
   a. **Incidence.** Although the condition is **rare,** it is a common cause of maternal mortality (1 in 50,000 pregnancies).
   b. **Etiology.** Amniotic fluid itself is innocuous, and amniotic fluid embolism is a systemic response to amniotic debris. "Anaphylactoid syndrome of pregnancy" is a suggested synonym.
   c. **Risk factors** include age greater than 30 years and multiparity. There is no relationship to the use of uterine stimulants, hyperstimulation, or fetal demise.
   d. The **mortality rate exceeds 85%.**

2. **Pathophysiology**
   a. **Amniotic debris** enters the pulmonary circulation from traumatized veins (cervical, uterine) or the disrupted placental site, leading to pulmonary vascular obstruction, pulmonary hypertension, and cor pulmonale.
   b. **Hypertonic contractions** are probably a secondary response, because uterine blood flow ceases with intrauterine pressures exceeding 40 mm Hg.
   c. **Biphasic response**
      (1) **Right heart failure.** Initially transient but intense vasospasm leads to severe pulmonary hypertension followed by right heart failure and hypoxia, resulting in neurologic injury.
      (2) **Left heart failure.** Hypoxia leads to in myocardial injury, resulting in left heart failure. This exacerbates pulmonary edema and adult respiratory distress syndrome and is followed by death.

3. **Clinical findings**
   a. **Symptoms** include dramatic, sudden onset of chest pain; respiratory distress; and cyanosis.
   b. **Signs** include hypotension and pulmonary edema, followed by cardiac arrest.
   c. **Maternal monitoring** shows hypoxia on ABG measurement and right ventricular strain on EKG. The chest radiograph may be non-specific, however.
   d. **Fetal monitoring** reveals bradycardia or repetitive late decelerations.
4. **Treatment** is largely supportive. **No type of intervention has changed the dismal maternal prognosis.**
   a. **Minimization of hypoxia** with supplemental oxygen and positive end-expiratory pressure (PEEP)
   b. **Maintenance of BP** with IV fluids and rapid digitalization
   c. **Placement of pulmonary artery catheter** if there is no coagulopathy
   d. **Treatment of associated coagulopathies** with selected blood products

B. **Asthma** is a disease of airway hyperreactivity with reversible obstruction of airflow.
   1. **Epidemiology**
      a. **Prevalence in pregnant women is 1%** (same as in general population). Pregnancy has no significant impact on asthma. During labor and delivery, 10% of patients experience a deterioration.
      b. **External allergens** include pollens, tobacco smoke, respiratory infections, and medications (especially NSAIDs).
      c. **Internal allergens** include cold weather or exercise.
   2. **Pathophysiology stages/sequence** (Table 4-3). ABG measurements reflect stages of clinical deterioration in asthma. Initially, hyperventilation compensates and PO_2 remains normal. As decompensation begins, PO_2 falls, leading to a rising PCO_2 and ultimately, acidosis.
   3. **Diagnosis**
      a. **Symptoms** include wheezing, dyspnea, chest tightness, and sometimes cough.
      b. **Signs** include tachypnea, tachycardia, prolonged expiratory phase, and use of accessory respiratory muscles.
      c. **ABG** measurements are essential to identification of the asthmatic phase. To interpret ABG measurements in asthma, remember the normal respiratory alkalosis of pregnancy: pH increased, PCO_2 decreased, and PO_2 increased.
      d. **Pulmonary function tests** give objective evidence of change in respiratory status. During pregnancy, normal parameters [e.g., forced expiratory velocity at 1 second (FEV_1)] are not significantly altered.
   4. **Treatment**
      a. **Searching for the inciting cause** such as allergy, bronchitis, pneumonia, or labor

Table 4-3. Arterial Blood Gas Measurements in Clinical Stages of Worsening Asthma

Stage	PO$_2$	PCO$_2$	pH
Mild respiratory alkalosis	Normal	↓	↑
Respiratory alkalosis	↓	↓	↑
Danger zone	↓	Normal	Normal
Respiratory acidosis	↓	↑	↓

   b. **Providing supplemental oxygen** by nasal prongs or face mask to maintain an oxygen saturation of ≥ 95%

   c. **Hydrating** with balanced crystalloid to liquefy secretions

   d. **Administering inhaled bronchodilators** (generally safe in pregnancy)

   e. **Administering systemic corticosteroids** (generally safe in pregnancy)

VI. THYROID DISORDERS

   A. Hypothyroidism

   1. **Epidemiology.** Prevalence in pregnant women is 1%.

      a. **Thyroid hormone deficiency** occurs predominantly as a primary thyroid defect.

      b. **Infertility** is a common result of overt hypothyroidism. Thus myxedema is seldom seen with pregnancy.

      c. **Untreated hypothyroidism** is associated with higher rates of miscarriage, stillbirth, preterm delivery, and preeclampsia.

      d. **If treated, hypothyroidism** has no impact on pregnancy outcome.

   2. **Etiology**

      a. **Autoimmune** causes **(most cases),** including **Hashimoto's thyroiditis** and **idiopathic myxedema**

      b. **Iatrogenic** causes, including radioactive iodine-131 (^{131}I) therapy and subtotal thyroidectomy

      c. **Drug-induced** causes, including iodide deficiency, excess lithium, or antithyroid drugs

   3. **Clinical findings and diagnosis**

      a. **Symptoms** include weakness, fatigue, cold intolerance, constipation, hair loss, weight gain, and amenorrhea.

      b. **Signs** include dry coarse skin, periorbital edema, thick tongue, decreased reflexes, hypertension, and bradycardia.

      c. **Laboratory values** include elevated thyroid-stimulating hormone (TSH) and decreased free thyroxine (T$_4$).

   4. **Treatment**

      a. **L-thyroxine** is the synthetic hormone replacement recommended regardless of the etiology. Lifetime replacement is generally required.

    b. Serial TSH and free T$_4$ levels should be monitored to identify the appropriate dosage.

B. Hyperthyroidism (thyrotoxicosis)

  1. Epidemiology. Prevalence in pregnant women is 0.2%.

    a. Thyroid hormone excess result is from a variety of causes, each of which is managed differently.

    b. Uncontrolled hyperthyroidism is associated with preterm delivery, low birth weight, and preeclampsia.

    c. Controlled hyperthyroidism has no impact on pregnancy outcome.

  2. Pathophysiology. Graves' disease and Plummer's disease account for most cases.

    a. Graves' disease is an organ-specific autoimmune disease in which thyroid-stimulating immunoglobulin (TSI) mimics TSH, resulting in thyroid hyperfunction. TSI activity usually declines in pregnancy.

    b. Toxic nodular goiter (Plummer's disease) is a condition in which a thyroid nodule produces thyroid hormones independently without regulation from the hypothalamic-pituitary axis.

  3. Clinical findings and diagnosis

    a. Symptoms include weakness, nervousness, heat intolerance, diarrhea, weight loss, emotional lability, and amenorrhea.

    b. Signs include goiter, warm smooth skin, eye stare, lid lag, exophthalmos, fine tremor, brink reflexes, tachycardia, and dysrhythmia.

    c. Laboratory values include decreased TSH, elevated free T$_4$, and presence of TSI (in Graves' disease).

  4. Treatment

    a. Antithyroid drugs are used for Graves' disease. **Propylthiouracil (PTU)** is the treatment of choice in pregnancy, using the minimum dose to restore euthyroidism. Serial free T$_4$ levels should be monitored. **Methimazole** is seldom used in pregnancy (associated with neonatal aplasia cutis of the scalp). Both medications cross the placenta and can cause fetal hypothyroidism and goiter. Remission may occur in one-third of patients.

    b. Radioactive ^{131}I ablation is the treatment of choice outside of pregnancy, but it is contraindicated in pregnancy because ^{131}I crosses the placenta and can ablate the fetal thyroid. Lifetime thyroid replacement is necessary.

    c. Thyroidectomy is seldom required except for failure of medical management. Lifetime thyroid replacement is necessary.

C. Postpartum thyroiditis

  1. Epidemiology. Prevalence in postpartum patients is 5%–10%.

  2. Pathophysiology. A destructive lymphocytic thyroiditis results in glandular release of hormone. The usual pattern is **hyperthyroidism** (1–4 months postpartum) followed by **hypothyroidism** (4–8 months postpartum). The majority of patients have positive **microsomal autoantibodies.**

3. **Clinical findings.** Symptoms and signs are typically nonspecific, including depression, carelessness, and impaired memory concentration.

4. **Treatment.** The hyperthyroid phase is usually managed conservatively, because antithyroid agents are ineffective. β-Adrenergic blockers may be used. The hypothyroid phase is treated with L-thyroxine replacement.

VII. LIVER DISEASE

A. **Cholestasis of pregnancy**

1. **Epidemiology.** Prevalence in pregnant women is 0.5%.

2. **Pathophysiology.** Intrahepatic cholestasis appears to be stimulated by high estrogen levels in genetically susceptible women. Bile acids are incompletely cleared by the liver and accumulate in the plasma. Mild jaundice may be seen. Resolution occurs after delivery.

3. **Clinical findings.** Troublesome generalized pruritus develops late in pregnancy with mild bilirubin elevation. Bile acids may be elevated in plasma up to 10- or 100-fold of normal. Mild elevation of serum aminotransferase levels (< 250 U/L) may occur. Cholestasis of pregnancy has no significant impact on maternal outcome, but preterm delivery and stillbirths may increase.

4. **Treatment.** Cholestyramine blocks enterohepatic circulation and absorption of bile acids. However, it may also impair absorption of fat-soluble vitamins, necessitating vitamin K supplementation. Oral antihistamines may provide symptomatic relief. Fetal antenatal testing and surveillance should be utilized.

B. **Acute fatty liver of pregnancy** is a life-threatening complication of pregnancy.

1. **Epidemiology.** Prevalence is 1 in 15,000 pregnant women.

2. **Pathophysiology.** The cause is unknown, but liver histology is similar to that seen with excessive doses of tetracycline. Grossly, the liver appears small, soft, yellow, and greasy. Histologically, microvesicular fat fills the swollen hepatocyte cytoplasm, but minimal necrosis is apparent. Lipid accumulation may also occur in renal tubular cells.

3. **Clinical findings.** Symptom onset is gradual over days to weeks in the third trimester, with flu-like symptoms, nausea, vomiting, epigastric pain, and jaundice. Proteinuria, hypertension, and edema may be confused with preeclampsia. Laboratory evidence of DIC may be apparent. Marked **hypoglycemia** is frequent with elevation of serum **ammonia** levels. Hepatic **encephalopathy** and coma may ensue, resulting in a maternal mortality rate up to 50% or more. Fetal death is common.

4. **Treatment.** Spontaneous resolution usually follows delivery if the mother survives. Intensive maternal, fetal, and neonatal care are critical.

C. **Viral hepatitis** is the **most common serious liver disease** identified in pregnancy. **Five types** have been diagnosed: **A, B, C, D,** and **E.** Acute hepatitis of any kind may be subclinical. Clinically, affected women present with nausea, vomiting, headache, and malaise. Symptoms typically improve after jaundice appears. At this point, elevation of liver enzymes peaks, with levels up to 4000 U/L. Liver tenderness may persist. Jaundice continues after liver enzymes have normalized. Mortality rates may approach 1%.

1. **Hepatitis A (HAV)**
   a. **Epidemiology.** Transmission of this RNA virus occurs by the oral-fecal route. Sexual transmission does not occur. No known carrier state has been identified.
   b. **Effect on pregnancy.** HAV is not teratogenic. The risk of transmission to the fetus is **negligible.** The preterm delivery risk may be increased.
   c. **Management.** The recommended mode of delivery is **vaginal.** The cornerstones of maternal therapy are a balanced diet and reduced activity.

2. **Hepatitis B (HBV)** [see Chapter 5 VII]
   a. **Epidemiology.** HBV is endemic in Asia and Africa. Transmission of this DNA virus occurs via any body fluids, and sexual transmission may occur. A chronic carrier state may exist.
   b. **Effect on pregnancy.** HBV is not teratogenic. Risk of transplacental transmission to the fetus is rare. However, **vertical transmission at delivery is significant:** 10% if the mother is hepatitis B surface antigen (HBsAg)–positive and 80% if the mother is both HBsAg- and hepatitis B e antigen (HBeAg)–positive.
   c. **Management.** Recommended mode of delivery is **vaginal.** Neonates of HBsAg-positive mothers should receive passive and active immunization within 48 hours of delivery.

3. **Hepatitis C (HCV)**
   a. **Epidemiology.** Transmission of this RNA virus occurs via any body fluids. Sexual transmission may occur, but it is not transmitted as readily as hepatitis B. HCV RNA serum titer is a marker for infectivity.
   b. **Effect on pregnancy.** HCV is not teratogenic. Perinatal outcomes are unchanged. The risk of transplacental transmission to the fetus is **negligible.** However, vertical transmission at delivery is significant. With HCV RNA–positive mothers, the mother-to-infant transmission rate at delivery is 10%.
   c. **Management.** The recommended mode of delivery is **vaginal.** Alpha-interferon may be used for persistently HCV RNA–positive patients or those with persistently elevated liver enzymes.

4. **Hepatitis D (HDV)** [delta hepatitis]
   a. **Epidemiology.** HDV involves a defective RNA virus that must coinfect with HBV and cannot persist in the serum longer than the HBV. Transmission is similar to HBV (by body fluids), but sexual transmission is less efficient than with HBV.
   b. **Effect on pregnancy.** Perinatal transmission is rare.
   c. **Management.** The recommended mode of delivery is **vaginal.**

5. **Hepatitis E**

a. **Epidemiology.** Transmission of this RNA virus is by the oral-fecal route (similar to HBV), but most cases occur with contaminated water in developing countries.

b. **Effect on pregnancy.** Vertical transmission and transplacental transmission can occur.

c. **Management.** The recommended mode of delivery is **vaginal.**

VIII. GLUCOSE INTOLERANCE

A. **Overview** (Table 4-4)

1. **Classification**

a. **Gestational diabetes mellitus (GDM).** GDM, the most common type of glucose intolerance in pregnancy, is usually diagnosed during the last half of pregnancy. Typically, management is with diet alone, but insulin may be needed. GDM usually resolves after delivery but may include new onset of type I or type II DM.

b. **Type 1 DM.** Pathophysiology involves autoimmune-mediated destruction of pancreatic islet cells leading to insulinopenia. Survival depends on insulin.

c. **Type 2 DM.** Pathophysiology involves cellular resistance to insulin or undersecretion of insulin. Oral agents may be used in the non-pregnant state but are contraindicated in pregnancy because of association with fetal/neonatal hypoglycemia. Pregnant women with overt diabetes should be treated with insulin.

2. **Incidence.** The overall incidence of diabetes in pregnancy is 3% (100,000 cases per year in the United States).

3. **Mechanism.** The diabetogenic effect of **human placental lactogen (hPL)** is the most significant factor in GDM. Placental insulinase, elevated free cortisol, and progesterone also act as mechanisms of glucose intolerance.

B. **Screening and diagnosis of GDM**

1. **Risk factors** are given in Table 4-5, but they are not used to determine which patients should be screened.

2. **Routine glucose screening** for all pregnant women includes the **1-hour oral glucose tolerance test (OGTT).**

a. **Procedure.** A 50-g oral glucose load is administered without the need for a fasting state. The test is performed at the first prenatal visit if patients meet risk criteria; otherwise, it is done between weeks 24 and 28.

b. **Results**

(1) If the screening value is 140 mg/dl or more, a 3-hr OGTT should be performed.

(2) If the screening value is 200 mg/dl or more, GDM is suggested.

c. **Nonvalid screening.** Tests **not used** for diabetic screening include urine glucose values and glycosylated hemoglobin.

3. **Definitive diagnosis** is achieved through the 3-hour OGTT.

Table 4-4.   Diabetes in Pregnancy

	Gestational Diabetes	Type 1 Diabetes	Type 2 Diabetes
Common name	Pregnancy-induced	Juvenile-onset	Adult-onset
When diagnosed	During pregnancy (usually in last half)	Onset prior to pregnancy	Onset prior to pregnancy
Mechanism	Insulin resistance	Pancreatic islet-cell destruction	Insulin resistance
Plasma insulin levels	High	Low	High
Increased risk of fetal anomalies	None	Possible	Possible
Therapeutic modalities	Diet (15% need insulin)	Insulin Diet Exercise	Insulin Diet Exercise
How diagnosed	≥ 2 abnormal values on a 3-hr 100 g OGTT	Unable to achieve nonpregnant euglycemia without insulin	May achieve nonpregnant euglycemia without insulin
How assess success	Home blood glucose monitoring	Home blood glucose monitoring	Home blood glucose monitoring
Blood glucose target values	FBS < 90 mg/dl 2-hr PP < 120 mg/dl	FBS < 90 mg/dl 2-hr PP < 120 mg/dl	FBS < 90 mg/dl 2-hr PP < 120 mg/dl
Fetal growth abnormalities	Macrosomia	Macrosomia IUGR (if small vessel disease)	Macrosomia
Neonatal hazards	Hypoglycemia Hypocalcemia Hyperbilirubinemia Polycythemia RDS	Hypoglycemia Hypocalcemia Hyperbilirubinemia Polycythemia RDS	Hypoglycemia Hypocalcemia Hyperbilirubinemia Polycycthemia RDS

OGTT = oral glucose tolerance test; *FBS* = fasting blood glucose; *2-hr PP* = 2 hour-postprandial/postmeal; *RDS* = respiratory distress syndrome.

  a. Procedure. A 100-g oral glucose load is administered following a fast for at least 8 hours but less than 14 hours. The test should be performed after 3 days of unrestricted carbohydrate diet.

  b. Fasting blood glucose. A value of 126 mg/dl or more is diagnostic of overt DM.

  c. Criteria. Two or more values equal to or greater than the following are necessary for positive diagnosis:

   (1) Fasting: 95 mg/dl

   (2) 1-hour: 180 mg/dl

Table 4-5. Risk Factors for Gestational Diabetes

Patient History	Clinical Clues
Family history of overt diabetes	Demographic clues • Obesity (> 130% of IBW) • Age > 25 years
Obstetric history • Unexplained stillbirth • Traumatic delivery • Shoulder dystocia	Obstetric clues • Polyhydramnios • Administration of terbutaline • Macrosomia
Neonatal history • Infant with congenital malformations • Infant with birth weight > 4000 g • Neonatal death from birth trauma	Medical clues • Hypertension • Recurrent candidiasis • Glycosuria

IBW = ideal body weight.

        (3) 2-hour: 155 mg/dl

        (4) 3-hour: 140 mg/dl

    4. The **"rule of 15s"** applies to GDM.

        a. 15% of gravidas have an abnormal 50-g screen.

        b. 15% of gravidas with a positive screen have an abnormal 3-hour OGTT.

        c. 15% of gestational diabetics require insulin.

        d. 15% of pregnant women with gestational diabetes have macrosomic infants.

  C. White's classification of diabetes in pregnancy (Box 4-3) is based on the age of diabetes onset and degree of end-organ involvement. In the past, this system was used to determine how prematurely to deliver infants of diabetic mothers to avoid fetal demise. Now, with the development of antenatal fetal testing and methods of assessing of fetal lung maturity, arbitrary premature delivery of these infants is no longer necessary.

  D. Fetal complications of diabetes

    1. GDM

        a. Macrosomia may occur from excessive transplacental glucose passage from **maternal hyperglycemia.**

Box 4-3. White's Classification of Diabetes in Pregnancy

A1	Normal fasting in gestational diabetes
A2	Abnormal fasting in gestational diabetes
B	Diabetes onset after age 20 years; duration < 10 years
C	Diabetes onset age 10–19 years; duration 10–19 years
D	Diabetes onset before age 10 years; duration ≥ 20 years
F	Presence of nephropathy
R	Presence of proliferative retinopathy
H	Presence of arteriosclerotic heart disease

    b. Anomalies are **not increased** because there is no hyperglycemia during **embryogenesis.**

  2. Type I and type II diabetes

    a. Macrosomia may occur as a result of maternal hyperglycemia.

    b. Asymmetric IUGR may occur as a result of **placental insufficiency** if the mother has small vessel vascular disease.

    c. Congenital anomalies may occur if **hyperglycemia** is present during **embryogenesis.** These include:

      (1) Neural tube defects (NTDs) [e.g., anencephaly, spina bifida]

      (2) Congenital heart defects (e.g., VSDs, transposition of great vessels)

      (3) Caudal regression syndrome/sacral agenesis, an anomaly that occurs 200 times more often in diabetic women

E. Clinical approach for gestational diabetes mellitus (GDM)

  1. Prenatal care. The **key objective is maternal euglycemia.**

    a. Frequency of prenatal visits

      (1) Every 1–2 weeks from diagnosis until 36 weeks

      (2) Every week from 36 weeks until delivery

    b. Dietary management. The cornerstone is the American Diabetes Association (ADA) diet.

      (1) Calories (generally 1800–2200 kcal/day)

        (a) Lean: 35 kcal/kg ideal prepregnancy weight (PPW)

        (b) Obese: 25 kcal/kg ideal PPW

      (2) Composition

        (a) Carbohydrates: 50%–60% (complex, high fiber)

        (b) Fat: 25%–30%

        (c) Protein: 10%–20%

      (3) Plan

        (a) Macronutrients and kilocalories should be spread evenly over three meals per day.

        (b) There should be a bedtime snack.

        (c) High-fiber foods should be encouraged.

        (d) Sweets should be avoided.

    c. Weight management

      (1) Steady, gradual weight gain is more important than total weight gain.

      (2) Third-trimester weight gain should be 1 pound per week.

    d. Management of maternal glycemic control is the central goal.

      (1) Daily self-monitoring of capillary blood glucose levels is performed, keeping a written record.

      (2) Blood glucose target values are:

        (a) Fasting: < 90 mg/dl

        (b) 1-hour postmeal: < 140 mg/dl

        (c) 2-hour postmeal: < 120 mg/dl

      (3) Outcomes

        (a) If the mother is normoglycemic, there is no increased risk of fetal jeopardy.

(b) If blood glucose values consistently exceed the target range, SQ injection of long-acting and short-acting human insulin is prescribed, using the same glycemic goals as in patients with overt diabetes.

e. **Fetal surveillance**

(1) **If risk factors are present** (e.g., prior stillbirth, hypertension, preeclampsia, macrosomia, insulin necessity), fetal well-being is not ensured. Twice-weekly NSTs and AFIs should be started at 32 weeks.

(2) **If no risk factors are present,** there is no risk of fetal jeopardy. Twice-weekly NSTs need not be started until 40 weeks.

2. **Delivery and postpartum management**

a. **Delivery management**

(1) **There is no need to induce labor** before 40 weeks' gestation in patients with glucose values in the target range.

(2) **Macrosomia risk** should be evaluated clinically and by ultrasound. A cesarean delivery should be considered if the estimated fetal weight exceeds 4000–4500 g. Operative vaginal delivery should be avoided.

(3) The **risk of shoulder dystocia** rises with increasing birth weight, especially in fetuses of diabetic mothers. The anterior fetal shoulder becomes impacted behind the symphysis pubis. Appropriate management should include:

(a) **Sharp flexion of maternal thighs** (McRoberts maneuver)

(b) **Suprapubic pressure** to disimpact the anterior shoulder

(c) **Rotation of the anterior shoulder** 180 degrees to disimpact the anterior shoulder (Wood's maneuver)

(d) **Delivery of the posterior arm** and rotation 180 degrees, bringing the anterior shoulder posteriorly

(4) **Blood glucose levels** should be monitored during labor (maintain between 80–100 mg/dl).

b. **Neonatal management.** Pediatric care should be available at time of delivery. Infants should be observed for:

(1) **Hypoglycemia** as a result of persistent hyperinsulinemia from in utero hyperglycemia

(2) **Hypocalcemia** as a result of immature parathyroid hormone function

(3) **Hyperbilirubinemia** as a result of liver enzyme immaturity and increased breakdown of polycythemic RBCs

(4) **Respiratory distress** as a result of delayed pulmonary surfactant production

(5) **Polycythemia** as a result of increased erythropoietin due to relative intrauterine hypoxia

c. **Postpartum follow-up.** Patients should receive the following:

(1) **Immediately after delivery,** observation for **postpartum hemorrhage** resulting from **uterine atony** (due to an overdistended uterus from a macrosomic infant)

(2) **6 weeks after delivery** (or after completing lactation), **evaluation** for **overt diabetes** using the 2-hour, 75-g OGTT. Normal

values are a fasting glucose of less than 126 mg/dl and postchallenge values of less than 200 mg/dl.

F. **Clinical approach to type I and type II diabetes mellitus (DM)**

1. **Preconception and prenatal management**

   a. **Preconception counseling.** The overall goal is **prevention of congenital malformations** by achieving euglycemia at the time of embryogenesis.

      (1) **Optimum glycemic control** should be achieved before conception.

      (2) **End-organ evaluation** should be performed (see VIII F 1 c).

      (3) An **effective contraceptive program** should be established.

      (4) **Rubella immunization** should be performed if the patient is susceptible.

      (5) **Folate supplementation** of 4 mg/day should be initiated to prevent fetal NTDs.

   b. **Prenatal care goals**

      (1) Elimination of intrauterine deaths

      (2) Prevention of iatrogenic prematurity and respiratory distress syndrome (RDS)

      (3) Prevention of immediate neonatal morbidity

   c. **End-organ evaluation in pregnant women with insulin-dependent DM**

      (1) **Renal status.** Creatinine clearance should be measured twice during pregnancy. Baseline 24-hour urine protein levels should be obtained, and then dipstick urine protein levels should be measured frequently. Pregnancy should not worsen nephropathy.

      (2) **Retinal status.** A retinal examination with the pupils dilated should be performed twice during pregnancy. Pregnancy does not worsen benign retinopathy, but it may increase active proliferative retinopathy.

      (3) **Neuropathy.** Long-standing DM can lead to an altered autonomic response to hypoglycemia, as well as to peripheral neuropathy and gastroparesis.

   d. **Detection and evaluation of malformations.** Identification of the population at greatest risk is important (i.e., those with elevated first-trimester glycosylated hemoglobin levels).

      (1) **13–14 weeks: sonography** to rule out anencephaly

      (2) **16–18 weeks: triple-marker screen** to rule out NTDs

      (3) **18–22 weeks: focused sonography** to identify other structural anomalies

      (4) **22–24 weeks: fetal echocardiography** to detect cardiac anomalies (only if the first-trimester glycosylated hemoglobin was elevated)

   e. **Regulation of maternal glycemia**

      (1) **Glycemic goals.** The following levels should be maintained:

         (a) **Fasting:** 60–90 mg/dl

         (b) **Before meals:** 60–105 mg/dl

         (c) **2-hour postprandial:** < 120 mg/dl

         (d) **2–6 A.M.:** > 60 mg/dl

(2) **Insulin therapy.** Insulin is administered via multiple injections or a SQ insulin pump. The morning dose is two-thirds the total dose (two-thirds NPH insulin, one-third regular insulin), and the evening dose is one-third the total dose (one-half NPH insulin, one-half regular insulin). Oral hypoglycemic agents are contraindicated in pregnancy.

(3) **Management team.** Optimal care is provided by a team consisting of a nurse educator, dietitian, social worker, and physician. Patients should have 24-hour access to a team member.

f. **Fetal surveillance**

(1) **Ultrasound biometry** is performed serially to assess fetal growth.

(2) **Maternal assessment of fetal activity** begins between 26–30 weeks and continues until delivery.

(3) **Twice-weekly NSTs** are performed starting **at 32 weeks** with no risk factors and **at 26 weeks** with risk factors (vasculopathy, hypertension, or poor glycemic control).

2. **Delivery care in patients with insulin-dependent DM**

a. **Timing.** Delivery can occur after 38 weeks' gestation if amniotic fluid analysis documents fetal pulmonary maturity (lecithin:sphingomyelin ratio ≥ 2.0, and presence of phosphatidylglycerol).

b. **Delivery method.** Determination of the optimum route of delivery is individualized based on the following criteria:

(1) Previous obstetric history

(2) Glycemic control

(3) Presence of vascular disease

(4) Status of fetal well-being

(5) Estimated fetal weight

(6) Cervical status

c. **Intrapartum glycemic control.** An IV infusion is started with 10 U of regular insulin in 1 L D_5W at 100 ml/hr and hourly capillary blood glucose measurements are made with a target range of 80–100 mg/dl.

d. **Postpartum glycemic control.** If the insulin infusion is not reduced after the placenta is delivered, postpartum hypoglycemia can occur from the loss of insulin resistance because of a rapid fall in hPL.

IX. ANEMIA

A. **Definition**

1. **Physiologically,** anemia can be defined as a condition in which the oxygen-carrying capacity of the blood is decreased.

2. **Practically,** anemia in pregnancy can be defined as a hemoglobin level of less than 10 g/dl. The normal female hemoglobin reference range changes from 13–15 g/dl in the nonpregnant state to 10–12 g/dl with pregnancy.

3. The **hemodilution of pregnancy** explains the physiologic anemia.

a. The plasma volume increases 50% above nonpregnant levels. This increase is greater with twins than with single fetuses. The degree of increase correlates directly with birth weight.

       b. The RBC mass increases only 30% above nonpregnant levels. This RBC expansion accounts for the majority of the increased iron demands of pregnancy.

       c. The smaller increase in RBC mass than plasma volume results in a 15% dilution effect on normal hemoglobin levels.

  B. Classification of anemias is based on etiology (Table 4-6).

      1. Nutritional anemias involve the **heme** part of the hemoglobin molecule. Examples include iron, folate, and vitamin B_{12} deficiencies.

      2. Inherited anemias involve the **globin** portion of the hemoglobin molecule. Examples include hemoglobinopathies and thalassemias.

  C. Risk factors help identify those groups of women for whom screening, diagnosis, and treatment are crucial (Table 4-7).

  D. Iron-deficiency anemia

      1. Incidence. This is the **most common form of anemia in pregnancy.** More than 90% of all cases of anemia in women are caused by iron defi-

Table 4-6.   Anemias in Pregnancy

	Iron Deficiency	Folate Deficiency*	Thalassemia	Sickle Cell
Etiology	Nutritional Chronic bleeding	Nutritional Decreased absorption: • oral contraceptive pills • pyrimethamine • trimethoprim-sulfamethoxazole Hemolytic states	Inherited as autosomal recessive	Inherited as autosomal recessive
Molecular pathology	Decreased production of heme molecule from iron deficiency	Decreased production of heme molecule from alteration of one-carbon transfers	Decreased production of normal globin chains	Production of abnormal globin chains leading to chronic hemolysis
Diagnosis	CBC: microcytic, hypochromic RBCs	CBC: macrocytic RBCs; hypersegemented neutrophils; low RBC folate level	CBC: microcytic, hypochromic RBCs; hemoglobin electrophoresis	Hemoglobin electrophoresis
Impact on fetus	None	None	Death in utero if homozygous α-thalassemia (no adult hemoglobins are produced)	Increased perinatal mortality
Management	Ferrous iron salts to normalize peripheral hemoglobin and replace bone marrow iron stores ($FeSO_4$ 325 mg PO tid)	Folic acid supplements (folate 1 mg PO per day)	Conservative	Folic acid supplement Avoidance of excess iron Avoidance of hypoxia, acidosis Possible transfusion

*Maternal folate deficiency at embryogenesis is associated with increased neural tube defects.

Table 4-7. Risk Factors for Anemia in Pregnancy

Iron Deficiency	Folate Deficiency	Sickle Cell Disease	Thalassemia
Obstetric factors • Frequent pregnancies • Multiple gestation	Obstetric factors • Frequent pregnancies • Multiple gestation	Racial heritage • African descent	Geographical ethnicity • Mediterranean • Africa • Southeast Asia
Nutritional factors • Poor dietary habits • Pica	Seizure medications • Phenobarbital • Phenytoin		
Chronic bleeding • Epistaxis • Rectum • Vaginal	Antibiotic medications • Pyrimethamine • Trimethoprim- sulfamethoxazole		
Adolescence	Chronic hemolytic anemias • Sickle cell disease • Hereditary spherocytosis		

ciency. This type of anemia is 10 times more common in women than in men and is related to menstrual losses and pregnancy requirements.

2. **Pathophysiology.** Iron, which is centrally located in the hemoglobin molecule, is the most common substrate deficiency limiting RBC production. Iron is stored in the bone marrow, where erythropoiesis occurs. Iron-deficiency anemia does not occur until iron stores in bone marrow are completely depleted. Iron requirements increase with pregnancy, increasing the likelihood of iron bone marrow deficiency and subsequent risk of iron-deficiency anemia.

3. **Diagnosis**

   a. **RBC indices** include:

      (1) Microcytic, hypochromic RBC

      (2) Low mean corpuscular volume (MCV)

      (3) Low mean corpuscular hemoglobin concentration (MCHC)

      (4) High RBC distribution width

   b. **Serum iron studies** are of minimal value because the normal changes of pregnancy mimic findings in iron-deficiency anemia, such as:

      (1) Increased total iron-binding capacity

      (2) Decreased serum iron and ferritin

   c. **Bone marrow aspiration,** if performed, shows decreased iron stores. This is seldom done in pregnancy.

4. **Fetal/neonatal complications** do not occur, because iron is actively transported across the placenta to the fetus. Iron deficiency is not found in the fetus or neonate.

5. **Maternal symptoms** include tiredness and weakness.

6. **Management goals** are correction of the peripheral hemoglobin deficit and replacement of iron stores in bone marrow.

   a. Any **ferrous iron salts** are effective. Ferrous sulfate (325 mg PO) administered **three times daily** achieves the maximum bone marrow response. Ferrous gluconate and ferrous fumarate are alternative forms. Treatment should be continued for **3–6 months** to restore iron stores in bone marrow.

    b. Parenteral iron is indicated only if the patient's gastrointestinal (GI) tract is nonfunctional or when compliance cannot be ensured. There is no difference in the rapidity of the bone marrow response whether the iron is given orally or parenterally.

    c. Laboratory response parameters include the following:

        (1) The **reticulocyte count,** the first indicator to change, should increase within 3 days.

        (2) The **hemoglobin/hematocrit** increase is slower, taking 10–14 days.

  7. Prevention. The normal requirements of pregnancy are met with a daily supplement of 30 mg elemental iron. One tablet of ferrous sulfate (325 mg) contains 60 mg of elemental iron.

E. Folate-deficiency anemia

  1. Incidence. Folate-deficiency anemia, the second most common form of nutritional anemia in women, has an incidence of 0.5%–15%.

  2. Pathophysiology. Folate is a requisite for single-carbon transfer during the building of molecular hydrocarbon hemoglobin skeletons. Normal body stores last 90 days. Lack of folate results in decreased production of the heme molecule carbon skeleton. Folate is found in green, leafy vegetables.

  3. Diagnosis

    a. RBC indices include macrocytic RBC with high MCV and MCHC.

    b. Peripheral smear findings include hypersegmented neutrophils.

    c. RBC folate levels are low.

  4. Fetal/neonatal complications include low birth weight and NTDs (if folate deficiency was present during early embryogenesis).

  5. Maternal symptoms include tiredness and weakness.

  6. Management

    a. Folic acid (1 mg daily) produces the maximum hematologic response and replaces body stores.

    b. Iron supplements may also be needed, because 70% of patients with folate deficiency also lack iron stores.

    c. Laboratory response parameters include the following:

        (1) The **reticulocyte count,** the first indicator to change, should increase within 3 days.

        (2) The **hemoglobin/hematocrit** increase is slower, taking 10–14 days.

  7. Prevention. A daily supplement of **0.4 mg** of folic acid satisfies the normal requirements of pregnancy. To prevent NTDs in **women at high risk** (e.g., DM, previous infant with NTDs, anticonvulsant medications), the recommended dose is **4 mg/day** starting 3 months before pregnancy and during early embryogenesis.

F. Sickle cell disease

1. **Incidence.** Sickle cell disease is a genetic disorder that occurs mostly in blacks. Approximately 10% of African Americans have sickle cell trait, and 0.2% have sickle cell anemia.

2. **Pathophysiology.** Sickle cell disease is an autosomal recessive disorder passed with equal frequency to both sexes. Sickle cell trait is present when an individual is **heterozygous (SA)** for hemoglobin S, whereas sickle cell disease only occurs when an individual is **homozygous (SS).** Hemoglobin S confers protection against malaria.

   a. SS and SA are both characterized by an **abnormal hemoglobin S** molecule with a valine substituted for glutamic acid on β-chains in the sixth position from the N-terminal end.

   b. **With reduction of oxygen tension,** RBCs with more than 50% hemoglobin S can undergo intravascular **sickling.** This abnormal RBC morphology leads to:

      (1) **Chronic hemolytic anemia** from shortened survival time because of RBC phagocytosis by the spleen and liver

      (2) **Sickle cell crisis** in which capillary occlusion causes ischemic pain in the joints and long bones. A crisis may be precipitated by dehydration, acidosis, infection, or hypoventilation during general anesthesia.

3. **Diagnosis**

   a. **Screening tests** identify only whether hemoglobin S is present. They do not differentiate between SS and SA states.

   b. **Definitive testing** requires hemoglobin electrophoresis to differentiate between homozygous states (> 40% hemoglobin S) and heterozygous states (< 40% hemoglobin S).

4. **Fetal/neonatal complications**

   a. **Sickle cell trait** is not associated with any increase in perinatal morbidity or mortality.

   b. **Sickle cell disease** is associated with increased early spontaneous abortions, preterm delivery, IUGR, and stillbirths.

5. **Maternal complications**

   a. **Sickle cell trait** is associated with increased urinary tract infections (UTIs) [see X] and asymptomatic bacteriuria (ASB).

   b. **Sickle cell disease** is associated with:

      (1) **Increased morbidity** from hemolytic and folic acid anemias, sickle cell crisis, congestive heart failure, preeclampsia, and infections

      (2) **Increased mortality,** in which the maternal death rate can reach 1%

6. **Management**

   a. **Adequate oxygenation** to avoid hypoxia and acidosis

   b. **Narcotics for analgesia** if there is a sickle cell crisis

   c. **RBC transfusions** (to keep total hemoglobin S < 50%) for patients with congestive heart failure, sickle cell crisis, and marked anemia

   d. **Folate supplementation** (routine iron supplementation should be avoided to prevent hemosiderosis)

    e. Serial ultrasound assessment of fetal growth

    f. Serial antepartum fetal testing

    g. Preterm labor education

7. Prevention. There is no prevention for sickle cell disease. However, all at-risk patients should be screened for the presence of hemoglobin S. Prenatal diagnosis is available on fetal amniocytes using DNA techniques.

G. Thalassemia

1. Incidence. Thalassemia is a genetic disorder found in individuals originating geographically from Africa, southeast Asia, and the Mediterranean. Approximately 0.2% of pregnant women have some type of thalassemia.

2. Pathophysiology. Impaired production of one or more of the peptide chains that are normal components of globin results in ineffective erythropoiesis, hemolysis, and varying degrees of anemia. The two major forms involve either impaired production of alpha peptide chains (which causes **α-thalassemia**) or of beta peptide chains (which causes **β-thalassemia**).

3. Diagnosis. Hemoglobin electrophoresis is necessary for identifying the nature of the hemoglobin chain deficiency.

4. Fetal/neonatal complications

    a. α-Thalassemia homozygous (four-gene deletion) results in **hemoglobin Bart disease** and is associated with nonimmune hydrops and either stillbirth or early neonatal death.

    b. α-Thalassemia minor (two-gene deletion) has no impact on the fetus but does cause mild microcytic, hypochromic anemia.

    c. β-Thalassemia minor and major both result in healthy-appearing neonates who become anemic to varying degrees as hemoglobin F levels decrease. With the milder disease, infants remain asymptomatic but have a mild anemia. With β-thalassemia major, also known as Cooley's anemia, children become severely anemic, show failure to thrive, and may die during childhood.

5. Maternal complications

    a. Women with **α-thalassemia minor** and **β-thalassemia minor** tolerate pregnancy well, other than developing a mild anemia.

    b. Women with **β-thalassemia major** who survive childhood are usually sterile, and pregnant women with this condition are rare.

6. Management

    a. Observation in patients with thalassemia minor states

    b. RBC transfusions in patients with β-thalassemia major who have congestive heart failure and marked anemia

    c. Folate supplementation (excessive iron supplementation should be avoided to prevent hemosiderosis)

    d. Serial ultrasounds for assessment of fetal growth

    e. Serial antepartum fetal testing for assessment of fetal oxygenation

7. Prevention. There is no prevention for thalassemia. However, all at-risk patients should be screened for the presence of thalassemia. Prenatal diagnosis is available on fetal amniocytes using DNA techniques.

X. URINARY TRACT INFECTIONS (UTIs)

A. Classification

1. **Lower tract disease** involves only the bladder and includes ASB and acute cystitis.

2. **Upper tract disease** involves the kidney and includes acute pyelonephritis.

B. Pathophysiology.
UTIs usually originate from organisms in the vagina or rectum that ascend from the urethra to the bladder and then to the kidney. The most common causative organisms are gram-negative enteric bacteria. ***Escherichia coli* is involved in 80% of infections,** with the remaining 20% of organisms comprised primarily of *Klebsiella, Pseudomonas, Enterococcus,* and *Proteus.*

C. Risk factors

1. **Mechanical obstruction** such as:
   a. Ureteropelvic junction
   b. Ureteral/urethral stenosis
   c. Calculi

2. **Functional obstruction** such as:
   a. **Pregnancy**
   b. Vesicoureteral reflux

3. **Systemic diseases** such as:
   a. DM
   b. Gout
   c. Sickle cell trait/disease
   d. Cystic renal disease

D. Asymptomatic bacteriuria (ASB)

1. **Incidence.** ASB occurs in pregnant women at a rate of 8%, with the highest incidence in women with sickle cell trait.

2. **Obstetric significance.** Pyelonephritis develops in 30% of patients with ASB who go untreated.

3. **Diagnosis.** ASB is determined by a positive urine culture in asymptomatic patients. The urine culture should contain more than 100,000 colony-forming units/ml of a single organism other than *Lactobacillus* (a normal vaginal contaminant).

4. **Management** involves outpatient treatment consisting of 7–10 days of appropriate oral antibiotics. Nitrofurantoin (100 mg bid) is effective. A repeat culture after the antibiotic therapy should be performed to confirm that the treatment was efficacious.

E. Acute cystitis

1. **Incidence.** The rate of acute cystitis in pregnant women is 1%.

2. **Obstetric significance.** Acute cystitis may progress to pyelonephritis if treatment is inappropriate or nonexistent.

3. **Diagnosis**

   a. **Symptoms** include urgency, frequency, dysuria, and suprapubic discomfort.

   b. **Physical examination** is generally unremarkable with absent systemic findings.

   c. **Laboratory findings** include a positive urine culture as described for ASB. Hematuria may be present on urinalysis.

4. **Management** is identical to that for ASB. Urinary tract analgesics may be indicated for the first 24–48 hours of therapy.

F. **Acute pyelonephritis**

   1. **Incidence.** The rate of acute pyelonephritis in pregnant women is 1%–2%.

   2. **Obstetric significance.** Acute pyelonephritis is the **most common serious medical complication of pregnancy. Preterm delivery** is a major perinatal concern. Maternal complications include anemia, sepsis, renal failure, and pulmonary dysfunction.

   3. **Diagnosis**

      a. **Symptoms** are often abrupt in onset and include dysuria, shaking chills, headache, flank pain, as well as anorexia, nausea, and vomiting.

      b. **Physical findings** include fever, costovertebral angle tenderness (more commonly on the right side), and evidence of dehydration. UCs are common.

      c. **Laboratory findings** include significant pyuria and bacteriuria, as well as white blood cell (WBC) casts. Bacteremia is found in 15% of gravidas with acute pyelonephritis.

   4. **Management**

      a. **Admission** to the hospital for therapy is standard.

      b. **IV fluid hydration** may be necessary to correct dehydration and offset insensible fluid loss.

      c. **Antipyretic agents** may be required.

      d. **Single-agent IV antibiotic therapy** (ampicillin or cephalosporin 1–2 g q6hr) is administered until a clinical response is apparent. Oral agents are continued for 7 days after discharge. Multiple antibiotic agents are indicated if patients appear septic.

      e. **Periodic reculture** of the urine helps detect any recurrence. Patients should be given long-term prophylactic antibiotic treatment with a single daily dose of nitrofurantoin.

G. **Types of UTI recurrences**

   1. **Relapse.** Reappearance of the same organism usually occurs within 2–3 weeks of initial diagnosis. Relapse is usually secondary to perineal colonization or inadequate treatment.

   2. **Reinfection.** Infection with a new organism usually occurs within 12 weeks of completing therapy. A reinfection indicates recurrent bladder bacteriuria.

   3. **Superinfection.** Appearance of a new organism while still on therapy

for a previous organism denotes a superinfection. A different species or a new strain of the same species may be the causative organism.

H. Prevention. All pregnant women should undergo **screening for ASB** on the first prenatal visit and receive appropriate antibiotic treatment if the screen is positive. Further testing is based on the development of symptoms.

XI. DERMATOSES OF PREGNANCY

A. *Pruritic Urticarial Papules and Plaques of Pregnancy* (PUPPP syndrome)

1. **Epidemiology.** PUPPP is the most common pruritic dermatosis of pregnancy. It has a prevalence of 1%. Usually seen in nulliparas, who often have a positive family history, this condition seldom recurs. PUPPP has no observed adverse impact on perinatal outcome.

2. **Symptoms.** Severe, intense itching usually develops late in the pregnancy.

3. **Signs.** Erythematous urticarial papules and plaques start periumbilically on the abdomen and then spread to the thighs and extremities. It may resemble herpes gestationis (see XI B), but no vesicles or bullae are apparent. The face is not usually involved, and excoriation seldom occurs.

4. **Treatment.** Oral antihistamines may provide some relief, but corticosteroids (topical or systemic) are almost always necessary. Complete recovery is expected within 1 month of delivery.

B. **Herpes gestationis** (pemphigoid gestationis)

1. **Epidemiology.** This condition rarely occurs, with a prevalence of 1 in 10,000 pregnancies. It frequently recurs in subsequent pregnancies, and often appears earlier and is more severe. The family history may be positive. The etiology is unknown, but herpes virus does not appear to be involved.

2. **Symptoms.** Severe, intense itching usually develops late in the pregnancy.

3. **Signs.** Widespread, pruritic lesions appear in the third trimester on the abdomen and extremities. Lesions range from erythematous, edematous papules to large, tense vesicles and bullae. Exacerbations and remissions are common with the majority of patients experiencing postpartum exacerbations. Scarring is rare.

4. **Complications.** Preterm delivery may occur, and IUGR may be apparent.

5. **Treatment.** Oral antihistamines may give some relief, but corticosteroids (topical or systemic) are almost always necessary.

C. **Impetigo herpetiformis**

1. **Epidemiology.** This rare condition probably represents an acute form of psoriasis that occurs during pregnancy. Most patients also either have chronic psoriasis or a family history of psoriasis.

2. **Symptoms.** Itching is usually mild. Systemic findings include fever, malaise, nausea, vomiting, and diarrhea.

3. **Signs.** The classic lesions are sterile pustules that form around the margins of the psoriatic patches. The pustules can become secondarily infected after rupture, and sepsis is a major concern. Mucous membranes are often affected. Hypocalcemia and hypoalbuminemia often occur.

4. **Complications.** Maternal sepsis is common. Impact on perinatal outcome is unclear.

5. **Treatment.** Systemic steroids may relieve the symptoms associated with skin lesions, and antimicrobials are required to treat secondary infections and sepsis. Correction of electrolyte imbalances is essential. The disease may persist for weeks to months after delivery.

D. **Papular eruptions of pregnancy** include **prurigo gestationis** (more common) and **papular dermatitis** (more rare).

1. **Epidemiology.** The etiology may involve allergic processes. These eruptions do not recur in subsequent pregnancies. It is not clear whether they have any impact on pregnancy.

2. **Symptoms.** Severe, intense itching usually develops in the third trimester of pregnancy.

3. **Signs.** Prurigo, which is usually milder, is characterized by small, pruritic lesions on the forearms and trunk. Papular dermatitis, generally more severe, is characterized by a generalized pruritic eruption of soft, reddish brown papules. These lesions become rapidly excoriated because they are so itchy, leaving hyperpigmented areas after healing.

4. **Treatment.** Oral antihistamines and topical steroids may provide some relief. In most cases, high-dose tapered steroids are effective.

Review Test

Directions: Each of the numbered items or incomplete statements in this section is followed by answers or by completions of the statement. Select the **ONE** lettered answer or completion that is **BEST** in each case.

1. Which one of the following conditions is the most prevalent risk factor for preeclampsia?

(A) Diabetes mellitus (DM)
(B) Chronic renal disease
(C) Nulliparity
(D) Multiple gestation
(E) Hydatidiform mole

2. The underlying pathogenesis of preeclampsia is

(A) leakage of protein into the urine
(B) thrombocytopenia from platelet destruction
(C) edema from increased interstitial fluid
(D) disseminated intravascular coagulation
(E) diffuse vasospasm

3. A 30-year-old primigravida at 39 weeks' gestation is admitted in spontaneous labor. The woman is in active labor at 6 cm dilation, making normal progress. The presentation is cephalic, with a station of 0. Her blood pressure (BP) has gradually risen to 155/93 mm Hg, and her protein on urine dipstick is 2+. Which one of the following medications is the agent of choice for prevention of eclamptic seizures?

(A) Phenobarbital
(B) Diazepam
(C) Magnesium sulfate
(D) Indomethacin
(E) Labetalol

4. The definitive treatment for preeclampsia is

(A) bed rest in the left lateral position
(B) pregnancy termination
(C) high-protein diet
(D) daily doses of aspirin
(E) magnesium sulfate

5. A 38-year-old woman (gravida 3, para 2) who is at 20 weeks' gestation has a history of tetralogy of Fallot that was surgically corrected at age 2 years. She has no symptoms at rest, but she has minor limitations with activity. Her functional classification of heart disease, according to the New York Heart Association, is

(A) Class I
(B) Class II
(C) Class III
(D) Class IV

6. A 21-year-old nulligravida has been diagnosed with Eisenmenger's syndrome. During a visit for preconception counseling, she asks about her risk from pregnancy. What is the maternal mortality rate associated with pregnancy and Eisenmenger's syndrome?

(A) 5%
(B) 10%
(C) 15%
(D) 25%
(E) 50%

7. A 35-year-old woman (gravida 4, para 3) comes to the office for a routine prenatal visit at 26 weeks' gestation. She received a diagnosis of gestational diabetes mellitus (GDM) during her last pregnancy, in which she delivered a 4200-g infant at term. Which one of the following screening tests is recommended to identify if she now has GDM?

(A) A 1-hour, 50-gram oral glucose tolerance test (OGTT)
(B) A 2-hour, 75-gram OGTT
(C) A 3-hour, 100-gram OGTT
(D) Serial observation for glycosuria
(E) Glycosylated hemoglobin

8. A 23-year-old nulligravida received a diagnosis of type 1 diabetes mellitus (DM) at age 13 years. She is planning to become pregnant and wants to do everything she can to optimize her pregnancy outcome. The reason for suggesting that she achieve euglycemia preconceptually is that this

(A) decreases complications of small vessel disease
(B) reduces the chance of fetal macrosomia
(C) prevents preterm delivery
(D) improves antenatal compliance
(E) diminishes teratogenic risks of hyperglycemia

9. Which one of the following statements regarding the need for prophylactic iron supplementation in pregnancy is true?

(A) The standard dose is of elemental iron is 60 mg three times a day.
(B) The average iron stores in the female bone marrow are 1000 mg.
(C) Maternal anemia in pregnancy results in fetal anemia.
(D) Most of the increased iron needed in pregnancy goes to the fetus.
(E) Iron supplementation does not maintain prepregnancy hemoglobin levels.

10. All of the following are criteria for mild preeclampsia EXCEPT

(A) increased deep tendon reflexes
(B) an increase in blood pressure (BP) of ≥ 15 mm Hg diastolic and/or ≥ 30 mm Hg systolic
(C) face and/or upper extremity edema
(D) BP increase ≥ 140/90 mm Hg absolute
(E) proteinuria ≥ 1–2+

11. A 29-year-old woman (gravida 3, para 2) underwent a 1-hour glucose screen at 27 weeks' gestation; the result was 150 mg/dl. A 3-hour 100 gram oral glucose tolerance test (OGTT) was positive for gestational diabetes. In considering whether to start twice-weekly fetal surveillance in this woman, who is now at 32 weeks' gestation, all of the following are indications EXCEPT

(A) history of stillbirth
(B) anemia
(C) hypertension
(D) macrosomia
(E) insulin requirement

12. All of the following conditions are risk factors for urinary tract infections (UTIs) in pregnancy EXCEPT

(A) diabetes mellitus (DM)
(B) gout
(C) chronic hypertension
(D) sickle cell disease
(E) vesicoureteral reflux

Directions: The set of matching questions in this section consists of a list of four to twenty-six lettered options (some of which may be in figures) followed by several numbered items. For each numbered item, select the ONE lettered option that is most closely associated with it. To avoid spending too much time on matching sets with large numbers of options, it is generally advisable to begin each set by reading the list of options. Then, for each item in the set, try to generate the correct answer and locate it in the option list, rather than evaluating each option individually. Each lettered option may be selected once, more than once, or not at all.

Questions 13–16

For each of the characteristics identified, select the category of hypertensive disease in pregnancy that applies.
(A) Mild preeclampsia
(B) Severe preeclampsia
(C) Eclampsia
(D) Chronic hypertension
(E) Chronic hypertension with superimposed preeclampsia

13. Worst perinatal outcomes

14. Associated with convulsions

15. May precede pregnancy

16. Most common with young primigravidas

Answers and Explanations

1. The answer is C [I C 1 b (1)].

Nulliparity is the most significant risk factor for preeclampsia, a hypertensive disorder of pregnancy, in terms of numbers of women involved. It is found in all countries of the world and is not restricted to any specific ethnic group, socioeconomic level, or dietary pattern. Diabetes mellitus (DM), chronic renal disease, multiple gestation, and hydatidiform mole are also risk factors for preeclampsia.

2. The answer is E [I C 3].

The sequelae of preeclampsia can affect nearly every organ system in the body, including the heart, lungs, kidneys, liver, central nervous system (CNS), and hematologic system. In its most severe form, life-threatening eclamptic seizures develop. The common pathophysiology is a diffuse vasospasm that results in increased capillary permeability and reduced systemic perfusion. Some of the pathologic findings include leakage of protein into the urine, thrombocytopenia from platelet destruction, edema from increased interstitial fluid, and disseminated intravascular coagulation (DIC).

3. The answer is C [I E a b (2)].

In the United States, prophylactic treatment of eclamptic seizures usually involves intravenous (IV) or intramuscular (IM) magnesium sulfate. Eclampsia is the gravest manifestation of the spectrum of hypertensive disorders of pregnancy. One-half of eclamptic seizures occur intrapartum, with the remainder divided equally between antepartum and postpartum periods. Phenobarbital and diazepam are effective anticonvulsants for nonpregnant seizure disorders. Indomethacin and labetalol are spurious distractors. Labetalol is used to preserve uteroplacental blood flow.

4. The answer is B [I E 1 b (3)].

The only certain cure for preeclampsia is termination of the pregnancy. Bed rest in the left lateral position may increase placental perfusion, daily doses of aspirin may prevent preeclampsia, and magnesium sulfate may prevent eclamptic convulsions. These management modalities may temporize but do not cure the condition. A high-protein diet has not been shown to be an efficacious prevention or treatment.

5. The answer is B [II B 1].

Class II indicates no symptoms at rest, but minor limitations with activity. Class I indicates no symptoms of heart disease, regardless of activity. Class III indicates no symptoms at rest, but major limitations with activity. Class IV indicates symptoms at rest.

6. The answer is E [II B 2 b (3)].

The mortality rate of women with Eisenmenger's syndrome who are pregnant is 50%. Eisenmenger's syndrome is a group of heart conditions in which the pulmonary vascular resistance exceeds the systemic resistance, and there is a communication between the right and left ventricles. Pulmonary vascular resistance exceeds systemic resistance if hypotension develops, leading to a drop in systemic pressure. A right-to-left shunt then develops that bypasses the pulmonary circulation, resulting in hypoxia and death.

7. The answer is A [VIII B 2].

A 1-hour, 50-g oral glucose tolerance test (OGTT) is correct because it is the standard screening test for gestational diabetes mellitus (GDM) in a 1-hour, 50-g oral glucose load. The 2-hour, 75-g OGTT is conducted in nonpregnant individuals. The 3-hour, 100-g OGTT is performed on pregnant women who have a 1-hour, 50-g screen greater than 140 mg/dl. Serial observation for glycosuria and glycosylated hemoglobin are not valid screens for GDM; glycosuria is poorly correlated with hyperglycemia, and glycosylated hemoglobin has poor sensitivity for GDM.

8. The answer is E [VIII F 1].

The primary purpose of securing euglycemia preconceptually is to prevent hyperglycemic teratogenic effects during early embryogenesis. Preconceptual counseling is directed at women with type I and type II diabetes mellitus (DM) who are at significantly higher risk for delivering babies with major congenital anomalies. The most common birth defects of infants of pregestational diabetic mothers are neural tube defects (NTDs) and congenital heart disease. Although it is possible that decreased complications of small vessel disease, decreased chance of fetal macrosomia, prevention of preterm delivery, and improved antenatal compliance may be improved by preconception counseling, they are not the main reasons for it.

9. The answer is E [IX D 6–7].

Although iron supplementation increases the maternal hemoglobin, compared with no supplementation, the increase is not sufficient to overbalance the dilution that occurs because of the volume expansion of plasma over that experienced by the red blood cells (RBCs). The standard prophylactic iron dose in pregnancy is 60 mg of elemental iron once daily. The average iron stores in the female bone marrow are 500 mg, not 1000 mg. Fetal hemoglobin is independent of maternal anemia because of active transport of iron across the placenta. The largest amount of iron demanded during pregnancy is for the increase in maternal RBC mass.

10. The answer is A [I B 1].

Increased deep tendon reflexes is the correct answer (but incorrect statement) because, although increased briskness of deep tendon reflexes is often found with preeclampsia, it is not part of the formal criteria for diagnosis. Mild preeclampsia is the mildest form of the hypertensive disorders of pregnancy. With appropriate management, the outcome of pregnancies with mild preeclampsia is no different than those that are unaffected by it. The triad of diagnostic findings for mild preeclampsia are hypertension, proteinuria, and edema. An increase in blood pressure (BP) of greater than or equal to 15 mm Hg diastolic and/or greater than or equal to 30 mm Hg systolic, face and/or upper extremity edema, BP greater than 140/90 mm Hg absolute, and proteinuria of 1–2+ are all criteria for mild preeclampsia.

11. The answer is B [VIII E 1 e (1)].

Maternal anemia is not associated with any adverse fetal outcome in women with gestational diabetes. History of stillbirth, hypertension, macrosomia, and insulin requirement are all associated with increased perinatal morbidity and mortality and are indications for early initiation of nonstress test (NST) surveillance.

12. The answer is C [X C].

Chronic hypertension is the correct answer (but incorrect statement) because it is not associated with pregnancy urinary tract infections (UTIs). Diabetes mellitus (DM), gout, sickle cell disease, and vesicoureteral reflux are all verified risk factors.

13–16. The answers are: 13-E [I B 5], 14-C [I B 3], 15-D [I B 4], 16-A [I B 1].

The worst pregnancy outcomes are in women who have chronic hypertension with superimposed preeclampsia. Eclampsia is the hypertensive disorder of pregnancy associated with convulsions. Chronic hypertension may precede pregnancy. Mild preeclampsia is the most common hypertensive disorder of pregnancy seen in young primigravidas.

5

Pregnancy: Perinatal Infectious Diseases

I. **PERINATAL INFECTIONS** account for 2%–3% of birth defects, which arise from a spectrum of organisms and have varying modes of transmission. Not all birth defects are routinely screened for during prenatal care, but all birth defects do pose a risk to the fetus or neonate. Table 5-1 summarizes the significant infections discussed in this chapter. The variation in residual status of the mother after primary infection should be noticed. Cesarean delivery is currently recommended only for mothers who have active genital herpes lesions at the time of delivery.

II. **TOXOPLASMOSIS** is a systemic infection by the protozoan *Toxoplasma gondii* that results in **lifelong immunity,** although reactivation can occur with immunosuppression.

    A. **Epidemiology.** Toxoplasmosis is one of the most common human infections worldwide.

        1. **Transmission** occurs via ingesting undercooked meat or unpasteurized goat milk or by exposure to an infected cat's feces.

        2. **Incidence.** Approximately 0.1% of pregnant women experience a primary infection during their pregnancy.

        3. **Seropositivity prevalence** is 10%–40% in reproductive-age women.

    B. **Clinical issues**

        1. **Significance.** Fetal infection requires a parasitemia.

            a. **Risk of fetal infection by trimester**

                (1) **First-trimester risk: 15%** (perinatal death rate is 75%)

                (2) **Second-trimester risk: 25%**

                (3) **Third-trimester risk: 65%** (all cases are mild or subclinical)

            b. **Consequences of fetal infection**

                (1) The **classic triad**—hydrocephalus, intracranial calcifications, and chorioretinitis—**is rarely seen.**

Table 5-1. Comparison of Perinatal Infections

	Toxoplasmosis	Rubella	Cytomegalovirus (CMV)	Herpes Simplex Virus	Syphilis	Hepatitis B	Human Immunodeficiency Virus (HIV)	Group B β Streptococcus (GBBS)
Organism involved	Parasite (*Toxoplasma gondii*)	Virus (RNA)	Virus (DNA)	Virus (DNA)	Spirochete (*Treponema pallidum*)	Virus (DNA)	Virus (RNA)	Bacterial
Mode of Transmission	Cat litter, raw meat, raw goat milk	Air droplets	Body fluids	Mucocutaneous contact	Mucocutaneous contact	Body fluids	Body fluids	Genital tract colonization; feces
Seropositivity in general population	[10%–40%]	85%–90%	50%	50%	N/A	1% chronic carriers	0.1%	35% genital colonization
Treatment in pregnancy	Pyrimethamine sulfadizaine	None	Ganciclovir	Acyclovir	Benzathine penicillin	Hepatitis B immune globulin	Zidovudine (AZT)	Penicillin
Routine screening?	No	Yes	No	No	Yes	Yes	Yes	No
Residual status	Lifelong immunity	Lifelong immunity	Lifelong latency	Lifelong latency	Lifelong latency (if not treated, but is curable)	Lifelong immunity with carrier status	Lifelong infection	Lifelong colonization
Transplacental infection risk	Yes*	Yes*	Yes	Yes*	Yes	Rare	Yes	Rare
Delivery (infection risk)	No	No	Rare	Yes	No	Yes	Yes	Yes
Recommended delivery route	Vaginal	Vaginal	Vaginal	Cesarean (only if lesions at delivery)	Vaginal	Vaginal	Vaginal	Vaginal
Maternal and infant immunization?	No	Yes (active only)	No	No	No	Yes (both active and passive)	No	No

*Fetal risk occurs only with a primary infection.

(2) **25% of infected infants are symptomatic,** with varying degrees of severity. Findings include mental retardation, seizure disorder, hepatosplenomegaly, and central nervous system (CNS) involvement.

(3) **75% of infected infants are asymptomatic.**

2. **Diagnosis is rarely made clinically,** because most infections are subclinical.

  a. **Overt infection** may appear as a **mononucleosis-like syndrome.**

  b. **Serologic testing** can be performed on **fetal** blood by percutaneous umbilical blood sampling (PUBS) or using cord blood. **Maternal** IgM antibodies may remain high for 4 months, and IgG antibodies may remain elevated for life.

  c. **Placental culture** is positive in 90% of cases if fetal infection is present.

3. **Treatment** of acute infection involves **pyrimethamine** (an antiparasitic agent) and **sulfadiazine plus folinic acid.**

4. **Route of delivery is vaginal.**

5. **Prevention** involves avoiding contact with cat litter and feces, wearing gloves when gardening, and avoiding the ingestion of raw meat and unpasteurized goat milk.

III. RUBELLA (GERMAN MEASLES) INFECTION is caused by an RNA virus that confers lifelong immunity.

  A. **Epidemiology.** Rubella is typically a childhood disease that affects children ages 5–14 years.

  1. **Transmission** occurs via **air droplets** (respiratory route).

  2. **Susceptibility** of adult women in the United States is **15%.**

  3. **Seropositivity** in the general population is **85%.**

  4. **Infectivity.** The rubella virus is highly contagious: 75% of infected patients become clinically ill. There is a 14–21-day incubation period. The period of infectivity is 7 days before the rash to 5 days after the rash appears.

  B. **Clinical issues**

  1. **Significance**

    a. **Course** of acute infection is unaltered during pregnancy.

    b. **Risk of fetal infection** is mostly affected by the gestational age at primary infection (Box 5-1).

    c. **Consequences of fetal infection** include the following:

      (1) **Spontaneous abortion**

      (2) **Seropositive, normal-appearing infant** (infection may remain subclinical for months)

      (3) **Overt congenital rubella syndrome** with the following findings:

        (a) **Congenital heart disease** (mostly affecting the great vessels)

        (b) Symmetric intrauterine growth restriction (IUGR)

        (c) Hepatosplenomegaly

<table>
<tr><td colspan="2" align="center">**Box 5-1.** Risk of Fetal Infection</td></tr>
<tr><td>**Gestational Age (weeks)**</td><td>**Fetus Infected (%)**</td></tr>
<tr><td align="center">< 11</td><td align="center">90</td></tr>
<tr><td align="center">11–12</td><td align="center">30</td></tr>
<tr><td align="center">13–14</td><td align="center">20</td></tr>
<tr><td align="center">15–16</td><td align="center">10</td></tr>
<tr><td align="center">> 16</td><td align="center">5</td></tr>
</table>

    (d) Thrombocytopenic purpura

    (e) CNS involvement, including:

        (i) Congenital deafness (most common sequelae)

        (ii) Cataracts, retinopathy, microphthalmia

        (iii) Microcephaly, panencephalitis, brain calcifications, mental retardation

2. Diagnosis

  a. Serologic testing of the neonate

    (1) A positive **IgM** titer in umbilical cord blood

    (2) A positive **IgG** titer in the infant's blood after 5 months of age (i.e., when maternal passive antibodies would have been metabolized)

  b. Serologic testing of the mother

    (1) The **IgM** titer begins at the onset of the rash and disappears in 4–8 weeks.

    (2) The **IgG** titer begins at the onset of the rash and remains elevated for life.

3. Treatment. There is no specific treatment for rubella.

4. Route of delivery is vaginal.

5. Prevention

  a. All pregnant women should be screened at their first prenatal visit with a rubella antibody titer.

  b. Pregnant women with a negative titer should be counseled to avoid exposure during pregnancy.

  c. Postpartum, women with a negative titer should be **vaccinated** with **attenuated live** rubella virus.

    (1) Approximately 90% of women acquire immunity.

    (2) The antibody titer should be checked after 6 weeks to ensure response.

    (3) Vaccination of the mother poses no hazard to the neonate, even to one who is breast-fed.

    (4) Pregnancy should be avoided for 3 months because of a possible increase in spontaneous abortion. Abortuses have had positive viral cultures, but no reported cases of congenital rubella syndrome in term liveborn infants have occurred.

IV. CYTOMEGALOVIRUS (CMV) INFECTION is a systemic DNA herpesvirus with a predisposition for lifelong latency. Reactivation possible with pregnancy and conditions of immunosuppression.

A. **Epidemiology.** CMV is the **most common congenital viral syndrome** in the United States.

1. **Transmission** may occur via **contact with infected blood** (transplacental or blood transfusion), **exposure to body fluids** (semen, vaginal secretions, saliva, urine, breast milk), or **organ transplantation.**

2. **Incidence.** CMV affects **1%–2%** of all liveborn infants in the United States.

3. **Seropositivity** prevalence is approximately **50%** in school-age children and pregnant women.

B. **Clinical issues**

1. **Significance**

a. **Risk of fetal infection**

(1) **50%** in all trimesters with **primary** infection

(2) **< 1%** with **recurrent** infection. Intrauterine infection can occur without a viremia.

b. **Consequences of fetal infection**

(1) **15% of infants are symptomatic** with varying degrees of severity. Findings include nonimmune hydrops, symmetric IUGR, hepatosplenomegaly, and CNS involvement (chorioretinitis, microcephaly, hydrocephaly, and calcifications).

(2) **85% of infants are asymptomatic.** Only 5% of these may later develop any of these symptoms: mental retardation, visual impairment, and progressive hearing loss.

2. **Diagnosis**

a. **Clinical infection (rarely seen)**

(1) **Symptomatic** infection may appear as a **mononucleosis-like syndrome** with hepatitis. Amniocentesis and then amniotic fluid culture should be considered to identify fetal infection.

(2) **Asymptomatic** infections are **most common,** with viral shedding persisting for months. Viral latency may occur in the salivary glands, renal tubules, and endometrium. Reactivation may occur years after the primary infection. Reinfection with a different viral strain is possible.

b. **Viral culture** of amniotic fluid, urine, or other body fluids

c. **Serologic testing** can be performed on **fetal** blood by PUBS or using cord blood. A positive IgG titer after the age of 5 months (i.e., when maternal passive antibodies would have been metabolized) is diagnostic. **Maternal CMV IgM peaks at 4 months, lasting up to 2 years,** making timing of infection difficult. CMV IgG antibodies peak rapidly, persist for life, and do not rule out persistent disease.

3. **Treatment** of overt, clinical CMV infection is with **ganciclovir.**

4. **Route of delivery is vaginal.**

5. **Prevention**
   a. **Counseling** the mother to avoid exposure during pregnancy
   b. **Using good hygiene in high-risk settings** such as neonatal intensive care units, day-care centers, and dialysis units
   c. **Avoiding transfusion with CMV-positive blood**

V. HERPES SIMPLEX VIRUS (HSV) INFECTION is caused by a DNA virus that establishes permanent, incurable latency in sensory nerve root ganglia. It is the **most frequent cause of genital ulcer disease in the United States.**

A. **Epidemiology**
   1. **Transmission** occurs via intimate mucocutaneous contact. HSV is one of the most highly contagious sexually transmitted diseases (STDs).
   2. **Incidence**
      a. **HSV type II (HSV-II)** causes 90% of infections, whereas **HSV type I (HSV-I)** causes the remaining 10%. HSV-I may protect against acquisition of HSV-II.
      b. HSV-II accounts for two-thirds of cases of genital herpes, and HSV-I for one-third.
   3. **Seropositivity** prevalence is approximately 50% in school-age children and pregnant women.

B. **Clinical issues**
   1. **Clinical findings**
      a. **Primary herpes**
         (1) **Symptoms.** Symptoms appear 3–7 days after exposure, beginning with prodrome. Mild paresthesias and burning occur.
         (2) **Physical findings**
            (a) **Evidence of systemic disease (100%** of patients), which includes low-grade fever, generalized malaise, and inguinal adenopathy
            (b) **Clear, painful, tender vesicles (100%** of patients) on the labia majora and minora, the vulvar vestibule, and the perianal skin
            (c) **Asymptomatic vesicular lesions (90%** of patients) in the vagina or on the ectocervix
         (3) **Clinical course**
            (a) **Vesicles rupture** after 1–7 days, forming shallow, painful, raised-edge ulcers that heal in 7–10 days and leave no scars.
            (b) **Dysuria and urinary retention** may occur if there is urethral or bladder involvement.
            (c) **Recurrent syndrome** develops in only 30% of patients with primary herpes.
            (d) During pregnancy, cervical shedding occurs in **10%** of women after their primary episode of HSV.
      b. **Recurrent herpes**
         (1) **Pathophysiology.** The **virus migrates up nerve fibers** to dor-

sal root ganglia; **remains dormant** until it is activated by stress, menses, or an upper respiratory infection; and then **travels down nerve fibers** to previously affected sites.

(2) **Physical findings** are **similar** to those in a primary infection but **lesions** are of **shorter duration, less severe,** and **more localized.** There are **no systemic findings or adenopathy.** In pregnancy, cervical shedding occurs in **0.5%** of women after a recurrent episode.

c. **Complications** include meningitis, hepatitis, radiculopathies, and transverse myelitis.

d. **Differential diagnosis** includes *Haemophilus ducreyi* (chancroid) and *Lymphogranuloma venereum.*

2. **Diagnosis**

a. **Culture** using fluid from a ruptured vesicle or a debrided ulcer **is the definitive method of diagnosis.**

b. **Cytology** of a smear from an ulcer base may show **multinucleated giant cells** (30% false-negatives).

3. **Significance**

a. **Primary herpes.** Viremia, which occurs only with primary herpes, markedly increases the risk of obstetric hazards and neonatal herpes.

(1) **Increased obstetric hazards** include spontaneous abortion, IUGR, fetal demise, and preterm labor. No malformation syndrome has been reported.

(2) **Neonatal herpes affects mostly premature infants,** leaving survivors with microcephalus, microphthalmos, mental retardation, and seizures.

(a) **Attack rate: 50%**

(b) **Mortality: 50%**

(c) **Permanent sequelae: 50%**

b. **Recurrent herpes.** Viremia does not occur in patients with secondary herpes.

(1) **Obstetric hazards are not increased.**

(2) **Neonatal attack rate is 4%.** The risk is related to passing through an infected birth canal.

4. **Management**

a. **Gynecologic management.** There is no effective cure.

(1) **Abstinence** from sexual contact is recommended **if lesions are present.**

(2) **Symptomatic relief** may be obtained from hot sitz baths and use of diluted Burow's solution.

(3) **Antiviral agents** include **acyclovir, famciclovir,** and **valacyclovir.**

(a) Primary HSV can be treated with either oral or IV routes depending on severity. Recurrent HSV is treated with oral route because of its mild course

(b) Recurrent infections are not prevented, but their frequency and severity may be decreased. **Suppression of recurrences may not decrease risk of sexual transmission.**

b. **Obstetric management**

(1) **Vaginal herpes cultures** do not predict neonatal outcome and are not recommended.

(2) **Route of delivery**

(a) **Cesarean** delivery is performed only if **active genital lesions** (primary or secondary) **are present** at the time of labor.

(b) **Vaginal** delivery is appropriate if **no genital lesions are present** or if an **intrauterine infection** has been documented through amniotic fluid cultures.

c. **Neonatal management.** It is not necessary to isolate the infant from the mother. Direct contact of the infant with lesions should be avoided. Breastfeeding is safe if there are no breast lesions.

VI. SYPHILIS is an STD that is caused by the motile spirochete *Treponema pallidum.*

A. Background

1. The **course** of syphilis is not affected by pregnancy.

2. **Transmission** is by contact with either intact mucous membranes or contact with broken skin. The most frequent entry sites in the female are the vulva, vagina, and cervix.

B. Clinical issues

1. Significance

a. **Risk of fetal infection** is 60% during primary disease, 60% during secondary disease, and unpredictable during tertiary disease because the longer syphilis exists in a woman before pregnancy occurs, the less likely the fetus is to be affected.

b. **Severity of fetal infection** is greater with primary and secondary disease than with tertiary disease.

(1) **Early congenital syphilis** is diagnosed at **birth** and has a **50%** perinatal mortality rate. **Findings** include nonimmune hydrops, anemia, thrombocytopenia, hepatosplenomegaly, hepatitis, macerated skin, and osteitis.

(2) **Late congenital syphilis** is diagnosed **after 2 years** of age. **Findings** include:

(a) **Hutchinson teeth,** which are notched and peg shaped

(b) **Mulberry molars,** which are more narrow at the crown than at the gingival margin

(c) **Saber shins**

(d) **Saddle nose** (from nasal septum destruction)

(e) **Interstitial keratitis**

(f) **Eighth cranial nerve deafness**

(g) **Failure to thrive**

2. Diagnosis

a. **Clinical findings with untreated disease** include the following:

(1) **Primary syphilis.** The **chancre is the classic lesion** localized at the site of entry (mouth, genitals, anus, or fingers).

        (a) Macular lesions appear 21 days after inoculation and become **papular,** progressing into firm, **painless** ulcers (with punched-out base and rolled edges) that spontaneously heal in 6 weeks.

        (b) Painless inguinal adenopathy is often noted.

    (2) Secondary syphilis is evidence of widespread dissemination of the spirochete.

        (a) Onset of systemic manifestations includes malaise, headache, anorexia, and sore throat. A generalized symmetric, asymptomatic maculopapular rash appears on the palms and soles (i.e., "money spots"). Generalized adenopathy occurs in 50% of cases.

        (b) Condylomata lata, the classic lesions, are highly contagious, exophytic broad excrescences that ulcerate. They may appear on the vulva, perianal skin, or upper thighs.

        (c) This stage spontaneously progresses into latent syphilis after 4 weeks.

    (3) Latent syphilis is diagnosed with absence of clinical manifestations but positive serologic tests.

        (a) Two-thirds of untreated patients remain in the latent phase. The duration of this stage lasts 2–20 years.

        (b) Positive serologies are most often detected in this phase.

        (c) Relapses of the secondary stage may occur in early latent phase.

    (4) Tertiary syphilis is diagnosed with diffuse organ system involvement, often with devastating, destructive effects.

        (a) One-third of untreated patients enter the tertiary phase, some up to 20 years after the chancre disappears.

        (b) Diffuse organ system involvement includes:

            (i) CNS effects: meningitis, tabes dorsalis, or paresis

            (ii) Cardiac effects: valvular disease or aortic aneurysms

        (c) Gummas are the **classic lesions,** consisting of a cold abscess with necrotic, ulcerative nodules.

  b. Laboratory tests include nonspecific screening serology, treponema-specific tests, and **darkfield** microscopy of lesion specimens. Findings include:

    (1) In **primary** syphilis, serology is **negative,** but darkfield microscopy is **positive.**

    (2) In **secondary** syphilis, serology is **positive** and darkfield microscopy is **positive.**

    (3) In **tertiary** syphilis, serology is **positive,** but **no lesions are seen.**

  c. Screening serology tests result in up to 15% false-positive rates.

    (1) Nonspecific tests include:

        (a) Venereal Disease Research Laboratory (VDRL) test

        (b) Rapid plasma reagin (RPR) test

    (2) False-positive screening serologies occur with the following conditions:

(a) **Autoimmune diseases** such as systemic lupus erythematosus and rheumatoid arthritis

(b) **Recent viral infections** such as rubeola, varicella, and early human immunodeficiency virus (HIV)

(c) **Other infections** such as malaria, Lyme disease, leptospirosis, and chancroid

(d) **Recent immunizations**

(e) **Recent febrile illness**

(f) **Chronic liver disease**

(g) **Pregnancy**

(3) **To confirm diagnosis** after a positive nonspecific screening test, a **treponema-specific test is used.**

(a) **Fluorescent titer antibody absorption (FTA-ABS)** test

(b) **MHA-TP (microhemagglutination assay for antibodies to *Treponema pallidum*)** test

3. **Management.** The treatment of choice is **benzathine penicillin.**

a. **Nonpregnant women**

(1) The dose is 2.4 million units intramuscularly (IM) once for primary, secondary, and latent syphilis (duration < 1 year). If latent syphilis has been present for more than 1 year, the dose is repeated three times at weekly intervals.

(2) In penicillin-allergic patients, **erythromycin** or **tetracycline** is administered orally for 14 days (500 mg qid).

b. **Pregnant women.** Benzathine penicillin crosses the placenta and treats the fetus in utero. The dose is 2.4 million units IM once. There is no satisfactory treatment alternative. Erythromycin and tetracycline cross the placenta poorly, and tetracycline is contraindicated in pregnancy. Therefore, women who are allergic to penicillin may be treated with penicillin after oral densensitization.

c. The **Jarisch-Herxheimer reaction** is an acute febrile reaction that occurs within the first 24 hours after any therapy for syphilis. Clinical findings include headache, myalgia, uterine contractions (UCs), and late decelerations. It occurs in 100% of women with primary syphilis and in 50% of women with secondary syphilis.

d. **VDRL titers should decrease** fourfold in 3 months and become negative 12 months after treatment. A spinal tap should be performed to rule out neurosyphilis if titers remain positive after 1 year.

e. **Sexual partners of infected patients should be treated.**

4. **Route of delivery is vaginal.**

5. **Prevention** follows the standard STD prevention principles (e.g., use of condoms).

VII. HEPATITIS B VIRUS (HBV) INFECTION is caused by a DNA hepadenavirus, type I.

A. **Background**

1. **Epidemiology**

a. **Distribution.** HBV is found worldwide but is endemic in certain areas. The virus causes 300,000 cases of acute hepatitis per year in the United States, where there are 1 million chronic carriers. There are 200 million chronic carriers worldwide. Carrier rates approach 35% in Asia and Africa.

b. **Transmission** is via body fluids such as blood, semen, vaginal secretions, oral secretions, and breast milk. **Mother–infant** transmission causes 40% of all chronic HBV infections.

2. **Types of infection**

a. **Asymptomatic.** Approximately 75% of all patients with HBV infections are asymptomatic.

b. **Acute hepatitis.** Acute disease is characterized by jaundice and elevated liver enzymes.

c. **Chronic hepatitis.** Chronic cases have the most serious consequences.

(1) **10%** of HBV-infected **adults** develop chronic hepatitis.

(2) **80%** of HBV-infected **infants** develop chronic hepatitis.

B. **Sequelae of chronic HBV infection**

1. **Cirrhosis** leading to liver failure causes 4000 deaths per year in the United States.

2. **Hepatocellular carcinoma risk** is increased up to 40-fold in patients with HBV, causing 800 deaths per year in the United States. HBV is second only to tobacco among human carcinogens.

C. **Immunologic markers for HBV**

1. Hepatitis B **surface antigen** (HBsAg) and **antibody** (anti-HBs). HBsAg is the marker that is most often sought in **screening tests.**

2. **Core antigen** (HBcAg) and **antibody** (anti-HBc). Core antigens usually present only in **overwhelming infections.**

3. Hepatitis B **e antigen** (HBeAg) and **antibody** (anti-HBe). HBeAg serves as an accurate predictor of **viral replication** and **infectivity.**

D. **Clinical issues**

1. **Significance**

a. **Course.** The course of acute infection is **unaltered during pregnancy.** Unless protein–calorie malnutrition is present, there is no increase in malformations or anomalies, spontaneous abortions, stillbirths, or IUGR.

b. **Fetal infection,** although uncommon, most often occurs with maternal infection in the **third trimester.** It may also occur in fetuses of mothers with active, acute hepatitis and with asymptomatic carriers.

c. **Impact of chronic active hepatitis**

(1) The **fetus or neonate** may suffer premature birth, low birth weight, or neonatal death.

(2) The **mother** may suffer cirrhosis, esophageal varices, or liver failure.

d. **Impact of asymptomatic HBsAg carrier state.** The significance for the mother is nil. However, the chance of acute newborn infection via vertical transmission at birth is:

(1) 10% if the mother is positive for **only HbsAg**

(2) 80% if the mother is positive for **both HBsAg and HBeAg**

2. **Diagnosis**

a. **All pregnant women should be screened for HBsAg at their first prenatal visit.**

b. **Patients in high-risk groups should be rescreened at 28 weeks if the first test was negative.** High-risk groups include:

(1) Patients with ethnic or geographic risk factors such as:

(a) Birth in Africa or Southeast Asia

(b) Descent from Asians, Pacific Islanders, or Eskimos

(2) Patients with environmental, occupational or domestic risk factors such as:

(a) Contact with a hemodialysis unit through work, treatment, or household contact

(b) Household contact with a hepatitis carrier

(c) Working or living in an institution for the mentally handicapped

(d) Occupational exposure to blood

(3) Patients with a history of multiple blood transfusions

(4) Patients with exposure to sexual transmission (e.g., those who have had repeated episodes of an STD, prostitutes)

(5) Abusers of IV drugs

3. **Management.** There is **no specific therapy for acute hepatitis. HBsAg-positive carriers** should be screened for liver involvement. Liver function tests and a complete hepatitis panel should be performed. Testing and vaccination should be offered to household members and sexual contacts.

4. **Route of delivery is vaginal.**

5. **Prevention**

a. **Neonates of HBsAg-positive mothers** should receive **passive immunization** with hepatitis B immune globulin (HBIg) and **active immunization** with hepatitis vaccine.

b. **HBsAg-negative mothers at high risk for hepatitis B** should receive **passive immunization** with HBIg and **active immunization** with hepatitis B vaccine. This vaccine can be administered during pregnancy, because it is a killed virus.

c. **Precautions to decrease vertical transmission** include avoiding scalp electrodes during labor and scalp needles after delivery, providing gentle resuscitation to eliminate pharyngeal mucosa trauma, and avoiding breastfeeding.

VIII. HUMAN IMMUNODEFICIENCY VIRUS (HIV) INFECTION

is caused by a single-stranded RNA retrovirus. HIV causes acquired immunodeficiency syndrome (AIDS).

A. **Background**

1. **Epidemiology.** The earliest identification of HIV was in 1959 in banked serum in the Congo (formerly Zaire). The first case of HIV in the United

States was reported to the Centers for Disease Control and Prevention (CDC) in 1981.

2. **Modes of transmission**
    a. **Sexual contact with an infected partner** (highest to lowest risk)
        (1) **Male-to-male: highest risk** (especially anal-receptive intercourse)
        (2) **Male-to-female: high risk**
            (a) The concentration of HIV in semen is high.
            (b) There are more breaks in introital mucosa than in penile skin.
        (3) **Female-to-male**
        (4) **Female-to-female: lowest risk**
    b. **Risk of HIV with various exposures**
        (1) **No risk** from Rh immune globulin (the virus is inactivated during processing)
        (2) **1 in 3** in neonates delivered to untreated HIV-positive mothers
        (3) **1 in 10** in neonates delivered to **zidovudine [azidothymidine (AZT)]**-treated HIV-positive mothers
        (4) **1 in 250** after needlestick exposure from a known seropositive patient
        (5) **1 in 153,000** after receiving one unit of HIV-screened packed red blood cells (RBCs)

3. **Microbiology**
    a. The **source of transmission** is virus-infected cells, not the free virus.
    b. The **virus attaches to CD4 helper cells** and makes a DNA copy of itself using a reverse transcriptase.
    c. **HIV integrates itself into the host genome,** and then it either goes into a latent state or begins to reproduce itself.

B. **Clinical issues**
    1. **Course of disease**
        a. **Primary effect.** The primary effect is profound and irreversible immunosuppression in a previously healthy person.
        b. **Early evidence of infection.** Approximately 90% of patients develop anti-HIV antibodies within 12 weeks of exposure and develop a mononucleosis-like illness within a few months.
        c. **Subsequent progression.** Patients gradually develop immune system dysfunction, with increasingly severe and diffuse systemic symptoms.
            (1) The risk of becoming symptomatic within 12 weeks of exposure is greater than 50%.
            (2) More than 50% of symptomatic patients have CNS symptoms.
            (3) The mortality of patients with AIDS is higher than 90%. Therapy with antiviral agents results in little improvement.
    2. **Diagnosis of AIDS.** HIV-infected persons with any of the following criteria may be diagnosed with AIDS.
        a. **Opportunistic infections**

       (1) *Pneumocystis carinii* pneumonia

       (2) CNS toxoplasmosis

       (3) Disseminated mycobacterial disease

       (4) Disseminated coccidioidomycosis, cryptococcosis, or histoplasmosis

       (5) CMV retinitis with loss of vision

       (6) Candidiasis of the esophagus, trachea, or bronchus

  b. Kaposi's sarcoma

  c. HIV encephalopathy

  d. Wasting syndrome

  e. CD4 cell count $\leq 200/\mu l$

  f. Invasive cervical carcinoma

3. Prevention of HIV and AIDS involves the following practices:

  a. Abstinence

  b. Mutually monogamous sex between HIV-negative partners

  c. "Safer" sex guidelines

       (1) Reduced number of sexual partners

       (2) Use of condoms for all coital activity

       (3) Use of Nonoxynol-9 spermicide to inactivate HIV

  d. Avoidance of contact with previously used needles

  e. Considering all body fluids HIV-infected (universal precautions)

  f. Avoidance of pregnancy in HIV-infected women

4. HIV testing

  a. Types of tests. Testing is usually aimed at detecting HIV-1 **antibodies.**

       (1) The **enzyme-linked immunosorbent assay (ELISA) is** used as a screen for antibodies. It uses antigens from disrupted viruses, and it is 99% specific and sensitive when repeatedly reactive. Detectable antibodies appear 12 weeks after exposure.

       (2) The **Western blot** test identifies the presence of HIV core and envelope antigens. Specific HIV antibodies are tested against three main HIV viral proteins. The Western blot test requires more antibody for a positive reading than the ELISA.

  b. Test interpretation

       (1) A negative test means either no HIV infection or a false-negative result (i.e., it is too early to detect the antibody).

       (2) Criteria for a positive test include the following:

           (a) The **ELISA is repeatedly reactive,** and the **Western blot assay is reactive.** False-negative results can occur if inadequate antibody titer is present. The false-positive rate is less than 1 in 10,000.

           (b) Identification of p24 core antigen indicates virus, not antibody.

5. Screening recommendations. According to the American College of Obstetrics and Gynecology (ACOG), HIV screening is recommended to all women, especially those with risk factors:

  a. Use of illicit drugs (especially IV drugs)

    b. Having multiple sexual partners (e.g., trading sex for drugs)

    c. Receipt of a blood transfusion before 1985 (i.e., onset of effective screening), as in hemophiliacs

    d. Living in HIV-endemic areas (e.g., Africa, Southeast Asia)

    e. Having symptoms of an HIV-related illness

    f. History of STDs

6. HIV in pregnancy

    a. Effect of pregnancy on asymptomatic, seropositive women. Progression to AIDS may be enhanced. Women who transmit HIV perinatally are at the highest risk for progressing to AIDS.

    b. Effect of asymptomatic seropositivity on pregnancy. There is no increase in preterm birth, low birth weight, or congenital malformations.

    c. Pregnancy management

        (1) Maternal counseling regarding the risks of continuing her pregnancy, including the risks of perinatal transmission and the effect of pregnancy on HIV (e.g., progressing to AIDS)

        (2) Maternal treatment for infectious diseases (e.g., other STDs, tuberculosis)

        (3) Maternal vaccination against HBV and influenza

        (4) Maternal antiviral prophylaxis with AZT should be administered to decrease the risk of HIV transmission to the fetus. AZT inhibits reverse transcriptase, is well tolerated in pregnancy, and has no teratogenic effects. This drug should be started at 14 weeks' gestation and continued throughout pregnancy, including intrapartum.

        (5) Multidrug antiviral therapy if the mother's HIV-RNA titer by polymerase chain reaction (PCR) is high and her CD4 count is low

        (6) Maternal prophylaxis for *P. carinii* pneumonia should be provided. This includes trimethoprim–sulfamethoxazole and aerosolized pentamidine.

        (7) Labor management. Scalp electrodes should be avoided to prevent HIV inoculation.

        (8) Mode of delivery. Spontaneous vaginal delivery is preferred with delayed rupture of membranes. The use of forceps, which may result in potential trauma to the fetal scalp and possible HIV inoculation, should be avoided. There is suggestive evidence that mother-to-infant HIV transmission may be decreased in some cases. It has not yet been clearly defined which pregnancies and fetuses would benefit from a cesarean delivery.

7. Pediatric HIV

    a. Perinatal HIV infection

        (1) Modes of transmission. Transplacental infection can occur as early as 13 weeks' gestation. Exposure of fetus and neonate to maternal genital secretions at delivery is significant. Breast milk is probably a minor risk.

        (2) Mother-to-neonate transmission rates vary as follows:

            (a) 10% with maternal AZT prophylaxis in pregnancy

(b) **30%** with no maternal prophylaxis in pregnancy

(c) **50%** with no maternal prophylaxis and previous delivery of an HIV-infected infant

(3) **Cesarean delivery.** Cesarean delivery may protect some infants from vertical transmission of HIV.

(4) **Risk factors**

(a) Maternal HIV RNA titer

(b) Maternal CD4 counts $\leq 700/\mu l$

(c) Delivery at < 34 weeks (risk is four times higher)

(d) Prolonged rupture of membranes

b. **Diagnosis.** HIV diagnosis may be confounded by passive newborn seropositivity from transplacental IgG transmission, which may persist for 18 months. Research is focusing on HIV IgM antibody.

c. **Clinical course.** AIDS is more aggressive in children than in adults. Approximately 50% of infants exposed to HIV develop AIDS in their first year of life; 85% by age 3 years. The mortality rate of children with AIDS is similar to that in adults (100%).

d. **Management of the newborn**

(1) Observe precautions with blood and body fluids

(2) Administer prophylactic AZT for 6 weeks

(3) Test for HIV RNA titer

IX. GROUP B β-HEMOLYTIC STREPTOCOCCUS (GBBS) INFECTION is part of the normal human bacterial flora with reservoirs of colonization in otherwise healthy individuals.

A. **Background.** The **gastrointestinal (GI) tract** is a major reservoir for GBBS, which can also be isolated from the vagina, cervix, throat, skin, urethra, and urine.

1. **Transmission** occurs via fecal contamination and sexual practices.

2. **Vaginal colonization rates** are 35% in all women, regardless of pregnancy, age, race, socioeconomic status, or parity. Only one-third of women are chronic carriers, whereas two-thirds of women are intermittent or transient carriers.

B. **Clinical issues**

1. **Significance**

a. **Transmission** of GBBS to neonates by colonized mothers at delivery is **50%.**

b. **Attack rate** of GBBS sepsis to neonates of colonized mothers is **1%.**

c. **Obstetric complications** include the following:

(1) Preterm labor/delivery

(2) Premature rupture of membranes

(3) Prolonged labor

(4) Intrapartum and puerperal fever

d. **Neonatal complications** include the following:

(1) **Early-onset infection,** which occurs within **48 hours** and has a **50% mortality rate**

(a) Prematurity places infants at the **highest risk.**

(b) The **mechanism** is direct mother-to-infant transmission at delivery.

(c) Onset is rapid with a fulminant course. **Pneumonia, meningitis, septicemia,** shock, and death are frequent manifestations.

(2) Late-onset infection, which occurs after the **first week of life** and has a **25% mortality rate**

(a) Prematurity is **not** a risk factor.

(b) The **mechanism** is nosocomial nursery infection.

(c) Meningitis is the **most common** presentation.

2. **Diagnosis.** GBBS is easily cultured on routine media. Rapid assays are available; they have low sensitivity but good specificity.

3. **Prevention of GBBS sepsis** involves **intrapartum antibiotic prophylaxis** by one of two methods, either of which prevents 70% of GBBS sepsis. Women may be selected by either **antepartum screening or intrapartum risk factors.**

   a. **General principles**

   (1) Penicillin G is the **antibiotic of choice,** because GBBS is highly sensitive to this drug. The dose is 2.5 million units IV q4hr. In penicillin-allergic patients, **erythromycin** or **clindamycin** may be used.

   (2) Women with a history of previous neonates diagnosed with GBBS sepsis should be treated intrapartum regardless of culture status.

   b. **Antepartum screening-based approach. Vaginal GBBS cultures should be obtained from all patients in the third trimester.**

   (1) No antibiotic prophylaxis is given if patients have negative GBBS cultures.

   (2) Penicillin G is administered if patients have positive GBBS cultures.

   c. **Intrapartum risk factor approach. No antepartum vaginal GBBS cultures are obtained.**

   (1) No antibiotic prophylaxis is given if gestation is term, membranes are ruptured for less than 18 hours, or the mother is afebrile.

   (2) Penicillin G is given if gestation is preterm, membranes are ruptured for more than 18 hours, or the mother is febrile.

Review Test

Directions: Each of the numbered items or incomplete statements in this section is followed by answers or by completions of the statement. Select the **ONE** lettered answer or completion that is **BEST** in each case.

1. Which one of the following perinatal infectious diseases has the highest risk of fetal infection in the first trimester?

(A) Hepatitis B virus (HBV)
(B) Syphilis
(C) Toxoplasmosis
(D) Herpes simplex virus (HSV)
(E) Rubella

2. Which one of the following perinatal infectious diseases can be prevented by prepregnancy immunization of susceptible women?

(A) Toxoplasmosis
(B) Rubella
(C) Human immunodeficiency virus (HIV)
(D) Cytomegalovirus (CMV)
(E) Herpes simplex virus (HSV)

3. Which one of the following perinatal infectious diseases is the most contagious?

(A) Toxoplasmosis
(B) Syphilis
(C) Human immunodeficiency virus (HIV)
(D) Cytomegalovirus (CMV)
(E) Herpes simplex virus (HSV)

4. Which one of the following perinatal infectious diseases can be prevented by postdelivery passive and active immunization of the neonate?

(A) Toxoplasmosis
(B) Syphilis
(C) Hepatitis B virus (HBV)
(D) Cytomegalovirus (CMV)
(E) Herpes simplex virus (HSV)

5. For which one of the following perinatal infectious diseases can transmission from mother to neonate be potentially prevented by cesarean delivery?

(A) Hepatitis B virus (HBV)
(B) Syphilis
(C) Toxoplasmosis
(D) Herpes simplex virus (HSV)
(E) Rubella

Directions: Each of the numbered items or incomplete statements in this section is negatively phrased, as indicated by a capitalized word such as NOT, LEAST, or EXCEPT. Select the **ONE** lettered answer or completion that is BEST in each case.

6. All of the following perinatal infectious diseases result in lifelong immunity after the primary infection EXCEPT

(A) hepatitis B virus (HBV)
(B) syphilis
(C) toxoplasmosis
(D) herpes simplex virus (HSV)
(E) rubella

7. All of the following perinatal infectious diseases are associated with fetal microcephaly and seizure disorders EXCEPT

(A) toxoplasmosis
(B) rubella
(C) human immunodeficiency virus (HIV)
(D) cytomegalovirus (CMV)
(E) herpes simplex virus (HSV)

8. A specific therapy is unavailable for all of the following perinatal infectious diseases EXCEPT

(A) human immunodeficiency virus (HIV)
(B) rubella
(C) hepatitis B virus (HBV)
(D) cytomegalovirus (CMV)
(E) syphilis

9. All of the following conditions are associated with false-positive syphilis screening serology tests EXCEPT

(A) hypertensive disease
(B) autoimmune disease
(C) renal disease
(D) recent immunizations
(E) viral infections

170

Directions: The set of matching questions in this section consists of a list of four to twenty-six lettered options (some of which may be in figures) followed by several numbered items. For each numbered item, select the **ONE** lettered option that is most closely associated with it. To avoid spending too much time on matching sets with large numbers of options, it is generally advisable to begin each set by reading the list of options. Then, for each item in the set, try to generate the correct answer and locate it in the option list, rather than evaluating each option individually. Each lettered option may be selected once, more than once, or not at all.

Questions 10–16

For each of the perinatal infectious diseases listed, select the appropriate mode of transmission.
(A) Air droplets
(B) Cat feces
(C) Body fluids
(D) Mucous membrane contact

10. Hepatitis B virus (HBV)

11. Syphilis

12. Human immunodeficiency virus (HIV)

13. Toxoplasmosis

14. Cytomegalovirus (CMV)

15. Herpes simplex virus (HSV)

16. Rubella

Answers and Explanations

1. The answer is E [III].

The risk of fetal infection with rubella is higher than 90% in the first 10 weeks of pregnancy. Hepatitis B virus (HBV), syphilis, toxoplasmosis, and herpes simplex virus (HSV) all have much lower first trimester attack rates. Toxoplasmosis, for example, has a fetal infection rate of only 15% in the first trimester.

2. The answer is B [III B 4].

Congenital rubella syndrome, a disease characterized by cataracts, deafness, and congenital heart disease, can be prevented by active immunization before conception in women who are rubella antibody–negative. The goal is to induce antibodies by injecting an attenuated live virus, thus preventing the possibility of a viremia of a primary infection that places the fetus at risk for congenital rubella syndrome. No current immunizations are available for toxoplasmosis, human immunodeficiency virus (HIV), cytomegalovirus (CMV), and herpes simplex virus (HSV).

3. The answer is E [V A 1, B 3].

Herpes simplex virus (HSV) causes a permanent, incurable latency in the sensory nerve root ganglia in the dermatome of involvement and is highly contagious. It is transmitted by intimate mucocutaneous contact in which one of the individuals must have symptomatic lesions. Prevalence of seropositivity is 50% in pregnant women in the United States. Active genital herpes places the fetus at risk for infection by delivery through an infected birth canal. Toxoplasmosis, syphilis, human immunodeficiency virus (HIV), and cytomegalovirus (CMV) are also contagious.

4. The answer is C [VII D 5 a].

Neonatal hepatitis B virus (HBV) can be prevented with a high degree of success through immunization of the infant immediately postdelivery. This is not true of toxoplasmosis, syphilis, cytomegalovirus (CMV), and herpes simplex virus (HSV). The rate of transmission of HBV at delivery from a mother who is a carrier to her infant is 10% if the mother is positive for only hepatitis B surface antigen (HBsAg), but it is 80% if she is positive for both HBsAg and hepatitis B e antigen (HBeAg).

5. The answer is D [V B 4 b].

Neonatal herpes can potentially be prevented by avoiding fetal contamination through an infected birth canal. This is not true of hepatitis B virus (HBV), toxoplasmosis, and rubella because they are not specific genital tract diseases. Although syphilis is a genital tract disease, it is of risk to the fetus primarily when the spirochete is carried through the blood stream with an active infection.

6. The answer is B [VI B 2 a (4)].

Syphilis can be contracted repeatedly despite previous successful exposures and treatment. No immunity results. Hepatitis B virus (HBV), toxoplasmosis, herpes simplex virus (HSV), and rubella each result in lifelong immunity, thereby protecting the host from secondary viremias or parasitemias. It is during the phase of blood stream dissemination in the maternal host that the placenta becomes infected, which secondarily seeds the fetal blood stream with the pathogenic organism.

7. The answer is C [VIII B 1–2].

Fetal human immunodeficiency virus (HIV) is not associated with known congenital anomalies. Toxoplasmosis, rubella, cytomegalovirus (CMV), and herpes simplex virus (HSV) are all associated with fetal microcephaly and seizure disorders in spite of being widely divergent in microbiological taxonomy. This is a consequence of the affinity of the varied organisms for the fetal central nervous system (CNS).

8. The answer is E [VI B 3].

Syphilis can be treated successfully with antibiotics in both the mother and the fetus in utero. Human immunodeficiency virus (HIV), rubella, hepatitis B virus (HBV), and cytomegalovirus (CMV) have no specific therapy available and are best addressed through primary prevention activities. Development of effective antiviral agents lags far behind antibiotics for bacterial or spirochete infections.

9. The answer is A [VI B 2 c (2)].

Hypertensive disease is not associated with a false-positive syphilis serology. Autoimmune disease, renal disease, recent immunizations, and viral infections are associated with false-positive Venereal Disease Research Laboratory/rapid plasmin reagin (VDRL/RPR) tests. The identification of a false-positive test rests on a negative follow-up test with a treponema-specific test such as fluorescent treponemal antibody absorption test (FTA-ABS) or microhemagglutination–*Treponema pallidum* (MHA-TP).

10–16. The answers are: 10-C [VII A 1 b], **11-D** [VI A 2], **12-C** [VIII A 2], **13-B** [II A], **14-C** [IV A 1], **15-D** [V A 1], **16-A** [III A 1].

Hepatitis B virus (HBV), human immunodeficiency virus (HIV), and cytomegalovirus (CMV) are associated with body fluid transmission. Syphilis and herpes simplex virus (HSV) are associated with mucous membrane contact. Rubella is associated with air droplet transmission. Toxoplasmosis is associated with cat feces–fomite transmission.

6

Labor and Delivery

I. NORMAL LABOR AND DELIVERY

A. Myometrial anatomy and physiology

1. **Cellular constituents of corpus.** Approximately 80% of the corpus consists of smooth muscle cells. The remaining 20% is a matrix of collagen and glycosaminoglycans.

2. **Myometrial cellular organization.** Myometrial cells are arranged in spiral bundles that allow three-dimensional strength. They are formed from the fusion of two müllerian tracts, which leads to two differently oriented spirals.

3. **Myometrial cell growth in pregnancy.** Myometrial cell growth occurs both by cell division and hypertrophy. Growth is induced by estrogen, progesterone, and mechanical distention.

4. **Formation of gap junctions.** Gap junctions between smooth muscle cells that form with advancing pregnancy have two purposes: facilitating synchronization of contractile activity among cells and permitting rapid transmission of electrical and chemical impulses between cells.

   a. **Promotors** of gap junctions: estrogens, prostaglandins (PGs), and mechanical distention

   b. **Inhibitors** of gap junctions: progesterone, and PG synthetase inhibitors (e.g., indomethacin)

B. Cervical physiology

1. **Cellular constituents of the cervix**

   a. **Smooth muscle** decreases from the proximal cervix to the distal cervix. There is 25% smooth muscle tissue at the internal os, compared with 10% at the external os.

   b. **Collagen** and **ground substance** are the main components of the cervix.

2. **Cervical ripening and effacement** (Figure 6-1)

   a. **Mechanism.** Collagen chains fracture and are solubilized. Insoluble

A. No Effacement

B. 50% Effacement

C. Full Effacement

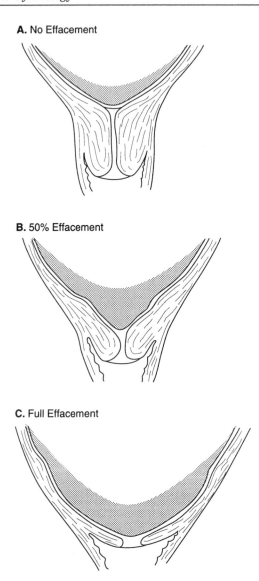

Figure 6-1. Degrees of cervical effacement. (Reprinted with permission from Hacker NF, Moore JG (eds): *Essentials of Obstetrics and Gynecology,* 2nd ed. Philadelphia, W.B. Saunders, 1992, p 120.)

glycosaminoglycans are replaced by more soluble hyaluronic acid, which increases the water content.

   b. Purpose. Increasing the water content of the cervix allows the cervix to become soft, distensible, and compliant.

   c. Softening of the cervix is promoted by relaxin, estrogen, prostaglandin E_2 (PGE_2), progesterone antagonists, and mechanical forces (e.g., stretch, Braxton-Hicks contractions).

C. Biochemistry of myometrial contractions

   1. Molecular components of the smooth muscle that slide over each other with contractions include myosin and actin.

2. **Mechanism.** Myosin is phosphorylated and reacts with actin. The critical enzyme is myosin light-chain kinase, which is dependent on calcium ions and calmodulin (calcium-dependent regulatory protein).

3. **Oxytocic agents** exert their action by mobilizing intracellular free calcium ions. These agents include oxytocin, which is produced by the posterior pituitary gland, α-adrenergic agonists, and PGs.

4. **Tocolytic agents** cause relaxation by decreasing intracellular free calcium ions. These agents include the following:
   a. **Calcium channel blockers,** which inhibit influx from the extracellular space
   b. **β-Adrenergic agonists,** which act through receptors involving adenyl cyclase and cyclic adenosine monophosphate (cAMP)
   c. **Magnesium sulfate,** which competes with calcium intracellularly
   d. **Oxytocin antagonists,** which block oxytocin receptors

D. Clinical issues

1. **Stages of labor** (Table 6-1). The three stages of labor identify changes over time in **cervical dilation, descent in station** of the fetus, and **placental separation.**
   a. **Stage 1 begins with** the onset of regular contractions and **ends with** complete cervical dilation. It is divided into two phases:
      (1) **Latent phase.** This begins with onset regular contractions and ends with acceleration of the cervical dilation slope, usually at 3–4 cm dilation.
         (a) **Purpose.** Coordination of contractions and softening and effacement of the cervix
         (b) **Duration.** No more than 14 hours in multiparas and 20 hours in primiparas
      (2) **Active phase.** This begins with acceleration of cervical dilation slope (3–4 cm) and ends at complete cervical dilation.
         (a) **Purpose.** As the cervix is completing dilation, the presenting fetal part descends into the birth canal. The fetus begins the cardinal movements of labor (see I D 3).
         (b) **Duration.** Cervical dilation rates should be ≥ 1.5 cm/hr in multiparas and ≥ 1.2 cm/hr in primiparas. Normally, the length is 4 hours in multiparas and 5 hours in primiparas.
   b. **Stage 2 begins with** complete cervical dilation and **ends with** delivery of the neonate. The descent of the presenting fetal part is completed, and the cardinal movements of labor are completed. The **duration** of stage 2 is normally 30 minutes for multiparas and 60 minutes for primiparas. Epidural anesthesia decreases the sensation of pelvic pressure and urge to push, thus lengthening the normal limits.
   c. **Stage 3 begins with** delivery of the neonate and **ends with** delivery of the placenta. Placental separation depends on uterine contractions (UCs) shearing the anchoring villi from their attachment to the decidual bed of the endometrium (Figure 6-2). The duration of stage 3 is normally less than 30 minutes.

Table 6-1. Characteristics of the Three Stages of Labor

| | Stage 1 | | Stage 2 | Stage 3 |
	Latent Phase	Active Phase		
Begins	Onset of regular uterine contractions	Acceleration of cervical diltation slope (≥ 3 cm)	Complete cervical dilation (10 cm)	Delivery of neonate
Ends	Acceleration of cervical dilation slope (≥ 3 cm)	Complete cervical dilation (10 cm)	Delivery of neonate	Delivery of placenta
Purpose	Coordination of contractions Cervical softening and effacement	Active cervical dilation Beginning of descent of presenting part Beginning of cardinal movements of labor	Completion of descent of presenting part Completion of cardinal movements of labor	Shearing of anchoring villi Delivery of placenta
Normal duration	< 14 hr in multipara < 20 hr in primipara	< 4 hr in multipara (cervical dilation ≥ 1.5 cm/hr) < 5 hr in primipara (cervical dilatation ≥ 1.2 cm/hr)	< 30 minutes in multipara < 60 minutes in primipara	< 30 minutes
Abnormalities	Prolongation disorders	Prolongation disorders Arrest of dilation disorders	Arrest of descent disorders	Prolongation disorders
Causes of disorders	Injudicious analgesics Hypo/hypertonic contractions	**Pelvis** (inadequate bony size) **Passenger** (abnormal orientation or excess size) **Power** (inadequate or ineffective contractions)	**Pelvis** (inadequate bony size) **Passenger** (abnormal orientation or excess size) **Power** (inadequate or ineffective contractions)	Inadequate contractions Abnormal placentation (accreta, increta, percreta)
Management	Therapeutic rest Sedation	Intravenous oxytocin Cesarean delivery	Forceps Vacuum extractor Cesarean delivery	Oxytocic agents Manual removal Uterine curettage Hysterectomy

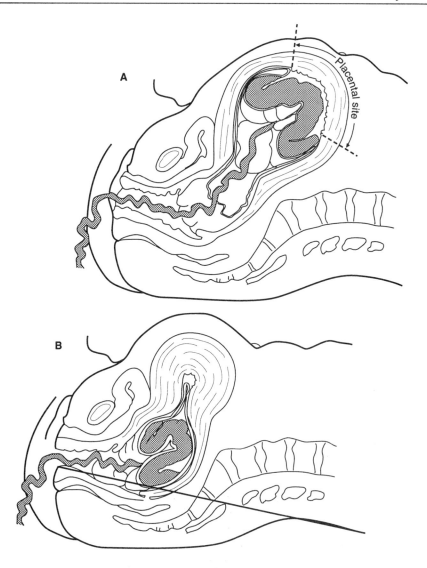

Figure 6-2. Relation of placenta to uterus in the third stage of labor. Notice that as the placental site contracts, the placenta is sheared loose. (Reprinted with permission from Scott JR, DiSaia PJ, Hammond CB, et al (eds): *Danforth's Obstetrics and Gynecology,* 6th ed. Philadelphia, J.B. Lippincott, 1990, p 185.)

2. **Obstetric anesthesia modalities must be simple and safe and must preserve fetal homeostasis** (Table 6-2).

    a. **Narcotics** may cause **neonatal respiratory depression.** Treatment is naloxone.

    b. **Paracervical block** may cause **fetal bradycardia.** Treatment is conservative, allowing spontaneous recovery of the fetal heart rate (FHR).

    c. **Regional anesthesia** may cause **maternal hypotension** from sympathetic blockade. Treatment is intravenous (IV) fluids, ephedrine, and change in maternal position.

    d. **Regional anesthesia** may cause **spinal headaches.** Treatment is hydration, caffeine, and blood patch.

Table 6-2. Obstetric Analgesia/Anesthesia

	Modality	Advantages	Disadvantages
Stage 1 of labor (involves nerve roots T_{10}–T_{12})	Narcotics	Ease of administration Inexpensive	Sedative effect Incomplete relief Neonatal respiratory depression
	Paracervical block	Requires moderate level of skill	Fetal bradycardia Variable pain relief
	Epidural block	Superior pain relief Can use for all stages of labor	Hypotension Patchy block Requires high level of skill Expensive Spinal headache if dural puncture
Stage 2 of labor (involves nerve roots S_2, S_3, and S_4)	Local infiltration	Ease of administration Inexpensive	Incomplete relief
	Pudendal block	Requires moderate level of skill	Variable pain relief
	Epidural block	Superior pain relief Can use for all stages of labor	Hypotension Patchy block Requires high level of skill Expensive Spinal headache if dural puncture
	Saddle block	Predictable complete block	Hypotension Requires high level of skill Expensive Spinal headache possible

3. The **cardinal movements** (also known as the **mechanisms of labor)** are changes in position and attitude of the fetal head during passage through the birth canal. Changes in position and attitude are necessary because of the asymmetrical shape of the fetal head and the maternal bony pelvis. The cardinal movements are required for an average-size fetus to pass through the average birth canal.

   a. **Mechanism.** The propulsive forces of UCs force the fetal head against the levator ani muscles through the path of least resistance. This causes the head to turn, rotate, flex, and extend.

   b. **Specific movements** are identified and described in Table 6-3.

II. ABNORMAL LABOR occurs when the duration of any stage or phase of labor is prolonged.

   A. **Criteria for adequacy of active labor**

   1. **Cervical dilation** must progress at least 1.2 cm or more per hour for primigravidas and 1.5 cm or more per hour for multiparas.

Table 6-3. Cardinal Movements of Labor

Movement	Definition	Purpose	Occurrence
Engagement	• Descent of BPD to below the plane of pelvic inlet • Head position is transverse to accommodate the widest diameter of pelvic inlet	Demonstrate adequacy of maternal bony pelvic inlet	• Prior to labor in primigravidas • After labor onset in multiparas
Descent	Movement of fetal head down through the curve of birth canal	Most important component of labor	• Begins gradually in latent phase • Most rapid in late active phase and stage II
Flexion	Placement of fetal chin on thorax	Allows narrowest AP diameter of fetal head (suboccipito-bregmatic) to present to the birth canal	Usually by beginning of the active phase
Internal rotation	Rotation of position of fetal head in the mid pelvis from transverse to AP	Allows the widest diameter of fetal head to present to the widest diameter of mid pelvis	Usually by the end of the active phase
Extension	Movement of fetal chin away from the thorax as the fetal head passes through the pelvic outlet	Directs the axis of the fetal head upward to the pelvic outlet	Begins with onset of stage II and ends with delivery of fetal head
External rotation	Rotation of fetal head outside the mother from AP to transverse after the head has been delivered	Allows the transverse diameter of fetal shoulders to present to the widest diameter of the mid pelvis	After the fetal head has been delivered but before the shoulders have been delivered
Expulsion	Delivery of the fetal shoulders and body	Completes the birth process of the fetus	Begins with delivery of fetal shoulders and ends with delivery of the body

AP = anterior-posterior; *BPD* = biparietal diameter.

   2. **Descent of the presenting part** must progress at least 1 cm or more per hour for primigravidas and 2 cm or more per hour for multiparas.

 B. **Classification of abnormal labor** (Figure 6-3)

   1. **Prolonged latent phase**

      a. **Criteria.** The latent phase is prolonged when it lasts more than 14 hours in multiparas and more than 20 hours in nulliparas.

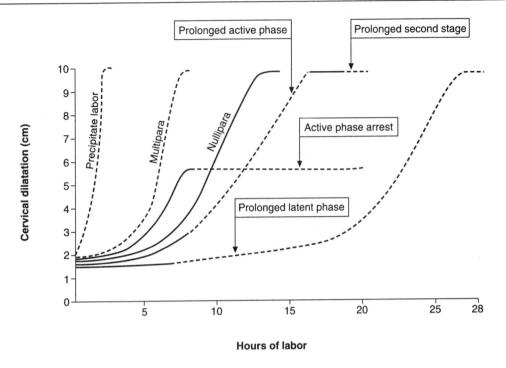

Figure 6-3. Abnormal labor curves. (Reprinted with permission from DeCherney AH, Pernoll ML (eds): *Current Obstetric and Gynecologic Diagnosis and Treatment*, 8th ed. East Norwalk, Conn., Appleton & Lange, 1994, p 218.)

  b. **Etiology.** Typically, women who enter labor without significant cervical effacement experience a prolonged latent phase, as do those with hypotonic or hypertonic contractions and those who receive analgesics injudiciously.

  c. **Management.** A prolonged latent phase is managed with therapeutic rest and sedation with 15–20 mg morphine. Amniotomy and cesarean delivery for "failure to progress" should be avoided.

2. **Protraction disorders of the active phase.** Dilation criteria are less than 1.2 cm/hr for primigravidas and less than 1.5 cm/hr for multigravidas.

3. **Arrest disorder of stage 1 (active phase arrest)** or **stage 2 (arrest of descent).** These diagnoses are made when there is either **no progression** in cervical dilation for at least 2 hours in stage 1 or **prolonged duration** of at least 2 hours in stage 2.

  a. **Etiology ("three Ps")**

   (1) *Pelvis.* Inadequate size of the bony pelvis or birth canal can contribute to arrest disorder (Table 6-4).

   (2) *Passenger.* Abnormal orientation of the fetus within the uterus (i.e., abnormal lie, presentation, position, attitude, synclitism) or excessive fetal size can contribute to arrest disorder (Table 6-5; Figure 6-4).

   (3) *Powers.* Inadequate or ineffective uterine expulsive forces can contribute to arrest disorder. Adequate UCs exhibit all of the following criteria:

Table 6-4. Pelvic Capacity

Pelvic Type	Pelvic Shape	Posterior Sagittal Diameter	Prognosis for Vaginal Delivery
Gynecoid	Round	Average	Good
Anthropoid	Long and oval	Long	Good
Android	Heart shaped	Short	Poor
Platypelloid	Flat and oval	Short	Poor

Table 6-5. Nomenclature for In Utero Fetal Orientation

Reference Category	Definition	Most Common Subcategory	Other Subcategories
Lie	Relationship between long axis of fetus and long axis of mother	**Longitudinal** (fetal body is vertical to the mother)—99%	Transverse (fetal body is horizontal to mother)—<1% Oblique
Presentation	Portion of fetus overlying pelvic inlet	**Cephalic** (fetal head lies closet to pelvic inlet)—95%	Breech (longitudinal lie with head in uterine fundus)—4% Compound (more than one fetal part is presenting)
Position	Relationship between a reference point on the presenting fetal part and maternal bony pelvis	**Direct occiput anterior (OA)** is most common at delivery with cephalic presentation*	Other OA positions: (ROA, LOA) Occiput transverse: (ROT, LOT) Occiput posterior: (OP, ROP, LOP)
Attitude	Degree of flexion or extension of fetal head	**Vertex** (complete flexion, chin against chest)	Military (partial flexion) Brow (partial extension) Face (complete extension)
Station	The degree of descent of the presenting part through the birth canal, expressed in cm; the presenting part is above or below the maternal ischial spine (i.e., station 0).	**Variable;** depends on descent of presenting part throughout the stages of labor	Prior to engagement the station will be −4, moving to +4 just prior to delivery of the head
Synclitism	Orientation of the fetal sagittal suture to the midline between maternal symphysis and sacral promontory	**Synclitic** (the sagittal suture is midway between the front and back of the pelvis)	Anterior or posterior asynclitism (when either the anterior or posterior parietal bone precedes the sagittal suture)

*Depends on the phase and stage of labor when assessed; varies with progression through the cardinal movements of labor.

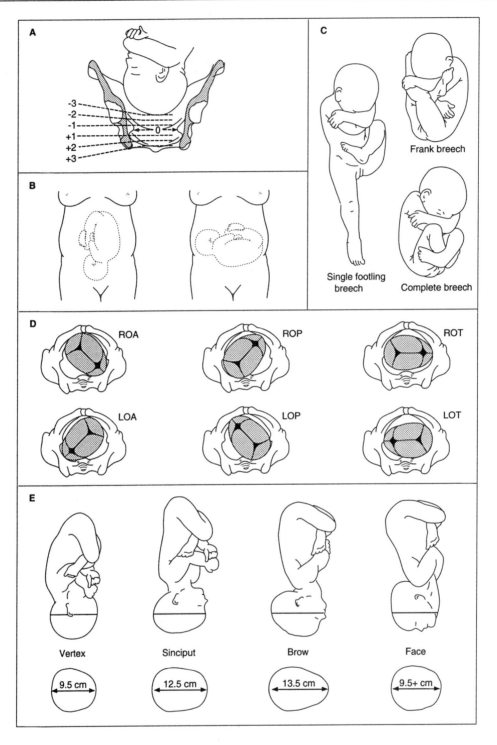

Figure 6-4. (A) Stations of the fetal head; (B) Longitudinal and transverse lies; (C) Types of breech presentation; (D) Various positions of the fetal head in a vertex presentation; (E) Types of cephalic presentation according to attitude of fetal head. After Beckmann CR, Ling FW, Barzansky BM, et al: *Obstetrics and Gynecology,* 2nd ed. Baltimore, Williams & Wilkins, 1995, p 172; DeCherney AH, Pernoll ML (eds): *Current Obstetrics and Gynecologic Diagnosis and Treatment,* 8th ed. East Norwalk, Conn., Appleton & Lange, 1994, pp 214, 411; Scott JR, DiSaia PJ, Hammond CB, et al (eds): *Danforth's Obstetrics and Gynecology,* 6th ed. Philadelphia, J.B. Lippincott, 1990, pp 168, 170).

          (a) Duration: 45–60 seconds

          (b) Frequency: every 2–3 minutes

          (c) Intensity: $\geq$ 50 mm Hg (with an intrauterine pressure catheter)

    b. Management. The causes of arrest disorder must be determined.

        (1) Problems with *pelvis* (size) **or *passenger*** (orientation or size)

          (a) In **stage 1 (active phase),** a cesarean delivery should be performed.

          (b) In **stage 2,** the delivery method may be either operative vaginal (forceps, vacuum extractor) or cesarean.

        (2) Inadequate *powers.* A dilute IV **oxytocin infusion** should be started and gradually increased until adequate contractions are achieved. **Potential complications** of oxytocin administration include uterine hyperstimulation or tetany, water intoxication (from antidiuretic hormone effect), or uterine atony (leading to postpartum hemorrhage).

III. INTRAPARTUM FETAL MONITORING

    A. Fetal response to labor depends on the following:

      1. Fetal reserve (jeopardized with fetal anemia)

      2. Umbilical blood flow (decreased with cord compression)

      3. Placental function (decreased with chorioamnionitis or placental aging)

      4. Intravillous blood flow (diminished with UCs)

      5. Uterine blood flow (reduced with maternal hypotension)

      6. Maternal environment (jeopardized with high altitude)

      7. Maternal cardiopulmonary function (decreased with pulmonary edema or heart failure)

      8. Fetal and maternal response to drugs (sedation from narcotics and local anesthetics)

    B. Clinical issues

      1. Methods for intrapartum monitoring of the FHR include the following:

        a. Intermittent auscultation of the FHR is equivalent to continuous electronic monitoring in assessing the fetal condition.

          (1) Direct. The FHR can be listened to directly by a DeLee fetoscope or a Doppler ultrasound device.

          (2) Standard practice. No data exist to define the optimal method. However, many practitioners listen during a contraction and for 30 seconds after the contraction every 15 minutes during the first stage of labor and every 5 minutes during the second stage of labor.

          (3) Nonreassuring findings

            (a) A baseline rate of $<$ 100 beats/min between contractions

            (b) A rate of $<$ 100 beats/min, 30 seconds after a contraction

(c) Unexplained baseline tachycardia of > 160 beats/min, 30 seconds after a contraction, especially in at-risk patients or in patients in whom tachycardia persists through more than three contractions despite corrective measures

b. **Continuous intrapartum electronic monitoring** involves two components: **FHR** and **UCs.**

(1) **Calculation.** The interval (in milliseconds) from one fetal heartbeat to the next is calculated and instantaneously converted into a rate per minute.

(2) **Electronic display.** The FHR and UCs are electronically displayed in a real-time fashion but are also recorded on a moving strip of paper for later review as well as storage.

(3) **Indirect and direct measurements.** Both the FHR and UCs can be obtained indirectly with external devices on the mother's abdomen or directly with devices placed in the uterus. Table 6-6 summarizes the details regarding the different methods that can be used in various tandem combinations.

(a) **External monitors** (sonocardiograph and tocodynamometer) are noninvasive and can be used prior to cervical dilation or membrane rupture but may have limited precision with obese patients.

(b) **Internal monitors** (fetal scalp electrode and intrauterine pressure catheter) have higher precision in all patients but can only be used after cervical dilation and membrane rupture.

(4) **Various combinations of heart rate (HR) and contraction monitoring**

(a) **General principles.** The most precise information is obtained from internal methods. Ideally, FHR and contraction data are obtained concurrently. External methods should be used if adequate tracing is obtained. Internal methods should be used if there are abnormal findings from external methods.

(b) **Combination methods**
(i) Sonocardiogram and external tocodynamometer
(ii) Fetal scalp electrode and external tocodynamometer
(iii) Fetal scalp electrode and intrauterine pressure catheter
(iv) Sonocardiogram and intrauterine pressure catheter

2. **Normal electronic fetal monitoring parameters** are baseline HR, beat-to-beat variability, and periodic changes. **There are many causes for abnormal fetal monitor patterns other than hypoxemia.** Table 6-7 summarizes these causes.

a. **Baseline HR** is the average rate between peaks and depressions.

(1) **Baseline rate criteria**
(a) Marked tachycardia: > 180 beats/min
(b) Moderate tachycardia: 161–180 beats/min
(c) **Normal rate: 120–160 beats/min**
(d) Moderate bradycardia: 100–119 beats/min
(e) Marked bradycardia: > 100 beats/min

(2) **Causes of abnormal HRs (note drug effects)**

Table 6-6. Methods of Intrapartum Continuous Electronic Monitoring

Modality	Device	What is Recorded	Risks	Advantages	Disadvantages
External-Indirect Fetal Heart Rate (FHR) Monitoring	Ultrasound sonocardiogram attached by belt to maternal abdomen	Fetal cardiac motion frequency	None	• Noninvasive • Can use with intact membranes	• Discomfort of belt • Poor signal quality if obese abdomen
Internal-Direct FHR Monitoring	Electrode attached to fetal scalp through a dilated cervix	Fetal cardiac electrical activity frequency	• Fetal scalp abscess • Inoculation of maternal genital tract infections (e.g., herpes, HIV)	• No belt discomfort • High-quality signal regardless of obese abdomen	• Membranes must be ruptured • Cervix must be dilated
External-Indirect Uterine Contraction (UC) Monitoring	Spring-loaded tocodynamometer strain gauge attached by belt to maternal abdomen	Uterine wall tautness and relaxation indicating beginning and end of contraction	None	• Noninvasive • Can use with intact membranes • Contraction frequency and duration are measured	• Discomfort of belt • Poor signal sensitivity if obese abdomen • Does not measure contraction intensity
Internal-Direct UC Monitoring	Intrauterine pressure catheter through a dilated cervix	Changing intra-uterine amniotic fluid hydrostatic pressure	• Passage into uterus of maternal lower genital tract organisms • Low-lying placenta could be perforated	• No belt discomfort • Measures contraction frequency, duration, and intensity	• Membranes must be ruptured • Cervix must be dilated

Table 6-7. Possible Causes of Abnormal Fetal Monitor Patterns

	Baseline Heart Rate		Baseline Variability	
	Tachycardia	Bradycardia	Increased	Decreased
Definition	> 160 beats/min	< 120 beats/min	> 10 beats/min	< 5 beats/min
Hypoxemia	+	+	+	+
Prematurity	+	−	−	+
Maternal fever	+	−	−	−
Fetal arrhythmia	+	+	+	−
Drug effect	+	+	−	+
Fetal movement	+	−	+	−
Fetal sleep	−	−	−	+
Technical artifact	−	−	+	−
Maternal hyperthyroid	+	−	−	−

+ factor **could be** associated with the specific abnormality.
− factor **is not** associated with the specific abnormality.

    (a) Baseline tachycardia (many nonhypoxemic etiologies). Causes include:

      (i) Hypoxemia

      (ii) Fever

      (iii) Prematurity

      (iv) Fetal arrhythmia

      (v) Prolonged fetal movements (merging of repetitive accelerations)

      (vi) Maternal hyperthyroidism

      (vii) Drugs (e.g., **scopolamine, atropine, β-adrenergic agonists)**

    (b) Baseline bradycardia (many nonhypoxemic etiologies). Causes include:

      (i) Hypoxemia

      (ii) Fetal arrhythmia

      (iii) Drugs (e.g., **local anesthetics, β-adrenergic blockers)**

  b. Beat-to-beat variability (small, rapid rhythmic fluctuations of 5–10 beats/min) is a sign of good autonomic interplay in the HR regulatory mechanism. The most predictive evidence of fetal well-being is HR variability. Short-term variability is controlled by the parasympathetic system, and long-term variability is controlled by the sympathetic system.

    (1) Baseline variability criteria

      (a) Absent: 0–2 beats/min

      (b) Minimal: 3–5 beats/min

      (c) Normal: 6–10 beats/min

      (d) Moderate: 11–25 beats/min

      (e) Marked: > 25 beats/min

    (2) Causes of increased baseline variability (many nonhypoxemic etiologies)

      (a) Early hypoxemia

      (b) Fetal movement

      (c) Fetal arrhythmia

      (d) Technical artifact

    (3) Causes of decreased baseline variability (many nonhypoxemic etiologies)

      (a) Chronic hypoxemia

      (b) Prematurity

      (c) Fetal sleep

      (d) Drugs (e.g., **parasympatholytics, sedatives, tranquilizers, narcotics)**

  c. Periodic changes are transitory FHR changes in relation to contractions. These include accelerations, early decelerations, variable decelerations, and late decelerations (Figure 6-5; Table 6-8).

    (1) Accelerations are always reassuring. They are indicated by an increase in the baseline of 15 or more beats/min that last for 15 seconds or more. Accelerations are mediated by **sympathetic stimulation** and can be a response to **fetal movement** or fetal stimulation.

A. Early deceleration

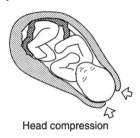

Head compression

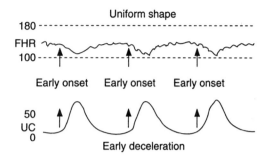

B. Late deceleration

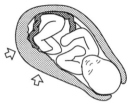

Uteroplacental insufficiency
(Compression of vessels)

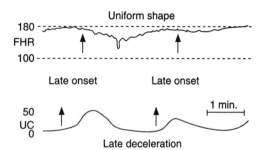

C. Variable deceleration

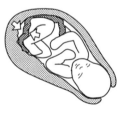

Umbilical cord compression

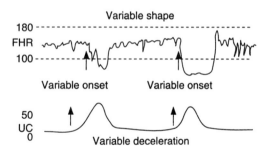

Figure 6-5. Deceleration patterns of the fetal heart rate. (Reprinted with permission from Hon EH: *An Atlas of Fetal Heart Rate Patterns.* New Haven, Conn., Harty Press, 1968.)

    (2) Early decelerations are not clinically significant. They appear as **mirror images of contractions** and are mediated by **vagal stimulation.** Early decelerations are caused by contraction **pressure on the fetal skull,** which is increased eightfold with membrane rupture.

    (3) Variable decelerations are **sudden decreases** in HR with a sudden return.

        (a) Clinical significance

            (i) Mild-to-moderate decelerations are not significant.

            (ii) Prolonged, repetitive, or **deep** decelerations are not reassuring.

Table 6-8. Periodic Changes With Electronic Fetal Monitoring

	Accelerations	Early Decelerations	Variable Decelerations	Late Decelerations
Appearance	Rise above baseline of ≥ 15 beats/min lasting ≥ 15 seconds	Drop below baseline appearing as mirror image of contraction	Sudden drop below baseline with sudden return	Gradual drop below base-line with gradual return after end of con-traction
Mediated by	Sympathetics	Vagal nerve	Vagal nerve	Vagal nerve; Myocardial depression
Response to	Fetal movement; Fetal stimulation	Pressure on fetal skull	Umbilical cord compression	Uteroplacental insufficiency
Interpret	Always reassuring	No problem	No problem if mild/moderate Not reassuring if severe	Not reassuring

> (iii) **Severe** variable decelerations are those that last longer than **60** seconds, drop to lower than **60** beats/min, or drop **60** beats/min below the baseline **(rule of "60s").**
>
> (b) **Characteristics.** Variable decelerations may occur at variable times during a contraction. They have variable, nonuniform shapes and variable amplitudes. They are mediated by **vagal stimulation** and occur in response to **umbilical cord compression.**
>
> (4) **Late decelerations** are **gradual decreases** in HR with a gradual return after the end of the contraction. They are not reassuring, especially if there is decreased variability. Late decelerations are mediated either by **vagal stimulation** from hypoxia or by **myocardial depression** caused by acidosis. They occur in response to **uteroplacental insufficiency.**

3. **Signs of fetal well-being** include all of the following:
   a. Normal baseline HR
   b. Normal baseline variability
   c. No late decelerations
   d. No severe variable decelerations

4. **Normal pH value for scalp/cord blood gases** exceeds 7.20.

5. **Nonreassuring intrapartum FHR** findings may include any of the following:
   a. Minimal or absent baseline variability (without explanation)
   b. Tachycardia or bradycardia (without explanation)
   c. Late or severe variable decelerations (regardless of variability)

6. **Generic intervention strategies for nonreassuring fetal monitor HR patterns include:**
   a. **Decrease in uterine activity.** Oxytocin infusion should be stopped, and a tocolytic agent should be administered [e.g., 0.25 mg terbutaline subcutaneously (SQ)].
   b. **Correction of hypotension.** A rapid IV bolus of 500 ml of isotonic fluids without dextrose should be administered.
   c. **Change in maternal position.** If the patient is supine, she should be placed on her left side. If the patient is lying on one side, she should be placed on the other side.
   d. **Administration of high-flow oxygen** (8–10 L/min)
   e. **Vaginal examination** to rule out a prolapsed umbilical cord
   f. **Stimulation of the fetus** (via scalp or vibroacoustic stimulation) to look for accelerations of 15 beats/min that last 15 seconds

IV. PREMATURE RUPTURE OF MEMBRANES (PROM), or the rupture of the membranes before the onset of labor. Preterm PROM (PPROM) occurs not only before the onset of labor but also before term. PROM is the **single most common diagnosis leading to neonatal intensive care unit admissions.**

A. **Background**
   1. **Amniotic fluid** is **hypotonic** to maternal plasma.
      a. **Sources** include **fetal urine output** (main source after the first trimester), fetal lung fluid, placental surfaces, and fetal membranes.
      b. **Functions**
         (1) Protects the fetus from blunt trauma
         (2) Provides space for fetal extremity and gross body movement
         (3) Provides space for chest wall breathing movements allowing lung development
         (4) Cushions the umbilical cord from compression
   2. **Tests of fetal pulmonary maturity** are based on measuring phospholipid surfactants that are secreted into the amniotic fluid from the fetal lung.
      a. **Surfactants** are surface-acting molecules that coat the membrane surface and lower the alveolar membrane surface tension when the alveolus diminishes in size with expiration.
      b. A **lung maturity profile** includes information on the levels of the following surfactants:
         (1) **Phosphatidylcholine** (lecithin), which increases dramatically between 34 and 36 weeks' gestation. A **lecithin:sphingomyelin ratio** ≥ 2 indicates lung maturity.
         (2) **Phosphatidylglycerol**
         (3) Phosphatidylinositol
         (4) Phosphatidylethanolamine
   3. **Functional anatomy of the fetal membranes** is described as follows:
      a. **Layers**

(1) The **inner layer (amnion)** is relatively **strong.**

(2) The **middle layer** is collagen-rich connective tissue that replenishes the amnion.

(3) The **outer layer (chorion)** is relatively **weak.**

b. **Strength.** The amnion and chorion together are stronger than either separately. The membranes are stronger when supported by a closed (rather than dilated) cervix. The relative collagen concentration decreases with advancing gestation.

B. **Clinical issues**

1. **Incidence and epidemiology.** PROM occurs in 10% of all pregnant patients and in 8% of term patients. Approximately 30% of preterm deliveries are associated with PPROM. PROM is more common in patients with a low socioeconomic status, teens, smokers, and patients with sexually transmitted diseases (STDs).

2. **Risk factors for PPROM**

a. Local defects within membranes

b. Serial damage to membranes from fetal growth and UCs

c. Ascending infections from lower genital tract flora

d. Cigarette smoking

3. **Causes of PROM and associated conditions**

a. **Causes**

(1) **At term.** Membranes undergo physical and biochemical weakening, which is probably a normal variant.

(2) **Preterm.** Inflammatory weakening of membranes may be local or intra-amniotic.

b. **Associations**

(1) Polyhydramnios

(2) Incompetent cervix

(3) Abruptio placentae

4. **Effects of PROM on maternal and neonatal outcome**

a. **Onset of labor** depends on gestational age.

(1) **Term gestation.** More than 90% of patients begin labor within 24 hours of PROM.

(2) **Preterm gestation.** More than 50% of patients begin labor within 24 hours of PPROM, and more than 85% of patients begin labor within 1 week.

(3) **Previable gestation.** Approximately 50% of patients begin labor within 1 week.

b. **Maternal infection** risk depends on gestational age.

(1) **At term.** Infection increases with the duration of PROM.

(2) **Preterm.** There is little relation between infection and the duration of PPROM.

(3) **Manifestations** include chorioamnionitis, endometritis, and sepsis.

c. **Perinatal hazards. Gestational age is the critical factor** in determining whether extrauterine or intrauterine life is best.

(1) With **delivery,** extrauterine life may result in the following:

             (a) **Respiratory distress syndrome (RDS)**

             (b) **Intraventricular hemorrhage (IVH)**

             (c) **Patent ductus arteriosus (PDA)**

             (d) **Necrotizing enterocolitis (NEC)**

             (e) **Retinopathy of prematurity (ROP)**

             (f) **Bronchopulmonary dysplasia (BPD)**

             (g) **Death**

       (2) With **conservative management,** intrauterine life may result in the following:

             (a) **Infection** ascending from maternal genital tract

             (b) **Deformations** from inability to move extremities

             (c) **Umbilical cord compression** from oligohydramnios

             (d) **Pulmonary hypoplasia** if gestational age is < 24 weeks

             (e) **Death**

C. Clinical approach to PROM

  1. Diagnosis

    a. Differential diagnosis. Urinary leakage, excess vaginal discharge, and bloody show must be ruled out.

    b. History. An accurate patient history leads to the correct diagnosis in 90% of patients. For example, did a sudden gush of fluid from the vagina go all over the floor or did the patient experience a minimal amount of perineal moistness?

    c. Digital examination. If the patient is not in labor, infection should be minimized by avoiding a digital intracervical examination.

    d. Speculum examination. PROM should always be confirmed by performing a sterile speculum examination unless fluid is grossly gushing from the introitus.

      (1) Specific parameters to look for include:

        (a) **Pooling** of amniotic fluid in the posterior fornix

        (b) **Nitrazine** paper turning blue when placed in alkaline amniotic fluid

        (c) **Ferning pattern** seen with a microscope when amniotic fluid is allowed to air dry on a glass slide

      (2) Gross cervical purulence should be ruled out by visual inspection.

      (3) Cultures or smears should be obtained to identify bacterial vaginosis, gonorrhea, *Chlamydia,* and group B β-hemolytic streptococcus (GBBS).

      (4) Cord prolapse should be ruled out.

    e. Ultrasound examination. Sonography can confirm decreased amniotic fluid, rule out fetal anomalies, and assess fetal well-being with a biophysical profile (BPP).

  2. Data. After the diagnosis is made, the following questions need to be answered:

    a. What is the gestational age? The accuracy of the date of the last menstrual period (LMP) must be determined. If an early sonogram was performed, it should be reviewed for verification of gestational age.

    b. Is the uterus infected?

      (1) Fever (most predictive clinical sign of overt chorioamnionitis)

      (2) Leukocytosis (left shift)

      (3) Tachycardia (maternal/fetal)

      (4) Uterine tenderness

      (5) Foul-smelling vaginal discharge

      (6) Positive cultures (late finding)

  c. Is the patient in labor? Regular, strong UCs are suggestive. **Digital cervical examination should be avoided** if labor is not confirmed. Examination with a sterile speculum to evaluate cervical change should be performed.

  d. Is the fetus in jeopardy? Repetitive variable decelerations (from cord compression) or late decelerations (from placental insufficiency) are not reassuring.

3. Management of PROM

  a. Term gestation (≥ 36 weeks). The goal is delivery. If the patient is in true labor, delivery is allowed. **If the patient is not in labor,** management is individualized as follows.

    (1) Chorioamnionitis. If the patient is not in labor but has chorioamnionitis, oxytocin administration should begin. Broad-spectrum antibiotics should be administered as soon as possible, and the pediatrician should be notified.

    (2) Fetal jeopardy. If the patient is not in labor but has a nonreassuring fetal monitor tracing, management is according to obstetric indications.

    (3) If the patient is not in labor, and **she and the fetus are stable,** oxytocin administration should begin immediately if the **cervix is favorable.** Management of a stable patient whose **cervix is unfavorable** is controversial. Induction of labor in such a patient is associated with a high cesarean delivery rate. Cervical ripening with PGE_2 may be helpful.

  b. Preterm gestation (25–35 weeks). The goal is to prolong the pregnancy.

    (1) If the patient is in labor, delivery should be allowed. The use of tocolytic agents is not beneficial. Routine cesarean delivery is associated with no improvement in neonatal outcome.

    (2) Chorioamnionitis should be ruled out.

      (a) If overt infection is present, IV broad-spectrum antibiotics should be started, and labor should be induced. Prompt delivery is indicated regardless of gestational age.

      (b) If no infection is detected, cervical cultures should be obtained and **prophylactic antibiotics** should be initiated (IV ampicillin and erythromycin for 2 days; then PO for 5 days). Conservative management is appropriate.

    (3) Fetal jeopardy should be ruled out using electronic FHR monitoring and BPP. The optimal frequency and duration for performing these tests are unknown.

    (4) Fetal lung maturity may be assessed. A vaginal pool specimen should be analyzed for surfactant. If the lungs are mature, delivery can be considered.

    (5) **Standard in-hospital management** includes the following:

        (a) **Bed rest** is recommended; however, hazards of prolonged immobilization include deep-vein thrombophlebitis and psychosocial separation from family.

        (b) **Frequent clinical examinations of the mother** should be performed to assess uterine tenderness and to check for perineal discharge.

        (c) **Frequent fetal heart testing** should be performed to watch for variable decelerations.

        (d) **Betamethasone** should be administered to the mother to accelerate fetal pulmonary maturity if gestational age is ≤ 32 weeks.

    (6) **Home management criteria** include a reliable patient with an acceptable home environment, a fetus with a cephalic presentation, and home nursing involvement.

    (7) **If the membranes "seal over,"** speculum examinations and sonograms should be repeated to confirm absence of fluid leakage and reaccumulation of amniotic fluid. The patient can be discharged home, but she should receive outpatient follow-up.

    (8) **If 36 weeks' gestation** is reached, the patient is managed as any term patient.

  c. **Previable gestation (< 25 weeks).** This gestational age is associated with **high risk of neonatal mortality and morbidity** from pulmonary hypoplasia, Potter's sequence, or deformation syndrome. These hazards are mediated through the resulting oligohydramnios.

    (1) **Cervical incompetency** may present as PPROM prior to viability and should be considered as a possible etiology.

    (2) **Management options** include induction of labor or expectant home management. Plans should include bed rest, pelvic rest, and instructions to return to the hospital if a fever occurs or if contractions begin.

V. PRETERM LABOR AND DELIVERY.

The leading cause of neonatal deaths in the United States is premature delivery. In spite of extensive use of tocolytic agents, no reduction in preterm birth rates has occurred in the past 50 years. Approximately 10% of all deliveries occur prior to 37 weeks' gestation.

  A. **Risk factors for preterm delivery** (Table 6-9). Patients with a statistically higher chance for delivering prior to 37 weeks' gestation should be identified. However, most patients who deliver prematurely have no identifiable risk factors.

  B. **Criteria for preterm labor (all must be present).** Not all patients with preterm contractions are in preterm labor.

    1. **Gestational age.** Between 20 and 37 weeks of gestation must have been completed.

    2. **Contractions.** Three or more contractions in 30 minutes must have occurred, and the duration of the contractions must have been 30 seconds or longer.

Table 6-9. Risk Factors for Preterm Delivery

Socioeconomic Factors	Lifestyle Factors	Medical History	Obstetric History
Low income	Smoking	Previous preterm birth* Uterine anomalies*	Multiple pregnancy*
Low educational level	Heavy physical labor; long work hours	Bacterial vaginosis*	Short cervix*
Maternal age extremes (i.e., < 16 years; > 40 years)	Anxiety	Second trimester abortion Diethylstilbestrol (DES) exposure	Hypertension Bacteriuria
	Poor nutrition	Renal disease	Hemorrhage
		Surgery	Polyhydramnios
		Sepsis	Dilated cervix
			Effaced cervix

*Most significant factors.

      3. Cervical dilation. The patient's cervix must be dilated 2 cm or more or there must be a change in cervical dilation and effacement.

  C. Management of a patient presenting with preterm contractions

      1. Documenting preterm labor

      2. Documenting gestational age

      3. Ruling out ruptured membranes by speculum examination

      4. Ruling out contraindications to tocolysis

      5. Establishing maternal and fetal well-being

  D. Contraindications for tocolysis. It is important to identify which patients in preterm labor would benefit from an attempt to suppress the contractions. Overall, 95% of patients who satisfy the criteria for preterm labor are not candidates for tocolysis. This may be because of fetal conditions, maternal hazards, or placental-membrane circumstances as outlined in Table 6-10.

  E. Methods of tocolysis (Table 6-11). The mechanism of action of most tocolytic agents is decreasing availability of intracellular calcium or interfering with action of PGs on smooth muscle. All tocolytic agents have potentially serious maternal or fetal side effects that limit their usefulness. No tocolytic agent has been shown to prolong pregnancy significantly. Methods with no proven value include sedation and hydration.

  F. Adjunctive interventions

      1. In utero corticosteroids have been confirmed to be highly efficacious.

          a. Mechanism. In utero corticosteroids induce pulmonary surfactant production by type II pneumocytes.

          b. Specific medications include betamethasone and dexamethasone, which cross the placenta. Prednisone should not be used because it does not cross the placenta.

Table 6-10. Contraindications for Tocolysis

Fetal Contraindications	Maternal Contraindications	Placenta/Membrane Contraindications
Fetal demise	Severe preeclampsia or eclampsia	SPROM
Fetal distress	Uncontrolled hyperthyroidism	Severe abruptio placentae
Severe IUGR	Advanced cervical dilation	Unstable placenta previa
Anomalies incompatible with life	Uncontrolled diabetes	Chorioamnionitis

IUGR = intrauterine growth retardation; *SPROM* = spontaneous premature rupture of membrane.

Table 6-11. Methods or Tocolysis

	β-Adrenergic Agonist	Magnesium Sulfate	Prostaglandin Synthease Inhibitors	Calcium Channel Blockers
Mechanism	Stimulate beta receptors to relax smooth muscle	Competes for calcium ions during depolarization	Inhibits prostaglandin synthesis and release	Decreases intra-cellular calcium ions
Agent	Ritodrine Terbutaline	Magnesium sulfate	Indomethacin	Nifedipine
Side effects	Cardiovascular Pulmonary Hypokalemia Hyperglycemia	Muscle weakness Respiratory depression Pulmonary edema	PDA closure in utero Oligohydramnios Increases NEC Gastrointestinal irritation	Tachycardia Hypotension Myocardial depression
Efficacy	Delay delivery 24–48 hrs	Delay delivery 24–48 hrs	Most effective	Delay delivery 24–48 hrs

NEC = necrotizing enterocolitis; *PDA* = patent ductus arteriosus

    c. The **greatest benefit** of these medications is realized if the gestational age is less than 34 weeks, if there is more than 24-hour latency from administration to delivery, and if the fetus is female, black, and singleton.

  2. **Neonatal surfactant administration** is highly efficacious but very expensive. It is administered via an endotracheal tube.

  3. **Cervical cultures** are recommended for gonorrhea, chlamydia, and GBBS. Patients should also be assessed for bacterial vaginosis.

  4. **Group B β streptococcus prophylaxis should be administered whenever preterm delivery is likely.**

  G. **Preventive measures**

    1. **Lifestyle changes** can help prevent preterm births. These changes include:

   a. Improving nutritional status
   b. Stopping the use of tobacco
   c. Reducing stress
   d. Reducing occupational fatigue
   e. Increasing daily rest
2. **Early detection of preterm labor** is enhanced by the following:
   a. **Patient education** regarding **subtle symptoms**
      (1) Menstrual-like cramps
      (2) New low back pain
      (3) Pelvic pressure
      (4) Change in vaginal discharge
   b. **Patient education** regarding **self-palpation of contractions**
   c. **Weekly digital cervical examinations** after 24 weeks to detect effacement or dilation
   d. **Serial ultrasound cervical length measurements** are reassuring if length is greater than 30 mm.
   e. **Open communication** with medical and nursing staff
   f. **Electronic UC monitoring**

VI. OPERATIVE DELIVERY refers to any obstetric procedure in which active measures are taken to accomplish delivery. This term includes forceps, vacuum extractor, and cesarean deliveries. The benefits of any operative delivery must be weighed against its risks to the mother and fetus.

   A. **Forceps delivery.** Two matched metal branches are maneuvered into appropriate relationship with the fetal head and then articulated. Traction with the forceps augments maternal expulsive efforts in delivering the head. Rotation of the fetal head position to anterior-posterior orientation may be performed.
   1. **Prerequisites**
      a. The operator must be experienced.
      b. The cervix must be fully dilated.
      c. The membranes must be ruptured.
      d. The head must be engaged.
      e. The head must present vertex or face.
      f. There must be no significant cephalopelvic disproportion (CPD).
      g. The mother's bladder should be empty.
      h. The orientation of the head must be determined.
   2. **Risks**
      a. **Maternal lacerations** may involve the cervix, vagina, perineum, or lower uterine segment. Classification of perineal lacerations is as follows:
         (1) **First degree:** involves only mucosa
         (2) **Second degree:** involves the perineal body but not the anal sphincter

         (3) Third degree: involves the anal sphincter but not the rectal mucosa

         (4) Fourth degree: involves the rectal mucosa

    b. Fetal trauma can result from poor forceps application or excessive traction.

  3. Classification of forceps is based on the station of the leading bony part of the fetal skull when the procedure is begun. Generally speaking, the higher the station, the higher the maternal and fetal risk. **High forceps are never appropriate in modern obstetrics.**

    a. Outlet forceps. The fetal skull has reached the pelvic floor and rotation will be less than 45 degrees.

    b. Low forceps. The fetal skull is below +2 station but not on the pelvic floor.

    c. Mid forceps. The fetal skull is below 0 station (engaged) but has not reached +2 station.

    d. High forceps. The fetal skull is above 0 station (unengaged).

B. Vacuum extractor delivery. A soft silastic cup is held on the fetal head by negative pressure from a vacuum pump. Traction is applied with contractions to augment the maternal expulsive efforts to deliver the fetal head.

  1. Requirements are the same as for the use of forceps with the following exceptions:

    a. A vacuum extractor is contraindicated in preterm delivery.

    b. A vacuum extractor should never be used for breech or face presentation.

  2. Complications include the following:

    a. Vaginal mucosa entrapment leading to lacerations

    b. Fetal scalp trauma: lacerations, bruising, hemorrhage, and cephalohematomas

    c. Neonatal hyperbilirubinemia

C. Cesarean section delivery

  1. Risks

    a. Maternal risks include the following:

      (1) Bleeding or hemorrhage

      (2) Infection in the abdominal wound, uterus, lungs, bladder, or kidneys

      (3) Visceral trauma to the bowel, bladder, or ureters

    b. Fetal risks include the following:

      (1) Traumatic delivery from elevating the impacted fetal head from the pelvis

      (2) Lacerating the fetus at the time of uterine incision

  2. Indications

    a. Primary cesarean

      (1) CPD, a generic descriptive term that denotes failure to follow a normal dilation curve during labor, **is the most common indication for a primary cesarean delivery.** CPD may involve any of the following specific causes:

(a) True disproportion of fetal size to the maternal pelvis
(b) Dysfunctional labor or uterine inertia
(c) Compound presentation
(d) Malposition of the fetal head
(e) Failure of flexion of the fetal head
(f) Asynclitism of the fetal head

(2) **Malpresentation** describes a presentation other than longitudinal lie, cephalic presentation. It may include breech presentation or transverse lie (see Figure 6-4).

(3) **Nonreassuring FHR tracing** describes a variety of conditions in which a lack of fetal well-being is presumed. This condition was formerly called **fetal distress,** a term that was neither accurate nor specific. It may include true fetal acidosis or hypoxia or a non-reassuring electronic fetal monitor pattern.

b. **Repeat cesarean**

(1) **Scheduled** procedures are performed **before** the onset of labor.

(2) **Emergency** procedures are performed **after** the onset of labor.

3. **Incisions**

a. **Abdominal wall incisions** (see Chapter 13 V D)

(1) **Transverse** incision

(a) **Pfannenstiel's** ("bikini" incision)
(b) **Maylard** ("muscle-splitting" incision)

(2) **Vertical midline** incision

b. **Uterine incisions** (Figure 6-6)

(1) **Low segment transverse, the uterine incision of choice.** This is a transverse incision in the noncontractile portion of the lower uterine segment.

(a) **Advantages.** Labor can be allowed safely in a subsequent pregnancy. There is a 1% risk of silent dehiscence of a previous incision. Maternal and perinatal mortality is negligible with this type of incision, and there is less blood loss.

(b) **Disadvantages.** The lower segment may not be adequately formed if there is no labor or the fetus is of preterm gestational age. A fetus in a position other than longitudinal lie may not be deliverable. There is a risk of bladder injury to the mother.

(2) **Low vertical.** Although this incision is technically in the noncontractile portion of the lower segment, in actuality, it may or may not extend into the upper fundal uterus. An operative report description of the incision is important to decide if subsequent labor is appropriate.

(a) **Advantages.** If the low vertical incision is limited to the lower segment, it has all the advantages of the low segment transverse incision. The possibility of extending laterally into the uterine vessels or broad ligaments is less.

(b) **Disadvantages.** If the low vertical incision extends into the contractile fundal portion of the uterus, it has all the disadvantages of the classical incision.

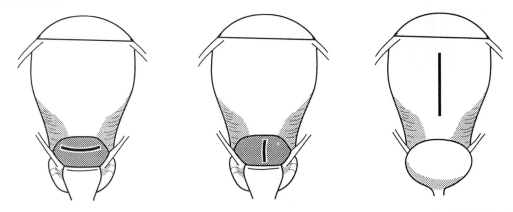

LOW SEGMENT TRANSVERSE	LOW SEGMENT VERTICAL	CLASSICAL
Advantages		
↓ Blood loss ↓ Adhesions VBAC okay after	↓ Blood loss ↓ Adhesions VBAC okay after	Any fetus(es) can be delivered regardless of orientation in uterus or gestational age
Disadvantages		
Risk of bladder injury Lower uterine segment must be formed Fetus must be in longitudinal lie	Risk of bladder injury Lower uterine segment must be formed May extend to upper segment Fetus must be in longitudinal lie	↑ Blood loss ↑ Adhesions VBAC unsafe Risk of uterine rupture

Figure 6-6. Comparison of uterine cesarean incisions. VBAC = vaginal birth after cesarean. (Adapted with permission from Gabbe SG, Niebyl JR, Simpson JL (eds): *Obstetrics: Normal and Problem Pregnancies,* 2nd ed. New York, Churchill Livingstone, 1991, p 646.)

    (3) Classical. This vertical incision is in the contractile fundal portion of the uterus.

        (a) Advantages. Any fetus(es), regardless of presentation(s), can be delivered via this incision. The classical incision can be used at any time during gestation.

        (b) Disadvantages

            (i) The **risk of uterine rupture** is 2% before or during labor with subsequent pregnancies. This is generally a catastrophic event with a 5% maternal mortality rate and 50% perinatal mortality rate.

            (ii) The **risk of blood loss and adhesion** is greater than with lower segment incisions.

  D. Vaginal delivery after a previous cesarean is possible in up to 85% of patients who attempt it. Prerequisites for a safe trial of labor include the following:

    1. Informed consent of the patient

    2. Previous lower segment transverse uterine incision

    3. Nonrepetitive indication for previous cesarean delivery

    4. No pelvic contracture

    5. Continuous electronic fetal monitoring

    6. Ability to perform an emergency repeat cesarean within 30 minutes of decision to operate

E. External cephalic version. This procedure, performed in a hospital setting, uses external uterine manipulation to change a breech presentation to cephalic presentation. The overall success rate is 65%. The **optimal gestational age** to attempt version is **37 weeks.** At an earlier gestational age, the spontaneous reversion rate is higher, whereas at a later time, the success rate is lower because of decreasing amniotic fluid.

    1. Methodology involves the following:

        a. Obtaining an ultrasound examination to confirm fetal orientation, localize placental implantation, evaluate amniotic fluid volume, and rule out fetal or uterine anomalies

        b. Confirming fetal well-being with a reactive nonstress test (NST)

        c. Administering SQ terbutaline to relax the myometrium

        d. Monitoring FHR and documenting version as the breech is displaced upward while the head is moved downward

        e. Discontinuing efforts because of excessive discomfort, persistent fetal bradycardia, or multiple failed attempts

        f. Administering Rh immune globulin if the mother is Rh negative

    2. Complications include the following:

        a. Fetomaternal hemorrhage

        b. Persistent fetal bradycardia

Review Test

Directions: Each of the numbered items or incomplete statements in this section is followed by answers or by completions of the statement. Select the **ONE** lettered answer or completion that is **BEST** in each case.

1. Which one of the following statements regarding myometrial anatomy and physiology is true?

(A) Uterine enlargement in pregnancy occurs by cellular hypertrophy alone.
(B) Myosin is the largest molecule responsible for myometrial contractility.
(C) Myometrial cell growth is inhibited by progesterone.
(D) Myometrial gap junctions are promoted by progesterone.

2. A 21-year-old multigravida at 39 weeks' gestation is 2 cm dilated on cervical examination. She has been experiencing regular, painful uterine contractions (UCs) for the past 15 hours, but her cervical dilation has not significantly changed from when she first came to the maternity unit. Which one of the following conditions is the most likely cause of her failure to dilate?

(A) Excessive fetal size
(B) Contracted pelvis
(C) Abnormal fetal lie
(D) Chorioamnionitis
(E) Injudicious analgesia

3. A 30-year-old primigravida at 41 weeks' gestation was admitted to the maternity unit 4 hours ago with a cervical dilation of 5 cm. Over the next 2 hours, it progressed to 8 cm. For the past 2 hours, her dilation has not changed. Which one of the following questions is the most significant in preparing a management plan for this patient?

(A) What is the estimated fetal weight?
(B) How adequate are the uterine contractions (UCs)?
(C) What are the dimensions of the pelvic inlet?
(D) What is the gestational age?
(E) What is the position of the fetal presenting part?

4. A 34-year-old multipara is in active labor. Her cervix has been dilated 5 cm for the past 3 hours without any change. Her uterine contractions (UCs) are being measured using external tocodynamometry. Which of the following parameters cannot be assessed using this monitoring modality?

(A) Onset of contractions
(B) End of contractions
(C) Intensity of contractions
(D) Frequency of contractions
(E) Duration of contractions

5. A 22-year-old multipara (gravida 2, para 1) presents for her first prenatal visit at 12 weeks' gestation. Her previous pregnancy was complicated by a preterm delivery at 31 weeks' gestation. Which one of the following conditions is the most significant risk factor for preterm delivery with this pregnancy?

(A) Bacteriuria
(B) Heavy maternal work
(C) Previous second-trimester abortion
(D) Previous preterm birth
(E) Uterine anomaly

6. A 24-year-old primigravida has just undergone a spontaneous vaginal delivery of a 4100-g male neonate with Apgar scores of 7 and 8 at 1 and 5 minutes, respectively. On inspecting the perineum, you note a laceration that extends from the vaginal introitus through the entire perineal body but does not involve the anal sphincter or rectal mucosa. The degree of obstetrical laceration described is

(A) first degree
(B) second degree
(C) third degree
(D) fourth degree

Directions: Each of the numbered items or incomplete statements in this section is negatively phrased, as indicated by a capitalized work such as NOT, LEAST, or EXCEPT. Select the ONE lettered answer or completion that is BEST in each case.

7. All of the following factors are associated with cervical ripening EXCEPT

(A) prostaglandin E_2 (PGE_2)
(B) estrogen
(C) mechanical stretching
(D) progesterone
(E) relaxin

8. All of the following statements are true regarding the cardinal movements of labor EXCEPT

(A) they allow descent of fetus using the path of least resistance
(B) they are dependent on force generated by uterine contractions (UCs)
(C) they involve all three stages of labor
(D) they result in internal and external rotation of the head
(E) they end with delivery of the entire fetus

9. All of the following are true statements regarding amniotic fluid EXCEPT

(A) it is supplied mostly from fetal urine production
(B) it protects the umbilical cord from compression
(C) it contains pulmonary surfactant
(D) it is secreted by fetal gastrointestinal (GI) tract
(E) it provides space for fetal movement

Directions: The set of matching questions in this section consists of a list of four to twenty-six lettered options (some of which may be in figures) followed by several numbered items. For each numbered item, select the ONE lettered option that is most closely associated with it. To avoid spending tco much time on matching sets with large numbers of options, it is generally advisable to begin each set by reading the list of options. Then, for each item in the set, try to generate the correct answer and locate it in the option list, rather than evaluating each option individually. Each lettered option may be selected once, more than once, or not at all.

Questions 10–14

For each of the following characteristics, select the stage of labor that is more appropriate.
(A) Stage I
(B) Stage II
(C) Stage III

10. Ends with delivery of the placenta

11. Starts with onset of regular contractions

12. Consists of two phases

13. Stage of maximum cervical dilation slope

14. Stage in which cardinal labor movements are completed

Answers and Explanations

1. The answer is B [I A].

Smooth muscle contraction occurs when the large myosin molecules and the smaller actin molecules slide over each other. To say that uterine enlargement in pregnancy occurs by cellular hypertrophy alone is incorrect, because both cellular hypertrophy and hyperplasia contribute to uterine enlargement in pregnancy. Progesterone enhances, not inhibits, myometrial cell growth. Progesterone inhibits myometrial gap junction formation.

2. The answer is E [II B 1].

The patient described in the question is, by definition, in the latent phase of the first stage of labor, which is the time period from the onset of regular contractions to the point where a change in the slope of cervical dilation is noted (usually 3–4 cm dilation). In this case, 15 hours have passed since the onset of contractions; when the latent phase lasts more than 14 hours in a multipara, it is said to be prolonged. The most common cause of a prolonged latent phase is administration of analgesics before the active phase of labor is well established. Excessive fetal size, contracted pelvis, abnormal fetal lie, and chorioamnionitis are incorrect, because they are associated with abnormalities of the active, not the latent, phase of the first stage of labor.

3. The answer is B [II B 3 b].

The patient described in this question has demonstrated active phase arrest of cervical dilation. The adequacy of uterine contractions (UCs) is the most important question to ask because inadequate UCs can be remedied most easily by administering oxytocin. Active phase labor arrest is diagnosed when there is no progression in cervical dilation for 2 hours or more. This problem may be related to the *p*elvis (i.e., size of the birth canal), the *p*assenger (i.e., the size, lie, presentation, or position of the fetus), or the *p*owers (i.e., intensity, frequency, or duration of UCs). Although the estimated fetal weight, dimensions of the pelvic inlet, gestational age, and position of the fetal presenting part may all be associated with active phase arrest, they are either not amenable to change or subject to only limited modification.

4. The answer is C [III B 1 b].

Measurement of contraction intensity cannot be standardized with an external monitor. The reason for this inability is that the mechanism of external tocodynamometry is based on a strain gauge that detects changes in the indentability of the maternal abdominal wall as the uterus undergoes the cycle of contracting and relaxing. However, the indentability is extremely variable, depending on the abdominal wall thickness and maternal obesity. Onset, end, frequency, and duration of contractions can usually be accurately measured by external tocodynamometry.

5. The answer is D [V B; Table 6-8].

Preterm delivery is the leading cause of perinatal morbidity and mortality in the United States. Approximately 10% of infants are born prematurely, and that percentage has changed little during the past 30 years. Prevention of preterm birth requires knowledge of the risk factors, the highest risk factor being previous preterm birth. Bacteriuria, heavy maternal work, previous second-trimester abortion, and uterine anomaly are also risk factors, but not as significant as previous preterm birth.

6. The answer is B [VI A 2 a].

The degree of laceration described by involvement of the perineal body is the second-degree type. First-degree lacerations involve only the mucosa. Third-degree lacerations extend through the anal sphincter, but not the anal mucosa, and fourth-degree lacerations that are either repaired poorly or that heal unsuccessfully can result in anal incontinence or rectovaginal fistulae.

7. The answer is D [I B 2 c].

Progesterone is the correct answer (but incorrect statement) because progesterone antagonists, not progesterone itself, are used for cervical ripening. Cervical ripening allows the cervix to become soft, distensible, and compliant in preparation for dilating and effacement. During this process, the collagen chains are fractured and solubilized. Various agents are available for accomplishing this purpose artificially. Prostaglandin E_2 (PGE$_2$), estrogen, mechanical stretching, and relaxin are all cervical ripening agents.

8. The answer is C [I D 2; Table 6-2].

The cardinal movements of labor do not involve all three stages of labor; the infant is already delivered by the time the third stage of labor begins. The cardinal movements of labor are changes in position and flexion that the fetal head goes through during its passage through the pelvis, which are necessary because of the asymmetry of the shape of the fetal head and maternal bony pelvis. All the other statements concerning the cardinal movements are correct: they allow descent of fetus using the path of least resistance, they are dependent on force generated by uterine contractions (UCs), they result in internal and external rotation of the head, and they end with delivery of the entire fetus are all correct statements.

9. The answer is D [IV A 1].

The fetal gastrointestinal (GI) tract decreases the amount of amniotic fluid by swallowing rather than increasing it by secretion. Amniotic fluid serves a vital function in the prenatal life of the fetus. The other options are correct because fetal urine production is the primary source of amniotic fluid, amniotic fluid protects the cord from compression, it is secreted by the fetal lung along with pulmonary surfactant, and it provides space for fetal movement within the uterus.

10–14. The answers are: 10-C, 11-A, 12-A, 13-A, 14-B [I D 1–3; Table 6-1].

Stage III of labor begins with delivery of the fetus and ends with placental delivery. Stage I begins with the start of regular uterine contractions (UCs) and ends with complete dilation of the cervix. Stage I has both a latent phase and an active phase. The active phase of stage I includes the period of maximum cervical dilation. The cardinal movements of labor begin in stage I but are completed in stage II.

7

The Puerperium

I. NORMAL PUERPERIUM

A. Background

1. **Formally, the puerperium** was usually considered to be the first 6 weeks after birth, beginning with delivery of the placenta and ending with return of the reproductive organs to their nonpregnant state.

2. **Actually, the puerperium** varies according to the organ system involved.

   a. Many pregnancy alterations have reversed **within 1 week.**

   b. Some alterations persist **past 6 weeks.**

   c. Other changes are **permanent.**

B. Involution of the reproductive tract

1. **Uterine corpus.** The number of myometrial cells is unchanged, but the size of the cells decreases to one-twentieth of that during pregnancy.

   a. **Immediately postdelivery,** the uterus weighs 1000 g and is at the umbilicus.

   b. **After 1 week,** the uterus weighs 500 g.

   c. **After 2 weeks,** the uterus weighs 300 g and once again becomes a pelvic organ.

   d. **After 3 weeks,** the uterus weighs 100 g.

2. **Endometrial regeneration**

   a. The **superficial layer of decidua** becomes necrotic and is sloughed off as **lochia.**

      (1) **Lochia rubra,** which is red, is sloughed off immediately after delivery.

      (2) **Lochia serosa,** which is pinkish-yellow, is sloughed off during the first postpartum week.

      (3) **Lochia alba,** which is whitish, is sloughed off after the second postpartum week.

   b. The **basalis layer** of the decidua is the source of new endometrial regeneration.

    c. Within 7 to 10 days, new epithelial regeneration is established. By the end of the third postpartum week, total regeneration is complete.

  3. Placental site involution. Within hours of delivery, multiple thrombosed vessels are seen at the site of placental implantation. Exfoliation of the site causes necrotic slough of infarcted tissues, which is followed by a reparative regeneration. Complete extrusion of the placental site takes up to 6 weeks. If the process is defective, **delayed puerperal hemorrhage** may occur (even weeks after delivery).

  4. Uterine vessels. Hypertrophied vessels undergo obliteration by hyalinization and are replaced by smaller caliber vessels.

  5. Cervix. After delivery, the cervix is a thin, collapsed, flabby structure that slowly contracts. Lateral lacerations are usually present at the external os (outer cervical margin).

    a. By the end of the first week, the external os admits only one finger.

    b. The cervix gradually thickens, and the canal reforms.

    c. The external os then is no longer round; it becomes fish-mouthed at old lacerations.

  6. Vagina. After delivery, the vagina gradually decreases in size, but it does not return to nulliparous dimensions. Rugae reappear by the third postpartum week, and the hymen converts to parous **myriform caruncles.**

  7. Abdominal wall. The soft and flabby abdominal wall takes weeks to return to normal. Exercise hastens recovery. **Diastasis recti abdominis** is found if the rectus muscles separate in midline.

C. Changes in nonreproductive organs

  1. Urinary system

    a. The **urinary bladder** is particularly susceptible to **urinary retention.**

      (1) Impact of labor and delivery. The bladder base may be traumatized by labor and delivery. Mucosa may be edematous and hyperemic. Epidural anesthesia may decrease the sensation of fullness, and perineal pain may inhibit normal voiding. Mobilization of third-space fluid may lead to polyuria. These factors may contribute to the following:

        (a) Bladder overdistention with myogenic decompensation leading to residual detrusor atony

        (b) Incomplete emptying with increased postvoid residuals

        (c) Susceptibility to urinary tract infections (UTIs)

      (2) Management of any complications involving the urinary bladder may include the following:

        (a) Intermittent catheterization every 6 hours

        (b) Use of an indwelling catheter if marked bladder distention occurs

        (c) UTI prophylaxis (i.e., acidification, antibiotics)

        (d) UTI therapy (i.e., antibiotic based on culture bacteriology)

        (e) Cholinergic medications to increase detrusor muscle tone

    b. Kidneys. Mild proteinuria is noted in 50% of women for 1–2 days. Creatinine clearance returns to prepregnancy values in 1 week. Dilation of ureters and renal pelves reverses within 6 weeks. Renal hypertrophy may persist for a few months.

2. **Fluid balance changes.** More than 10 L of fluid is lost during the puerperium. Approximately 2 L of fluid is lost during the first week, and approximately 1.5 L is lost during each of the next 5 weeks.

3. **Metabolic changes**
   a. **Lipid values.** Total and free fatty acids become normal 2 days after delivery. Cholesterol and triglycerides return to normal values in 6–8 weeks.
   b. **Blood glucose.** Fasting and postprandial values decrease rapidly, reaching a nadir on the third day. Stabilization of insulin and glucose values requires approximately 1 week. Diabetic insulin requirements decrease rapidly. Early puerperal glucose tolerance tests are of limited value.

4. **Blood volume changes**
   a. **Normal delivery blood loss values**
      (1) **Vaginal delivery: 500 ml**
      (2) **Cesarean delivery: 1000 ml**
      (3) **Cesarean hysterectomy: 1500 ml**
   b. **Total blood volume** is normalized by 3 weeks postdelivery, with most change occurring during the first week.
      (1) In **normal patients,** the hematocrit value increases within the first week.
      (2) In **patients with preeclampsia,** the hematocrit value may decrease as a result of the resolution of peripheral vasoconstriction or of the mobilization of excess extracellular fluid into the intravascular space.
      (3) **Delivery of the placenta** removes a low-resistance shunt, decreases the maternal vascular bed size by 15%, and ends placental hormonal stimulus of vasodilation.

5. **Cardiac work changes.** Immediately after delivery, cardiac work values peak at 80% higher than prelabor values because of the **autotransfusion of uteroplacental blood.** Peripheral vascular resistance (PVR) rises because of the loss of the low-resistance placental shunt, which results in a 15% decrease in the size of the maternal vascular bed. PVR returns to prepregnancy levels within 3 weeks.

6. **Respiratory changes**
   a. **Rapid normalization** of residual volume (RV) and functional residual capacity (FRC) occurs. Decreases in uterine size allow abdominal organs to return to their prepregnancy position and allow increased thoracic cage capacity (i.e., increased RV, increased FRC).
   b. **Slower normalization** of other pulmonary parameters (e.g., expiratory reserve volume, inspiratory capacity, vital capacity) occurs.

7. **Endocrine changes**
   a. A precipitous **decrease** in the following placentally produced **plasma hormone concentrations** occurs.
      (1) **Human placental lactogen (hPL)** is undetectable 1 day after delivery.

(2) **Human chorionic gonadotropin (hCG)** is undetectable by day 14 postdelivery.

(3) **Estradiol** levels decrease 90% within 3 hours, with a nadir at postpartum day 7. The decrease in estradiol level coincides with breast engorgement on postpartum days 3 and 4. There is a variable latent period of estradiol return to follicular phase levels in women who are:

(a) Nonlactating: 20 days

(b) Lactating with menses: 70 days

(c) Lactating but amenorrheic: 180 days

b. Maternal **prolactin** concentrations normalize within 2 weeks in non-lactating women. Lactating women experience a gradual decrease, but basal levels remain increased.

c. **Spontaneous menstruation** occurs earlier in nonlactating women than in lactating women. However, 75% women in both groups are ovulating within 9 months (Table 7-1).

D. Conduct in the normal puerperium

1. Emotional response

a. After delivery, most women experience joy and happiness on seeing their healthy infant. The negative and abnormal emotional responses of **postpartum blues, postpartum depression, and postpartum psychosis** are summarized in Table 7-2.

b. **Mother–infant bonding** is the physical and emotional contact that nurtures normal mothering responses.

(1) **Bonding may be adversely affected by the following factors:**

(a) Delayed contact with neonate because of prematurity or neonatal illness

(b) Lack of social support (e.g., spousal rejection, distant friends and family)

(2) **Management** involves counseling to assist mothers in working through the issues that are affecting them.

2. Bladder care. Overdistention of the bladder should be avoided. Intermittent catheterization should be used if necessary.

a. Indwelling catheterization should be used if the bladder contains more than 1000 ml urine.

b. Prophylactic urine acidification or antibiotics should be considered.

c. A postvoiding residual of less than 250 ml is the goal before leaving

Table 7-1. Percentage of Women Spontaneously Menstruating Postpartum

Weeks Postpartum	Nonlactating (%)	Lactating (%)
6	45	15
12	70	30
36	75	75

Table 7-2. Postpartum Emotional Responses

Category	Findings	Incidence	Relationship to Self and Infant	Postpartum Time Frame	Management
Postpartum blues	Feelings of inadequacy, tearfulness, mood swings, fatigue, and headache	50%–80%	Personal appearance with care of self and infant maintained	• Day 3–10 • Often history of PMS	• Reassurance • Rooming-in • No medications needed
Postpartum depression	More severe symptoms with feelings of despair, hopelessness, and anxiety	5%–25%	Personal appearance with care of self and infant neglected	• Weeks 2–6 • Can last for months • High recurrence rate	• Psychotherapy • Antidepressants often helpful • Seldom needs hospitalization
Postpartum psychosis	Impairment of reality perception with hallucinations and delusions	1–2 per 1000 deliveries	May express ideation to harm self and/or infant	• Within first 3 weeks • High recurrence rate	• Psychotherapy • Antipsychotic medications are necessary • Hospitalization required

PMS = premenstrual syndrome

the hospital. If this is not achieved, patients may need to go home with an indwelling catheter.

3. **Bowel care**
   a. **Puerperal constipation** is common.
      (1) **Contributing factors** include:
         (a) Decreased puerperal gastrointestinal (GI) motility
         (b) Reflex ileus from perineal pain
         (c) Loss of excess fluid
      (2) **Management** includes oral hydration and stool softeners.
   b. **Hemorrhoids** are a common complaint, and they are related to the length of the second stage of labor. Management includes stool softeners and sitz baths.

4. **Bathing hygiene.** A sitz bath is safe the second day after delivery. Water does not enter the vagina.

5. **Episiotomy and laceration care**
   a. **Ice packs** (first 24 hours) decrease perineal edema.
   b. **Dry heat** (lamp) [after the first day] promotes mobilization of tissue fluid. Gentle washing with soap and water is recommended after voiding and defecation.
   c. **Daily inspection** should be performed to rule out hematoma or infection.

6. **Rh$_o$(D) immune globulin** is administered when indicated to prevent maternal isoimmunization.

    a. Criteria for Rh$_0$(D) immune globulin administration (both must be present)

        (1) The mother is Rh negative (D−) without active anti-D antibodies [a low titer is noted if 28-week prophylactic Rh$_0$(D) immune globulin was given].

        (2) The infant is Rh positive (D+) or Du positive.

    b. Management includes intramuscular (IM) administration of 300 mg Rh$_0$(D) immune globulin within 72 hours of delivery to block antigens on 15 ml of fetal red blood cells (RBCs) [see Chapter 3 VI]. If a larger fetomaternal bleed occurs, multiple vials of Rh$_0$(D) immune globulin should be administered.

7. Rubella immunization is administered to induce active immunity in rubella-susceptible women. An IM vaccine of live attenuated rubella virus results in seroconversion in 90% of women. Lactation is not a contraindication, but pregnancy should be avoided for 3 months. Arthralgia or rash are common side effects.

8. Sexual relations

    a. Normalization of the sexual response cycle may be delayed up to 3 months. Genital vasocongestion and lubrication may be delayed for 2 months.

    b. Penis-in-vagina intercourse may be resumed by week 3 postdelivery, if desired. Approximately 50% of women report return of sexual desire by week 3.

    c. Complicating factors of sexual relations after delivery include the following:

        (1) Perineal pain from episiotomy and lacerations

        (2) Fatigue and weakness from lack of sleep

        (3) Vaginal atrophy from hypoestrogenic lactational state (vaginal estrogen cream may be used to combat this)

        (4) Milk ejection during sexual relations (nursing the infant before intimate relations can help minimize this response)

9. Contraception

    a. Breastfeeding is epidemiologically significant in decreasing the birth rate, but it is not a reliable method alone for individuals. There is an 8% pregnancy rate in women with lactational amenorrhea and a 36% pregnancy rate in women with lactation and menses. Ovulation is unusual in breastfeeding women for 3 months following delivery.

    b. Vaginal diaphragm. Fitting should be delayed until the 6-week postpartum visit to allow vaginal involution. A larger size may be needed than was appropriate prior to pregnancy.

    c. Hormonal contraception

        (1) Mini-pills (progestin-only) may be started immediately. There is no impact on thromboembolic complications, and milk yield is not decreased.

        (2) Combination oral contraceptive pills should not be started until at least week 3 to allow reversal of the hypercoagulable state of pregnancy. The estrogen component may diminish milk production.

(3) Injectable methods. A 150-mg IM injection of depomedroxyprogesterone acetate (DMPA) may be administered in the hospital. There is no impact on thromboembolic complications, and milk yield is not decreased.

d. Intrauterine contraceptive device (IUD). Placement is best deferred until the 6-week postpartum visit. With IUD placement immediately postdelivery, the expulsion rate is up to 20%.

II. POSTPARTUM HEMORRHAGE (PPH). Excessive blood loss (i.e., > 500 ml during the first 24 hours postpartum) after the delivery of an infant is known as PPH. It can occur before, during, or after delivery of the placenta.

A. Epidemiology

1. The **incidence** of PPH is 10%.

2. **Pathophysiology** follows a predictable sequence:
   a. In healthy women, vital signs undergo only a only minimal change, even with significant blood loss.
   b. With continued bleeding, only gradual deterioration is noted.
   c. Decompensation occurs suddenly, manifested by tachycardia, hypotension, dyspnea, and diaphoresis.

3. **Sequelae** include the following:
   a. **Acute blood loss,** if not stopped, leads to death.
   b. **Chronic blood loss** results in anemia, which weakens patients, lowers resistance, and predisposes to puerperal infection.
   c. **Sheehan's syndrome** is a hazard of PPH that results in **anterior pituitary insufficiency** in women of childbearing age.
      (1) Mechanism. The pregnancy-associated increase in vascularity renders the pituitary gland susceptible to hypoperfusion. Massive obstetric hemorrhage leads to severe shock, resulting in pituitary ischemia and necrosis. The onset of symptoms may be rapid or can develop gradually over many years.
      (2) Symptoms. Because necrosis can be partial or total, symptoms may vary.
         (a) Failure to lactate is the most common presentation because of decreased prolactin levels.
         (b) Weakness, lethargy, and cold hypersensitivity result from a decreased level of adrenocorticotropic hormone (ACTH).
         (c) Excessive uterine involution, genital atrophy, and menstrual disorders result from decreased levels of follicle-stimulating hormone (FSH) and luteinizing hormone (LH).

B. General supportive measures

1. **Volume expansion** is the key to successful treatment.
   a. Blood that is transfused should be equivalent to replace at least the amount lost.
   b. Plasma expanders (i.e., crystalloids, colloids) should be used until blood is available.

    c. If the response to volume expansion is unsatisfactory, the following possibilities should be considered:

        (1) Continued unappreciated oozing

        (2) Blood collection into an atonic uterus, behind a uterine pack, or silently filling the vagina

        (3) Hematoma formation not identified

        (4) Intraperitoneal bleed (e.g., ruptured uterus)

        (5) Disseminated intravascular coagulopathy (DIC)

        (6) Bacteremic shock

2. The foot of the bed should be elevated to enhance venous return and maintain perfusion of vital organs.

3. General anesthesia should be discontinued, and high-flow oxygen should be administered by face mask to maintain tissue oxygenation.

4. Warm blankets should be used to maintain body heat and to minimize oxygen requirements.

5. Patients should be sedated with morphine to relieve anxiety and decrease cardiopulmonary stress.

C. Uterine atony is the most common cause of PPH (50%) and it should be suspected if the uterus is boggy and enlarged (Table 7-3).

    1. Mechanism. Contraction of interlacing myometrial fibers and retraction of myometrial blood vessels cut off blood flow to the placental site, which controls uterine bleeding. Failure of myometrial contraction, from any cause, results in ongoing hemorrhage from the placental site vessels.

Table 7-3. Approach to Postpartum Hemorrhage

Diagnosis to Consider	Clinical Finding	Management Plan
Uterine atony **(most common cause)**	Uterus is boggy and enlarged on palpation	• Uterine massage • Bimanual uterine compression • Remove intrauterine clots • Administer oxytocin, methergine, or prostaglandins
Undiagnosed tears involving episiotomy, cervix, vagina, or uterus	Bleeding is present from genital tract lacerations	Repair lacerations and extensions
Retained placental fragments	Placenta is not complete on examination	• Manual uterine exploration • Uterine curettage
Disseminated intravascular coagulopathy	Generalized bleeding, purpura, petechiae	• Remove all placental tissue • Intensive care unit support • Selective blood product replacement
Uterine inversion	Uterus is not palpable on abdominal examination	Uterine replacement by elevation of vaginal fornices
All else has failed	Persistent, unexplained, uncontrollable bleeding	• Uterine artery ligation • Internal iliac artery ligation • Hysterectomy

2. **Risk factors** include primary myometrial dysfunction, pharmacologic causes, and uterine overdistention (Table 7-4).

3. **Management**
   a. **External uterine massage may help reverse uterine atony.** The myometrial smooth muscle fibers contract in response to tactile stimulation.
   b. **Bimanual uterine compression** provides twice the uterine stimulation as uterine massage alone. The atonic uterus is elevated and anteverted with one hand placed in the vagina, and the other hand is placed on the abdomen and used to bring the uterus down over the symphysis pubis. The uterus is massaged with both hands while compression is maintained.
   c. **Uterotonic medications** should be administered promptly to obtain and maintain myometrial contractions.
      (1) **Oxytocin:** 20–40 U in 1 L of crystalloid should be given by intravenous (IV) infusion at a rate of 1–15 ml/min.
      (2) **Methylergonovine:** 0.2 mg can be administered IM unless the patient is hypertensive.
      (3) **Prostaglandin 15-methyl F_{2a}** (dinoprost): Up to three vials can be administered IM.
   d. **Manual exploration of the uterus** ensures that all placental parts have been delivered and that the uterus is intact. A freshly gloved hand is placed through the cervix, and the fingers are swept across the entire surface of the uterus from the fundus to the lower segment.
   e. **Uterine packing** was widely used in the past with the goal of tamponading bleeding placental vessels. However, this technique is no longer recommended because the uterus can passively distend, thereby allowing a large volume of blood to accumulate behind the packing.

Table 7-4.   Risk Factors for Postpartum Hemorrhage

Uterine Atony	Genital Tract Lacerations	Retained Placenta	Disseminated Intravascular Coagulopathy	Uterine Inversion
Primary myometrial dysfunction • Rapid and protracted labor • Chorioamnionitis • Grandmultipara	Uncontrolled vaginal delivery Forceps delivery Vacuum extractor delivery	Accessory placental lobes Abnormal trophoblastic invasion • Placenta accreta • Placenta increta • Placenta percreta	Abruptio placentae Severe preeclampsia Amniotic fluid embolus Prolonged fetal demise	Fundal placental implantation Partial placenta accreta
Pharamcologic • Magnesium sulfate • Halogenated general anesthetics	Internal podalic version			Congenital or myometrial weakness
Uterine overdistention • Fetal macrosomia • Multiple pregnancy • Polyhydramnios				Previous uterine inversion

    f. Uterine or internal iliac artery ligation requires exploratory laparotomy and is used when conservative measures fail.

    g. Emergency hysterectomy is used only as a last resort but can be effective and lifesaving if performed in time.

D. Genital tract laceration. The second most common cause of PPH is genital tract laceration (20%), which most often occurs after either an uncontrolled spontaneous vaginal delivery or an instrumental delivery.

    1. Clinical findings

        a. Bright red bleeding is noted in the presence of a well-contracted uterus.

        b. Laceration of vaginal or vulvar vessels can cause unrecognized concealed hemorrhage, resulting in large hematomas.

        c. Episiotomy bleeding can occur with retraction of the large vessels beyond the apex or when large varicosities are involved.

        d. Cervical lacerations occur mostly at three and nine o'clock on the cervix.

        e. Spontaneous rupture of the uterus is rare. It is important to differentiate a true transmural laceration from dehiscence of a previous cesarean scar (see Chapter 3 III A 4).

    2. Risk factors include uncontrolled vaginal delivery, forceps or vacuum extractor delivery, and internal podalic version (see Table 7-4).

    3. Management

        a. Adequate analgesia or anesthesia should be ensured.

        b. Lacerations should be sutured promptly.

        c. Hematomas should be explored and evacuated. Bleeding vessels should be identified and ligated, leaving the cavity open to drain.

        d. Uterine rupture can often be repaired leaving reproductive potential intact. Emergency hysterectomy may be required if repair is not feasible.

E. Retained placenta. The third most common cause of PPH is retained placenta (10%), which can usually be identified by careful examination of the placenta. Persistently attached placenta prevents complete implantation site retraction. There is no correlation between the amount of placenta remaining and the severity of hemorrhage.

    1. Clinical findings

        a. On examination of the maternal surface of the placenta, the absence of one or more cotyledons may be noted.

        b. On examination of the fetal surface of the placenta, vessels may be found extending past the placental disk onto the membrane surface, suggesting an **accessory (succenturiate) lobe.**

        c. The third stage of labor may be prolonged. When manual placental removal is attempted, a cleavage plane cannot be identified in the presence of abnormal trophoblastic invasion.

    2. Abnormal trophoblastic invasion

        a. Incidence. Abnormal trophoblastic invasion occurs in 1 in 50,000 deliveries.

b. **Mechanism. Nitabuch's layer** is either defective or absent in the uterine decidua basalis, which allows deeper penetration of the villi to varying degrees into the uterine wall (Figure 7-1). A presumptive diagnosis must be made clinically, because a definitive diagnosis is made only on histologic examination of the uterus.

   (1) **Placenta accreta** is the most common type (80%) with villi invading the decidua basalis but not the myometrium.

   (2) **Placenta increta** is uncommon (15%) with villi invading the myometrium (but not the full thickness).

   (3) **Placenta percreta** is the rarest type (5%) with villi penetrating the full myometrium into the uterine serosa or the bladder.

3. **Risk factors** include accessory placental lobes and abnormal trophoblastic invasion (see Table 7-4).

4. **Management**

   a. **Manual uterine exploration** is imperative immediately to detect any retained placental cotyledons or accessory lobes.

   b. **Uterine curettage** under simultaneous ultrasound guidance should be performed to ensure complete removal of placental fragments. Excessive curettage, particularly in an infected uterus, can result in focal complete removal of the endometrium, resulting in **Asherman's syndrome.**

   c. **Emergency hysterectomy** must be undertaken to save the mother's life if hemorrhage continues unabated with presumed placenta accreta. This is particularly true if the placenta is implanted over a previous cesarean scar.

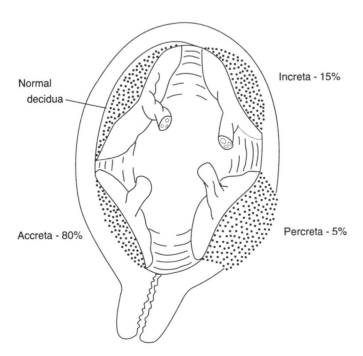

Normal decidua

Increta - 15%

Accreta - 80%

Percreta - 5%

Figure 7-1. Uteroplacental relationships found in abnormal placentation: placenta accreta, placenta increta, placenta percreta. (Reprinted with permission from Gabbe SG, Niebyl JR, Simpson JL (eds): *Obstetrics: Normal and Problem Pregnancies,* 2nd ed. New York, Churchill Livingstone, 1991, p 588.)

F. Disseminated intravascular coagulopathy (DIC), an uncommon cause of PPH, is a secondary phenomenon resulting from an underlying disease state.

1. Mechanism

a. Inappropriate activation of the coagulation cascade within the maternal systemic circulation results from:

(1) Endothelial cell injury

(2) Release of tissue thromboplastin from autolysis of the decidua and placenta

(3) Release of phospholipid from RBC or platelet injury

b. If widespread, DIC can lead to:

(1) Increased platelet aggregation, with resulting thrombocytopenia

(2) Consumption of coagulation factors, leading to prolonged prothrombin time (PT) and partial thromboplastin time (PTT)

(3) Secondary activation of the fibrinolytic system, leading to hypofibrinogenemia and an increased level of fibrin split products

(4) Deposition of fibrin into multiple organ sites, resulting in ischemic damage

2. Diagnostic findings

a. DIC should be suspected in the presence of risk factors and the finding of generalized bleeding, purpura, or petechiae.

b. Histologic findings of **fibrin deposits** provide the only **definitive diagnosis** of DIC.

c. Laboratory tests may provide indirect evidence of DIC as follows:

(1) Prolonged PT, PTT, and bleeding time

(2) Decreased platelet count (< 100,000/ml) and serum fibrinogen level (< 150 mg/dl)

(3) Increased levels of fibrin split products

(4) Peripheral blood smear showing schistocytes, fragmented RBCs, and helmet cells

3. Risk factors include abruptio placentae, severe preeclampsia, amniotic fluid embolus, and prolonged fetal demise (see Table 7-4).

4. Management

a. Removal of placental tissue from the uterus is the only way to alleviate obstetrically caused DIC.

b. Supportive intensive care involves correction of shock, acidosis, and tissue ischemia.

c. Blood component therapy should be initiated only if clinically indicated. Even with massive hemorrhage, most obstetrical DIC can be managed without transfusion.

d. Heparin therapy is generally ineffective for treatment of obstetric DIC, with the exception of cases related to prolonged fetal demise.

G. Uterine inversion. The prolapse of the fundus to or through the cervix is known as uterine inversion, resulting in the uterus essentially being turned inside out. It is a rare cause of PPH.

1. Clinical findings

a. Shock is often out of proportion to estimated blood loss.

    b. With **complete inversion,** a dark, beefy-appearing bleeding mass is visible inside the vagina or outside the introitus.

    c. With **incomplete inversion,** the mass may be only palpable or visible at the cervix.

2. Risk factors include fundal placental implantation, partial placenta accreta, congenital or myometrial weakness, and previous uterine inversion (see Table 7-4).

3. Management (Figure 7-2)

    a. Acute inversion is diagnosed shortly after delivery while the cervix is still dilated. The uterus can be manually repositioned by elevating the fornices and pushing upward in the axis of the uterus using general anesthesia if necessary.

    b. Chronic inversion is not diagnosed until after cervical contraction has occurred around the prolapsed uterus, trapping it in the vagina. Uterine replacement requires exploratory laparotomy. A vertical posterior lower uterine segment incision is made, the uterus is repositioned by pulling from above, and the uterine wound is sutured in the usual fashion.

H. Prevention

1. Antepartum measures

    a. Every woman should know her blood type and Rh factor.

    b. Antepartum anemia should be identified and treated.

    c. Risk factors for PPH should be identified.

    d. If significant risk factors are noted, adequate units of packed RBCs should be cross-matched and available before delivery.

2. Intrapartum measures

    a. An IV infusion should be started before delivery.

    b. Oxytocin should be added via IV to ensure adequate uterine contractility after the placenta is expelled.

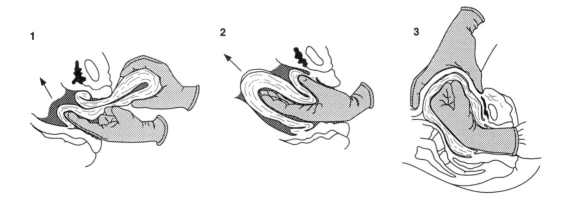

Figure 7-2. Replacement of an inverted uterus. (Reprinted with permission from DeCherney AH, Pernoll ML (eds): *Current Obstetric and Gynecologic Diagnosis and Treatment,* 8th ed. Norwalk, Conn., Appleton & Lange, 1994, p 582.)

3. Postpartum measures

a. Excessive and prolonged inhalation anesthesia should be avoided, because it can prevent myometrial contractions that close the venous sinuses at the placental site.

b. Squeezing or kneading the uterus before the placenta has separated should be avoided.

c. As soon as the placenta has separated, it should be expelled from the uterus to allow closure of the venous sinuses at the placental site.

d. Oxytocin should be administered after delivery of the placenta.

e. Patients should be observed carefully for at least 1 hour postpartum. The oxytocin infusion should continue as should palpation of the uterus to prevent it from filling with blood.

III. PUERPERAL INFECTION

A. Epidemiology

1. The **incidence** of postpartum infection after vaginal delivery is 1%–3%. After cesarean delivery, the incidence is 15%–30%.

2. **Bacterial pathogenesis** in pregnant women involves the same polymicrobial genital tract flora as in nonpregnant women.

a. **Anaerobes** constitute the **majority** of organisms (70%), including:

(1) Anaerobic cocci

(2) Peptococci, streptococci, and peptostreptococci

(3) Bacteroides species, including *Bacteroides fragilis*

b. **Aerobes** constitute the **minority** of organisms (30%), including:

(1) Enteric bacilli, including *Escherichia coli*

(2) Enterococci

(3) Streptococci, including α- and β-hemolytic species

3. **Criteria for postpartum febrile morbidity** include a temperature of 100.4°F (38°C) or higher that occurs on two separate occasions at least 24 hours apart after the first 24 hours after delivery (Table 7-5).

4. **General risk factors** include prolonged rupture of membranes, prolonged labor, multiple intrapartum vaginal examinations, and emergency cesarean section.

B. General approach

1. A thorough physical examination, including a pelvic examination, should be performed.

2. Treatment must be initiated early without waiting for culture results.

3. Antibiotic therapy selection should be based on the presumptive diagnosis and should be continued for a period appropriate for the source of infection identified.

C. Endometritis is the most common cause of puerperal infection. Findings are usually noted on the **second or third postpartum day.**

1. Pathophysiology

Table 7-5.   Diagnosis to Rule Out in Patients with Puerperal Fever

Mnemonic	Diagnosis	Postpartum Day
Wind	Atelectasis pneumonia	0
Water	Urinary tract infection	1–2
Womb	Endomyoparametritis	2–3
Wound	Surgical incision infection	4–5
Walk	Septic pelvic thrombophlebitis	5–6
Wonder drugs	Drug fever	5–6
"Watermelons"	Congestive mastitis	2–3
	Infectious mastitis	7–10

  a. Postdelivery lochia is an excellent culture medium for normal genital flora ascending from the vagina.

  b. Devitalized tissue after a cesarean delivery and suture foreign bodies provide an even more optimal environment for contamination by sources of infection.

  c. Polymicrobial bacteria infect the endometrium initially, causing an **endometritis.** The organisms can rapidly invade the myometrium and broad ligament through lymphatic channels, causing an **endomyometritis** and **endomyoparametritis.** The end result of untreated or inadequately treated infections may be a **pelvic abscess.**

2. Risk factors emergency cesarean section, prolonged membrane rupture, prolonged labor, multiple intrapartum vaginal examinations, and intrauterine manipulation procedures (Table 7-6).

3. Clinical findings

  a. Fever ranges from 100.4°F (38°C) to 104°F (40°C) but is seldom in the upper end of the range.

  b. Uterine tenderness is exquisite, and the uterus is usually poorly contracted.

  c. Abdominal findings are usually minimal, although decreased peristalsis may be noted with more extensive infection.

  d. Adnexal examination is usually unremarkable unless an abscess has formed.

4. Diagnosis (see Table 7-5). Initial diagnosis is based on clinical findings alone.

  a. Lochial cultures are not routinely performed, because the flora is routinely polymicrobial.

  b. Blood cultures are not routinely obtained unless patients appear septic. Cultures are positive in up to 30% of patients, with anaerobes being the most frequently identified organisms.

Table 7-6. Risk Factors for Puerperal Infection

Endometritis	Urinary Tract Infection	Atelectasis and Pneumonia	Wound Infection	Septic Pelvic Thrombophlebitis	Mastitis
Emergency cesarean section	Indwelling Foley catheter	General anesthesia	Emergency cesarean section	Emergency cesarean section	Nipple trauma
Prolonged rupture of the membranes	Multiple catheterizations during labor	Smoking	Prolonged rupture of the membranes	Prolonged rupture of the membranes	
Prolonged labor	Multiple intrapartum vaginal examinations	Obstructive lung disease	Prolonged labor	Difficult vaginal delivery	
Multiple intrapartum vaginal examinations	Untreated asymptomatic bacteriuria		Multiple intrapartum vaginal examinations	Prolonged labor	
Intrauterine manipulative procedures			Obesity		

5. **Management**

   a. Most patients need to be admitted for **parenteral therapy.**

   b. **Broad-spectrum antibiotics** covering both aerobic and anaerobic species should be used.

      (1) **Clindamycin and gentamicin** are a standard first-line, **two-drug regimen** for uncomplicated endometritis, although **single-agent,** second- or third-generation cephalosporins are also appropriate choices.

      (2) A **three-drug regimen** (adding ampicillin to cover enterococci) should be used for complicated endometritis or for lack of rapid defervescence after single- or double-agent initial therapy.

      (3) **Parenteral antibiotics should be continued** until patients have been **afebrile for 48 hours.** Follow-up oral antibiotics are not needed.

      (4) **Additional diagnoses should be considered** if a satisfactory clinical response is not seen after 48 hours of a three-drug regimen:

         (a) Pelvic abscess

         (b) Wound infection

         (c) Septic pelvic thrombophlebitis

D. **Urinary tract infection (UTI),** which affects 2%–4% of gravidas, is the second most common cause of puerperal infection. Findings are usually noted on the **first or second postpartum day.**

1. **Pathophysiology**

   a. Frequent intrapartum catheterizations, multiple vaginal examinations, and perineal contamination provide UTI-causing bacterial innoculum that ascend from the perineum to the bladder.

   b. Trauma to the bladder and to the lower urinary tract from labor and delivery results in increased residual volume, detrusor hypotonia, and urinary reflux.

   c. Preexisting, untreated asymptomatic bacteriuria and undiagnosed urinary tract anomalies can predispose patients to urinary infections.

2. **Risk factors** include indwelling Foley catheter, multiple catheterizations in labor, multiple intrapartum vaginal examinations, and untreated asymptomatic bacteriuria (see Table 7-6).

3. **Clinical findings**
   a. **Lower tract disease** characteristically is localized in extent.
      (1) **Common symptoms** include urinary urgency, frequency, and dysuria.
      (2) **Common signs** include low-grade fever and suprapubic tenderness.
   b. **Upper tract disease** usually has systemic involvement.
      (1) **Common symptoms** include sweats, chills, nausea, and vomiting.
      (2) **Common signs** include high fever, malaise, and costovertebral angle tenderness.

4. **Diagnosis**
   a. **Urinalysis** reveals pus cells and bacteria in centrifuged catheterized urine specimens.
   b. **Urine culture** confirms the diagnosis and identifies the specific bacteria. In 75% of cases, *E. coli* is the offending organism.

5. **Management.** Women with **lower UTIs** can be treated as outpatients, but those with **upper UTIs** (particularly if systemic findings are present) should be admitted to the hospital.
   a. **Single-agent antibiotics** should be administered to cover the organism identified effectively. Antibiotic coverage should continue until patients are afebrile for 24 hours. Then oral antibiotics should be continued until a 10-day course is completed.
   b. **Multiple-agent IV antibiotic therapy** is indicated if patients appear septic.
   c. **Generous hydration** with high intake of oral or IV fluids should be encouraged. Febrile patients with pyelonephritis have high insensory fluid losses.

E. **Pneumonia and atelectasis** are complications of the very early puerperium in cesarean patients and are usually noted within the **first 24 hours postpartum.**

1. **Pathophysiology**
   a. Postoperative abdominal pain and the decreased FRC of the supine position both contribute to underexpansion of the lungs and resultant atelectasis.
   b. The airway collapse leads to capillary drainage from atelectatic areas carrying unoxygenated blood, which results in shunting and hypoxia.
   c. Infected secretions from preexistent bronchitis can lead to the development of pneumonia in the atelectatic areas.

2. **Risk factors** include general anesthesia, smoking, and obstructive lung disease (see Table 7-6).

3. **Clinical findings**
   a. **Mild atelectasis** may manifest with mild fever in the immediate

postoperative period as the only finding. Chest auscultation and radiographic appearance may be unremarkable.

b. Extensive atelectasis is associated with increased temperature, pulse, and respiratory rate. Chest examination shows dullness to percussion with inspiratory rales. Radiographic findings may reveal patchy opacities.

c. Pneumonia may follow unresolved atelectasis with higher temperatures and evidence of systemic involvement. Lung sounds may reveal pulmonary consolidation and coarse rales. Radiographic appearance may later show diffuse patchy infiltrates, although the radiographic findings often lag behind the clinical findings.

4. Management

a. Atelectasis responds to ambulation and pulmonary exercises. Adequate analgesia and inspiratcry spirometry allow patients to expand the lungs and resolve the atelectasis.

b. Pneumonia requires specific antibiotic therapy based on sputum culture and sensitivities obtained from induced sputum specimens.

F. Wound infection occurs in 5%–10% of cesarean patients. Findings are usually identified on the **fourth or fifth postpartum day.**

1. Pathophysiology. The microbiologic etiology arises from either skin flora (e.g., *Staphylococcus aureus*) or from the polymicrobial genital tract bacteria that had colonized the amniotic cavity during labor.

2. Risk factors include emergency cesarean section, prolonged membrane rupture, prolonged labor, multiple intrapartum vaginal examinations, and obesity (see Table 7-6).

3. Clinical findings

a. Unexplained, spiking puerperal fevers that persist despite adequate antibiotic therapy are common (see Table 7-5).

b. Wound erythema, edema, tenderness, or fluctuance are often found.

c. Spontaneous purulent drainage from the wound is pathognomonic.

4. Management

a. If the findings suggest cellulitis, IV antibiotics should be administered. However, if the findings reveal purulence and fluctuance, the entire wound must be opened and explored to break up any loculations, as well as to confirm the integrity of the fascia. This allows drainage of infected material.

b. If the fascia is not intact, patients must be taken to the operating room so the wound can be debrided to the fascial level and the defect can be repaired.

c. Cultures should be obtained from the wound drainage, and appropriate broad-spectrum antibiotic coverage should be initiated. If patients are febrile, they should receive parenteral antibiotics until the fever resolves.

d. The primary therapeutic approach in treating puerperal wound infections is saline-soaked packing twice a day. Packing prevents the wound from forming infected loculations. Removing the dried dressing enhances the removal of nonviable debris.

e. Once the wound has a clean granulation tissue base, it can be brought together by delayed closure or allowed to close spontaneously by secondary intention.

G. **Septic pelvic thrombophlebitis** occurs in fewer than 1% of cesarean patients. Findings are usually identified on the **fifth or sixth postpartum day.**

   1. **Pathophysiology**
      a. The intimal lining of the pelvic veins is injured by a variety of puerperal processes. The ovarian vein is the most common site.
      b. Thrombi form on the damaged intima, and bacteria, gaining access from an infected uterus via endometrial and myometrial lymphatics, invade the blood clots.
      c. The infected clots may fragment resulting in septic emboli.

   2. **Risk factors** include emergency cesarean section, prolonged membrane rupture, difficult vaginal delivery, and prolonged labor (see Table 7-6).

   3. **Clinical findings**
      a. The diagnosis of puerperal septic pelvic thrombophlebitis is often a diagnosis of exclusion after wound infection and abscess have been ruled out. Unexplained, spiking puerperal fevers that persist despite adequate antibiotic therapy suggest septic pelvic thrombophlebitis (see Table 7-5).
      b. A **picket-fence fever** curve with wide swings from normal to as high as 105.8°F (41°C) is often found. Patients typically feel fine otherwise.
      c. Pelvic and abdominal examinations are frequently unremarkable, although worm-like, thrombosed veins may be palpated in the adnexae, and thrombosed ovarian veins may be detected.

   4. **Management**
      a. Patients have usually been on multiple-agent, broad-spectrum antibiotic coverage. This should be continued while they receive IV heparin at rates that are sufficient to prolong the PTT to double the baseline values.
      b. Resolution of the fever should occur in 48–72 hours. Heparin administration should be continued for a total of 10–14 days with no further anticoagulation required.

H. **Puerperal mastitis** (see Chapter 15 II D) usually develops 1 week or more postdelivery. The mechanism involves introduction of *S. aureus* from the infant's nostrils into traumatized nipples. Breastfeeding is continued, and antibiotic treatment (cloxacillin or dicloxacillin) is begun.

Review Test

Directions: Each of the numbered items or incomplete statements in this section is followed by answers or completions of the statement. Select the **ONE** lettered answer or completion that is **BEST** in each case.

1. Which of the following organ systems undergoes increased stress in the puerperium immediately following delivery?

(A) Cardiac
(B) Pulmonary
(C) Renal
(D) Gastrointestinal (GI)
(E) Endocrine

2. Which of the following conditions is the most common complication of defective involution of the placental site?

(A) Leiomyoma formation
(B) Late hemorrhage
(C) Infertility
(D) Adenomyosis

3. Which of the following characteristics is evidence of postpartum depression?

(A) Feelings of inadequacy to take care of the infant
(B) Verbalizing a desire to harm the infant
(C) Lack of concern from the mother about her appearance
(D) Not wanting to breastfeed the infant

4. Within what period of postdelivery should $Rh_o(D)$ immunoglobin (RhoGAM) be given to appropriate candidates to prevent anti-D isoimmunization?

(A) 12 hours
(B) 24 hours
(C) 36 hours
(D) 72 hours
(E) 96 hours

5. Which of the following contraceptive methods should be delayed until 6–8 weeks postpartum?

(A) Condoms
(B) Oral steroid contraceptives
(C) Medroxyprogesterone acetate
(D) Spermicidal agents
(E) Diaphragm

6. The answer to which of the following questions is most significant when preparing a management plan for a patient with postpartum hemorrhage?

(A) How much did the infant weigh?
(B) What are maternal vital signs?
(C) What was the level of hemoglobin before delivery?
(D) What is the mother's blood type?
(E) Is blood available for possible transfusion?

7. Which of the following conditions is the most common cause of postpartum hemorrhage (PPH)?

(A) Uterine atony
(B) Retained placenta
(C) Perineal lacerations
(D) Disseminated intravascular coagulopathy (DIC)
(E) Uterine rupture

8. Which of the following conditions is the most common cause of puerperal fever?

(A) Abscess
(B) Endometritis
(C) Urinary tract infection (UTI)
(D) Pelvic septic thrombophlebitis
(E) Pulmonary etiology

Directions: Each of the numbered items or incomplete statements in this section is negatively phrased, as indicated by a capitalized word such as NOT, LEAST, or EXCEPT. Select the ONE lettered answer or completion that is best in each case.

9. All of the following agents are indicated for a patient with uterine atony EXCEPT

(A) oxytocin
(B) methergine
(C) prostaglandin 15-methyl F_{2a}
(D) calcium gluconate
(E) halothane

10. All of the following statements regarding lochia are true EXCEPT

(A) it derives from sloughing of superficial decidual layers
(B) it appears as dark red lochia rubra immediately after delivery
(C) it is replaced by endometrial regeneration from zona basalis
(D) it changes to pinkish lochia serosa at the end of week one
(E) it takes 6 weeks to convert to whitish lochia alba

11. All of the following conditions adversely affect the return of female sexual functioning postpartum EXCEPT

(A) perineal lacerations
(B) return of ovulation
(C) lactational effect of the vagina
(D) fatigue and exhaustion
(E) milk ejection with stimulation

Answers and Explanations

1. The answer is A [I C 5].

The puerperium is associated with multiple and profound changes as the organ systems return to a nonpregnant state. Most changes are decreases in the increased workload of pregnancy. An exception to this is the heart, in which cardiac output increases immediately after delivery up to 80% higher than prelabor values. Patients with heart disease can expect the risk of complications to increase after the placenta is delivered, regardless of whether the delivery was vaginal or cesarean.

2. The answer is B [I B 3].

The vessels of the placental site on the uterine surface normally undergo physiologic thrombosis to decrease bleeding. This normal process is followed by reparative regeneration. If this process is defective, the most common sequelae is late puerperal hemorrhage.

3. The answer is C [I D 1 a; Table 7-2].

Lack of concern on the part of the mother regarding her appearance is typical of postpartum depression. Postpartum emotional responses can include the postpartum "blues" or feelings of inadequacy, which resolve with minimal intervention. Having a desire to harm the infant is characteristic of psychosis, which necessitates psychiatric intervention. Not wanting to breastfeed the infant is not necessarily related to any postpartum emotional problems.

4. The answer is D [I D 6].

Prevention of maternal isoimmunization through passive immunization with anti-D antibodies is an important postpartum intervention for susceptible patients. Failure to give the $Rh_o(D)$ immunoglobin (RhoGAM) within 72 hours may result in maternal lymphocytes being activated, after which they produce anti-D antibodies.

5. The answer is E [I D 9].

Contraceptive planning is important because ovulation can return rapidly after delivery in some patients. Fitting a diaphragm before completion of vaginal involution at 6–8 weeks could result in loose fit and a high failure rate. Condoms can be used anytime. Combination oral contraceptives, because of their estrogen component, should be deferred for 3 weeks to allow reversal of the hypercoagulable state of pregnancy. Oral progestin ("minipill") and injectable medroxyprogesterone acetate, both hormonal contraceptives, can be started immediately postpartum. Spermicidal agents are appropriate whenever intercourse is resumed.

6. The answer is B [II A 2 a, 3].

Stabilization of the mother's vital signs is of the utmost importance in managing a patient with postpartum hemorrhage. Adequate intravenous (IV) access should be ensured with an isotonic solution infusing at a rapid rate. The infant's birth weight, the predelivery hemoglobin level, the mother's blood type, and the availability of blood for possible transfusion are all appropriate considerations after the mother has been stabilized.

7. The answer is A [II C].

Uterine atony is by far the most common cause of postpartum hemorrhage (PPH), which occurs in up to 10% of deliveries. The primary mechanism of postpartum hemostasis of the placental site is contraction of myometrial fibers and retraction of myometrial blood vessels. Retained placenta, perineal lacerations, disseminated intravascular coagulopathy (DIC), and uterine rupture are also causes of PPH but are not as common as atony.

8. The answer is B [III C; Table 7-5].

Endometritis is correct, because infection of the uterus is the most common etiology of puerperal fever. The pathophysiology is usually dissemination of ineffective organisms from the uterus outward via lymphatic spread mostly involving normal genital flora. Both aerobic and nonaerobic bacteria are involved. Although abscess, urinary tract infection (UTI), pelvic septic thrombophlebitis, and pulmonary etiology such as pneumonia are all other causes of puerperal fever, none occurs as often as endometritis.

9. The answer is E [II C 3 c].

The fundamental basis for treatment of uterine atony is administration of agents that contract the uterine muscle. Halothane is the correct answer (but incorrect agent to give) because, as a relaxant, it relaxes the myometrium and therefore is contraindicated. Oxytocin, methergine, prostaglandin 15-methyl F_{2a}, and calcium gluconate are potent uterotonic agents; therefore, they are indicated.

10. The answer is E [I B 2 a].

Lochia is the dark, bloody-appearing vaginal discharge that appears after the delivery of the placenta. Lochia is derived from sloughing of superficial decidual layers. Immediately after delivery, the dark red lochia rubra, appears. It is replaced by endometrial regeneration from the zona basalis, and it changes to pinkish lochia serosa at the end of the first postpartum week. By the end of the second (not the sixth) postpartum week, whitish lochia alba appears.

11. The answer is B [I D 8].

Return of ovulation is the correct answer (but completes an incorrect statement), because it tends to improve sexuality due to a normalization of estrogen levels. Normalization of the female sexual response may be delayed up to 3 months postpartum. Sexuality is a complex process mediated by higher brain centers, and inhibition can easily result from a variety of factors. Perineal lacerations such as episiotomy, lactational atrophy of the vagina, fatigue and exhaustion, and milk ejection with sexual stimulation may all diminish sexuality and libido.

8

Common Gynecologic Complaints

I. GYNECOLOGIC HISTORY

A. Identifying information should include:

1. **Age** is important because the differential diagnosis and the treatment approach vary with the patient's stage of life.

2. The **last normal menstrual period** establishes a baseline for evaluating subsequent complaints.

3. **Gravidity** describes the total number of confirmed pregnancies (regardless of gestational age when the pregnancy ended). Gravidity should be confirmed by a:

   a. Positive pregnancy test

   b. Sonogram showing gestational sac or embryo

   c. Embryo/fetus that was passed

   d. Pathology report showing trophoblastic villi

4. **Parity** describes pregnancies that continue for more than 20 weeks' gestation (regardless of the number of fetuses and whether they were live births or stillbirths).

5. **Abortions** describes pregnancies that terminated spontaneously (unintentionally) or through induction (intentionally) at less than 20 weeks' gestation. The duration of the pregnancy should be determined (i.e., first or second trimester).

6. **Reproductive history "shorthand"** may use two different formats, one with three numbers and one with five numbers. The following examples describe the same reproductive history: five pregnancies that resulted in three term deliveries (with three children currently alive), one preterm delivery of triplets (with one stillborn fetus and two children currently alive), and one spontaneous abortion.

   a. **Three-number method: $G_5P_4A_1$** [G = gravidity, P = parity, and A = abortions (see I A 3–5)]

b. Five-number method: G_5P_{3115} [G = gravidity; the four numbers following "P" can be remembered as TPAL where T = term pregnancies, P = preterm pregnancies, A = abortions, and L = living children (see I A 3–5)]

B. Chief complaint and presenting illness should be determined.

1. The **patient's description** of her concern in her own words is important. She should be asked, "What brought you to the office?"

2. **Details should be obtained systematically.**

    a. Date and time of onset of complaint

    b. Description of complaints

       (1) Course of symptoms (i.e., getting worse or better)

       (2) Location and duration of complaints

    c. Modifying factors (i.e., what makes symptoms worse or better)

    d. Impact of complaint on daily life

C. Reproductive history includes menstrual history, contraceptive history, gynecologic history, and obstetric history (Table 8-1).

D. Social history includes sexual history, social history, and domestic violence or abuse history (see Table 8-1).

E. Family history includes the health status of immediate relatives, familial diseases or conditions, and genetic screening history (see Table 8-1).

F. Medical history includes history concerning allergies, medications, substance use, surgeries, and medical problems (see Table 8-1).

II. THE GYNECOLOGIC EXAMINATION

A. Breast examination

1. **Visual inspection**

    a. **Use a good light** when looking for **lumps, dimpling, or wrinkling of the skin on the breast and axillae.**

    b. **Place the patient in a sitting position** first with arms at her sides, then with arms pressed on her hips while tensing her pectoralis muscles, and finally with arms held above head.

2. **Bimanual palpation of breasts.** The patient should be examined in the following positions:

    a. **Sitting position,** leaning forward with hands on knees

    b. **Supine position,** with arms relaxed at side

3. **Palpation of the axillae and breasts** is performed using fingers.

4. **Palpation of the nipples** is performed using the thumb and forefinger.

5. **Palpation of the supraclavicular areas** is performed using fingers.

B. Abdominal examination. The patient should be supine and relaxed, with knees flexed. The examination consists of the following actions performed in the order listed:

1. **Inspection** for contour and skin color

Table 8-1. Histories Taken During the Initial Gynecologic Interview

Reproductive History	Social History	Family History	Past Medical History
Menstrual Onset of menarche Intermenstrual interval Flow duration and character Intermenstrual bleeding Severity and character of cramping Premenstrual symptomatology	**Sexual** Currently sexually active? Sex with men, women, or both? How many partners? Is the relationship satisfying? If not, why? Pain with intercourse? Difficulty lubricating?	**Health status of immediate relatives** Children Parents Grandparents Siblings	**Allergies** Medication Environmental **Medications** Prescription Nonprescription
Contraceptive Type and duration of methods Side effects or complications Oral (e.g., amenorrhea, thromboembolic disorders) IUD (e.g., dysmenorrhea, menorrhagia, PID)	**Social** Educational level Occupation Marital/partner history Health and relationship with husband/partner Nature and quality of	**Familial diseases or conditions** Heart disease Hypertensive, renal, or vas- cular disease Hirsutism Breast and	**Substance use** Recreational drugs Smoking Alcohol **Surgeries** Gynecologic Nongynecologic
Gynecologic STDs (types, treatments, complications) Abnormal Pap smears (severity, colposcopy/biopsy findings, treatments) Pelvic pain (onset, description, radiation, course, worsening or improving factors) Urinary incontinence Vaginal discharge (onset, description, symptoms, odor) Vulvar complaints	support systems Knowledge/practice of healthy lifestyle **Domestic violence/abuse** Has partner ever in- flicted verbal, emotional, or physical abuse? Is information about help and shelters desired?	ovarian carcinoma **Genetic screening** Mental retardation Stillbirths Neonatal deaths Birth defects	**Medical problems** Diabetes Hypertension Others
Obstetric Pregnancies in chronologic order Prenatal course (duration, complications) Intrapartum course (labor, anesthesia, mode of delivery, complications) Perinatal outcome (sex, weight, morbidity, mortality)			

IUD = intrauterine device; PID = pelvic inflammatory disease; STD = sexually transmitted disease.

    2. Auscultation for peristalsis

    3. Palpation for rigidity, guarding, masses, and tenderness (palpation should begin gently, with increasing firmness and deepness)

    4. Percussion for organ enlargement, masses, and ascites

  C. Pelvic examination

    1. General principles

      a. Take an unhurried history, setting the tone for the examination.

      b. Ensure general relaxation by noting if the abdomen is soft.

   c. Ensure a chaperone is in the room.

   d. Warm instruments prior to use.

   e. Explain each step while giving positive reinforcement.

   f. Obtain specimens for wet mount or culture if an abnormal discharge is present.

2. External genitalia inspection

   a. Escutcheon should be inspected for normal female hair distribution.

   b. Pubic skin should be inspected for lesions.

   c. Clitoris and prepuce should be inspected and palpated for tenderness and assessment of normal size.

   d. Labia minor and majora should be inspected and palpated for symmetry and lesions.

   e. Bartholin's and vestibular glands should be palpated for tenderness and masses.

   f. Perianal area should be inspected for hemorrhoids, fissures, inflammation, and lesions.

3. Hymen. Inspect and palpate for **imperforate status** (in a virginal woman) and **carunculae myriformes** (in a sexually active woman).

4. Perineal support. The patient should be asked to bear down while the physician spreads the labia apart and inspects for **cystocele, rectocele,** and **uterine prolapse.**

5. Urethra. The physician should inspect, palpate, and strip the **urethral and Skene's glands** for tenderness and discharge. The urethra should also be inspected for a **caruncle** or **urethrocele.**

6. Vagina examination

   a. Use the smallest speculum that affords adequate visualization.

     (1) The **Pederson speculum** has narrow, parallel blades.

     (2) The **Graves speculum** has duck-billed, distally wider blades.

   b. Lubricate the warmed speculum with water to obtain a cervical Papanicolaou (Pap) smear.

     (1) **Obtain scrapings of transformation zone** cells with a spatula.

     (2) **Obtain endocervical cells** with a swab or brush.

     (3) **Fix the specimens** on a glass slide immediately to avoid air-drying artifacts.

   c. Inspect the vaginal walls as the speculum is being withdrawn. The walls should be palpated with the index and middle fingers for lesions and tenderness.

7. Cervix. The cervix first should be visually examined first looking for cervicitis, discharge, and lesions. Obtain cultures for chlamydia and gonorrhea as indicated.

8. Bimanual examination

   a. The **cervix** should be palpated for **masses** and **motion tenderness.**

   b. The **uterus** should be palpated between two fingers of the vaginal hand and the fingers of the abdominal hand. **Size, shape, consistency, mobility,** and **position** (i.e., anteverted, mid-position, retroverted) should be assessed.

    c. The **adnexae** should be palpated between two fingers of the vaginal hand and the fingers of the abdominal hand. **Ovarian size, mobility,** and **tenderness** should be assessed; however, the ovaries may not be palpable in obese or postmenopausal women. Any **abnormal adnexal masses** should be described.

9. **Rectovaginal examination.** The patient should be instructed to hold her breath and bear down, so that the anal sphincter relaxes. A well-lubricated middle finger is placed in the rectum, and the index finger is placed in the vagina to palpate for **uterosacral ligament tenderness and nodularity.**

10. **Rectal examination.** The patient should be instructed to bear down to relax the anal sphincter. A well-lubricated forefinger is placed through the anus reaching high as possible into the rectum. The physician should palpate for **anal lesions** and **rectal tumors.** If stool remains on the glove, a **guaiac examination** should be performed to detect **occult blood.**

III. ABNORMAL PAPANICOLAOU (PAP) SMEAR

A. **Normal developmental changes in cervical topography**

    1. **Embryonic development in utero.** The cervix and upper vagina in utero are covered with columnar epithelium. With advancing development, vaginal columnar epithelium progressively is replaced by squamous epithelium.

    2. **At birth**
        a. In most normal girls, the region of columnar epithelium is limited to the endocervix and the central ectocervix.
           (1) **Adenosis** is found in 4% of normal girls and 30% of diethylstilbestrol (DES) daughters. The columnar epithelium extends onto the vaginal fornices.
           (2) **Gross examination** shows orange-red tissue that is only one cell layer thick. Blood vessels in the underlying stroma are apparent (thus the orange-red color).
        b. **The original squamocolumnar (SC) junction** is found where the original (native) squamous and columnar epithelia meet (see Figure 1-5).

    3. **During adolescence and first pregnancy,** a **new SC junction** is formed through squamous metaplasia of the columnar epithelium to stratified squamous epithelium.
        a. The new SC junction is more proximal to the external os than the original SC junction.
        b. The **transformation (T) zone** is the area between two SC junctions.

B. **Abnormal changes in cervical topography**

    1. **Abnormal maturation begins at the T zone.** Approximately 95% of **squamous intraepithelial neoplasia** occurs within the T zone.

    2. **Carcinogens** may contribute to abnormal cervical changes

    a. Cigarette smoke, which is secreted through endocervical glandular mucus

    b. Intercourse at a young age (with an immature T zone)

    c. Human papilloma virus (HPV) types 6 and 11 but especially **16 and 18**

C. Papanicolaou (Pap) smear screening for cervical intraepithelial neoplasia (CIN). Inadequate cytologic sampling or inappropriate processing results in false-negative Pap smears. The false-negative rate for Pap smears is 20%.

    1. Defer screening if the cervix is <u>infected or inflamed</u>, because early dysplastic changes may be obscured <u>by inflammatory cells</u>.

    2. Scrape exfoliated cells from the cervix with a spatula. The entire T zone must be sampled. Incomplete sampling (i.e., failure to include any abnormal cells present on the cervix in the smear sample) of the T zone could produce a false-negative smear.

    3. Sample the endocervical canal with a swab or cytobrush to screen for lesions in the endocervical canal.

    4. Streak specimens immediately onto a glass slide. A sample is incomplete without both specimens (i.e., cells from the cervix and from the endocervical canal).

    5. Fix the smears immediately to avoid air-drying cytologic artifacts.

D. Pathologic appearance of cervical dysplasia (disordered growth)

    1. Cytologic changes include increased nuclear-cytoplasmic ratio, prominence of nuclear chromatin, and multinucleation.

    2. Histologic changes

        a. Dysplasia is a continuum of **intraepithelial neoplastic transformation,** arising from **basal cells,** in which abnormal, immature, disorganized cells replace normal cells. Histologic abnormalities are reported as follows:

            (1) Mild. The deeper cell layer is minimally involved.

            (2) Moderate. Involvement is significant, but not full thickness.

            (3) Severe. The entire thickness is involved except for a few surface layers, which show maturation

            (4) Carcinoma in situ (CIS). There is complete loss of cellular polarity when CIS is involved.

        b. Invasive carcinoma has three forms.

            (1) Minimal microscopic stromal invasion. The basement membrane is penetrated by tumor cells but just barely so (< 3 mm).

            (2) Microscopic invasion. The basement membrane is penetrated but less than 5 mm, and there is no vascular or lymphatic involvement.

            (3) Frank (gross) invasion. The basement membrane is penetrated more than 5 mm or vascular or lymphatic involvement is found.

    3. Association with vulvar dysplasia. The "field effect" states that patients with CIN are at a higher risk for <u>vulvar intraepithelial neoplasia</u> (VIN).

E. **Comparison of terminology in different Papanicolaou (Pap) smear systems** (Table 8-2). The newest system of Pap smear terminology, which has changed over time, is the **Bethesda system.**

F. **Natural history of cervical dysplasia** (Box 8-1). Prediction of lesion behavior is unpredictable with current technology.

G. **Risk factors for cervical dysplasia and carcinoma**

 1. **Sexually related practices** (e.g., early age of sexual intercourse, multiple sexual partners)

 2. **Pregnancy-related factors** (e.g., early age of pregnancy, high parity)

 3. **Social factors** (e.g., low socioeconomic status, divorce)

 4. **Cigarette smoking**

 5. **HPV,** especially **types 16 and 18**

 6. **Immunocompromised host**

H. **Clinical approach**

 1. **Onset and frequency of obtaining cervical Pap smears**

  a. Pap smear screening should **initially** be started at onset of sexual activity or age 18 years.

  b. Patients **with risk factors** should have annual Pap smears.

  c. Patients **without risk factors** should undergo annual Pap screening until negative smears are reported for 3 consecutive years, then undergo screening every 3 years.

  d. Patients who have undergone **total hysterectomy** (uterine corpus and cervix removed) for benign reasons do not require Pap screening. However, if the reason for hysterectomy was cervical neoplasia, they should have annual vaginal cuff smears.

  e. Patients who have undergone **subtotal hysterectomy** (uterine corpus removed, but cervix left in place) should undergo Pap screening annually or every 3 years based on risk factors as if they had no surgery.

 2. **Colposcopy and directed biopsies.** A Pap smear is only a screening test. A **definitive diagnosis** requires inspection of a well-illuminated

Table 8–2. Comparison of Terminology in Different Pap Smear Systems

Class System	CIN System	Bethesda System
Class I: Normal	Normal	Within normal limits
Class II: Inflammation	Inflammatory	Inflammatory with or without atypia
Class III: Mild/moderate dysplasia	CIN I or II	Low-grade SIL
Class IV: Severe dysplasia/CIS	CIN III	High-grade SIL
Class V: Suggestive of cancer	Suggestive of cancer	Squamous cell cancer

CIN = cervical intraepithelial neoplasia; *CIS* = carcinoma-in-situ; *SIL* = squamous intraepithelial lesion.

Box 8-1. Variations in Natural History of Cervical Dysplasia

• **Complete involution**	75% of cervical dysplasia in pregnancy
• **Gradual regression**	65% of mild dysplasia
• **Remaining static for years**	20% of mild dysplasia
• **Slow progression**	15% of mild dysplasia

---

cervix with a low-power, short–focal length binocular **colposcope** with **biopsy** of abnormal areas.

   a. The cervix is painted with a 3% aqueous **acetic acid solution** to enhance surface alterations and vascular changes.

   b. The colposcopic evaluation is considered **"adequate"** or **"satisfactory"** if the complete T zone and the full extent of the lesion(s) are visualized. If either the complete T zone or the lesion cannot be visualized, the evaluation is considered **"inadequate"** or **"unsatisfactory."**

   c. Visualized areas of abnormality (e.g., **white epithelium, mosaicism, punctation,** and **abnormal vessels**) are selectively punch biopsied.

3. Endocervical curettage (ECC)

   a. If part of the T zone extends into the endocervical canal **("inadequate" or "unsatisfactory"** colposcopy), an unseen lesion may be present, necessitating scraping or curetting of the canal. If the ECC specimen comes back abnormal, a follow-up deep, diagnostic cone biopsy is required for definitive histologic diagnosis of the site of the abnormal cells.

   b. Routine versus indicated ECC. Some clinicians perform routine ECC, regardless of adequacy of the colposcopy. Other clinicians perform ECC only if the colposcopy was **"inadequate"** or **"unsatisfactory."**

   c. Pregnant patients. Most clinicians do not perform routine ECC during pregnancy (because of increased vascularity of the cervix, enlargement of the area covered by columnar epithelium, and the increased risk of excessive bleeding).

4. Agreement between cytology and biopsy. Colposcopic-directed biopsy should come from the same site as do dysplastic cells on the Pap smear. A similar degree of abnormality can be expected on the two specimens. If the histology of the biopsied tissue is less severe than the Pap smear (more than a one-stage difference), it is assumed that the biopsy specimen did not come from the same location as the dysplastic Pap smear cells.

5. True intraepithelial lesions. Lesions that are intraepithelial but may look like invasive carcinoma include the following:

   a. Involvement of the endocervical glands below the basement membrane

   b. Tangential sections, which look like basement membranes that have been penetrated

6. **Management of CIN.** This includes all histologically diagnosed dysplastic lesions that have not penetrated the basement membrane including mild, moderate, and severe dysplasia as well as CIS.

    a. **Observation.** The majority of mild dysplasias regresses over time. In reliable patients, repeat Pap smears every 3 months (with colposcopy to ensure lesion regression) for 2 years is appropriate. Patients, even with mild dysplasia, who are not candidates for extended follow-up, should be managed with ablative therapy.

    b. **Ablative therapy.** These methods destroy, or excise the dysplastic epithelium. **Lesions confined to the epithelium** can be treated with various methods of **excision, ablation, or resection** (Table 8-3).

        (1) **Cryotherapy.** Liquid nitrogen is used to cool an **acorn-shaped** cervical probe to −40°F (−20° C). The probe is placed blindly on the ectocervix and distal endocervical canal creating an "ice-ball"

Table 8-3. Selecting the Appropriate Mode of Excision, Ablation, or Resection

Mode	Advantages	Disadvantages
Cryotherapy	Painless, inexpensive outpatient procedure No scarring	Cannot selectively target only dysplastic areas Copious vaginal discharge as destroyed epithelium sloughs off SC junction moves into endocervical canal No histologic specimen 10%–20% failure rate
LEEP	Provides histologic specimen, but surgical margins are difficult to evaluate Relatively painless, inexpensive outpatient procedure	Risk of cervical stenosis Risk of cervical amputation
Carbon dioxide laser	Precise destruction of only dysplastic areas Minimal scarring SC junction remains unchanged	Painful, requiring expensive operating room procedure and general anesthesia No histologic specimen 5%–10% failure rate
Electrocautery	Low failure rate (5%)	Painful, requiring expensive operating room procedure and general anesthesia May cause cervical stenosis No histologicl specimen
Conization	Provides histologic specimen High cure rate	Bleeding and infection Risk of cervical incompetence Risk of cervical stenosis
Hysterectomy	Provides histologic specimen High cure rate	Significant risks associated with expensive, major surgery Elimination of reproductive function

LEEP = loop electrodiathermy excision procedure

4 mm deep. The thermal injury results in sloughing of a circular area of dysplastic (as well as normal) epithelium over the next 1–2 weeks. Reepithelialization with stratified squamous epithelium follows. This **common procedure** may be performed on an outpatient basis with minimal discomfort. No surgical specimen is obtained.

(2) **Loop electrodiathermy excision procedure (LEEP).** An electric current, which heats a curved wire at the end of a probe, is used to excise areas of visually identified dysplastic epithelium. The excised tissue is sent for microscopic examination. This **common procedure** may be performed on an **outpatient** basis with minimal discomfort.

(3) **CO$_2$ laser.** A highly focused high-energy laser beam is used to vaporize visually identified dysplastic epithelium. This expensive and thus **uncommon procedure** must be performed in an **operating room** under anesthesia because of the inherent pain involved. No histologic specimen is obtained.

(4) **Electrocautery.** An electric current, which heats the tip of a probe, is used to scorch visually identified dysplastic epithelium. This, too, is an expensive and thus **uncommon procedure**. Because of the inherent pain involved, it must be performed in an **operating room** under anesthesia. No histologic specimen is obtained.

(5) **Conization.** A cold scalpel is used to widely excise a cone-shaped area of cervical epithelium and underlying stroma. A shallow cone is performed for ectocervical lesions, whereas a deep cone is used for lesions believed to be in the endocervical canal. This costly procedure is performed for specific indications (see III H 7). Because of the inherent pain involved, it must be performed in an **operating room** under anesthesia. A complete histologic specimen is obtained.

c. **Hysterectomy.** This is the most costly method for management of CIN. This major surgical procedure is used to remove the uterine corpus and cervix by either vaginal or abdominal routes. Indications are high-grade dysplasia or CIS in women who have completed their reproductive goals.

d. **Follow-up evaluations** should be scheduled every 4 months for 2 years, then every 6 months for the next 3 years.

7. **Indications for a diagnostic cone biopsy**

   a. A cervical lesion that cannot be fully visualized

   b. A positive ECC

   c. Significant discrepancy between the Pap smear and the biopsy

   d. Microinvasive squamous cell carcinoma on cervical biopsy

   e. Adenocarcinoma in situ on cervical biopsy

8. **Invasive cervical carcinoma**

   a. **Epidemiology**

      (1) Cervical carcinoma is the **third most common** female reproductive malignancy, and it accounts for 20% of gynecologic cancers.

      (2) The most common tumor type is **squamous cell carcinoma**

(80%), with adenocarcinoma accounting for the majority of remaining cancers.

   (3) Average age at diagnosis is **45 years.**
   (4) **Risk factors** are the same as those for cervical dysplasia.

b. Clinical findings and diagnosis

   (1) The most common symptoms are **abnormal vaginal bleeding** and discharge, but most early stage I disease is asymptomatic.
   (2) **Definitive diagnosis requires a biopsy.**
   (3) Primary spread is by **local extension.**
   (4) **Lymphatic spread** involves the pelvic nodes then the **para-aortic** nodes.

c. Staging is clinical but intravenous pyelography (IVP) can be used (Table 8-4). **Cervical cancer is the only gynecologic malignancy that is not surgically staged.**

d. Management. The overall 5-year survival is 55%. Treatment options include the following:

   (1) **Simple total hysterectomy** is the treatment for stage Ia1 (minimally invasive) disease. Cone biopsy may be selectively performed if a young woman wants to preserve her reproductive function.
   (2) **Modified radical hysterectomy** is the treatment of choice for stage Ia2 (microinvasive) disease. Cone biopsy may be selectively performed if a young woman wants to preserve her reproductive function.
   (3) **Radical hysterectomy** (with bilateral pelvic lymphadenectomy) as well as **radiation therapy** give similar cure rates for stage Ib and stage II disease.

Table 8-4.   Clinical Staging for Cervical Carcinoma (FIGO,* 1994)

Stage	Description
Stage 0	**Carcinoma-in-situ; confined to the epithelium only**
Stage I	**Invasion is strictly confined to the cervix.**
IA1	Minimal microscopically evident stromal invasion < 3 mm deep
IA2	Microscopic invasion ≤ 5 mm, with horizontal spread ≤ 7 mm
IB	All others
Stage II	**Invasion is beyond the cervix but not to the pelvic wall or lower third of the vagina.**
IIA	Parametria is not involved.
IIB	Parametria is involved.
Stage III	**Invasion is to the pelvic wall or lower third of vagina.**
IIIA	Pelvic wall is not involved.
IIIB	Pelvic wall is involved; hydroenphrosis or nonfunctioning of the kidney may occur because of tumor.
Stage IV	**Invasion is beyond the true pelvis or to the mucosa of the bladder or rectum.**
IVA	Spread is to adjacent organs.
IVB	Spread is to distant organs.

FIGO = International Federation of Gynecologists and Obstetricians.

(4) Radiation therapy alone is recommended for extension beyond the adnexae or significant vaginal involvement.

(5) Chemotherapy has traditionally been of minimal value except as an adjunct to primary radiation therapy. New data suggest that chemotherapy given concurrently with radiotherapy may be efficacious.

IV. VAGINAL DISCHARGE

A. Characteristics of the normal vaginal ecosystem

1. **A dynamic equilibrium** exists involving intact stratified squamous epithelium, normal colonizing microorganisms, and local secretory and cellular immune factors.

2. **Vaginal pH is low** (i.e., 3.8–4.2), which helps create an unfavorable environment for pathogens.

   a. **Normal pH mechanism.** Estrogen increases vaginal epithelial glycogen content. The glycogen is metabolized by **lactobacilli** into glucose and then into lactic acid, which helps maintain a normal acidic pH.

   b. **Abnormal pH.** Increases in vaginal pH that may alter the normal ecosystem are caused by epithelial desquamation, trauma, low estrogen, menses, and alkaline seminal fluid.

3. **Normal vaginal flora composition**

   a. **Lactobacilli** (mainly hydrogen peroxide producers) in concentrations of 10^5 to 10^8/ml

   (1) These gram-positive rods are found in 96% of women with normal flora.

   (2) Hydrogen peroxide–producing strains are found in 100% of women with normal flora.

   (3) These organisms protect against bacterial and candidal infection by interfering with adherence to epithelial cells.

   b. **Facultative organisms** (low, nonpathogenic concentrations)

   (1) Diphtheroids

   (2) Coagulase-negative staphylococci

   (3) Streptococci (including groups B and D)

   (4) *Escherichia coli*

   (5) *Ureaplasma urealyticum*

   (6) *Mycoplasma hominis*

   c. **Anaerobic organisms** (low, nonpathogenic concentrations)

   (1) *Peptostreptococcus* species

   (2) *Bacteroides* species

   (3) *Fusobacterium* species

B. Terminology and definitions

1. **Vaginitis** causes a significant inflammatory response in the vaginal wall. It is accompanied by an increased number of leukocytes in the vaginal fluid. It is most commonly found in women with **trichomoniasis** and **candidiasis**.

2. **Bacterial vaginosis (BV)** causes a minimal inflammatory response

with only a few leukocytes found in the vaginal wall. Concentrations of bacteria (other than lactobacilli) increase 100- to 1000-fold compared with normal women. Previous terms for BV include nonspecific vaginitis, *Haemophilus* vaginitis, *Corynebacterium* vaginitis, *Gardnerella vaginalis* vaginitis, and anaerobic vaginosis.

C. Clinical approach

1. The **source of the discharge** must be determined. Sources of perineal discharge include the vagina, cervix, urinary tract, and rectum.

2. **Symptoms** may include odor, burning, and itching.

3. **Physical findings** may include the gross appearance of discharge, erythema or edema of the vaginal mucosa, and an increased pH level.

4. **Diagnostic tests** that may be helpful include the following:

    a. **Vaginal pH,** which is easily performed by using pH-sensitive (Nitrazine) paper

    b. **Wet preparation (wet prep),** in which vaginal discharge in sodium chloride medium is examined microscopically for **"clue cells."**

    c. **Potassium hydroxide preparation (KOH prep),** in which vaginal discharge in potassium hydroxide medium is examined microscopically. The potassium hydroxide dissolves cellular debris leaving **pseudohyphae** visible.

    d. **"Whiff" test.** The vaginal discharge of patients with BV has a characteristic **fishy odor,** which is the result of high concentrations of anaerobic species. The addition of potassium hydroxide may exaggerate the odor.

    e. **Culture** is not usually performed for initial evaluation.

5. **BV**

    a. **Epidemiology.** BV is the **most common cause of vaginal complaints,** although 50% of affected women are asymptomatic.

    b. **Microbiology.** There is a marked decrease in the concentration of lactobacillus and a marked increase in pathogens that cause BV (e.g., *Bacteroides, Peptostreptococcus, G. vaginalis*).

    c. **Diagnosis**

        (1) **Gray, homogeneous** discharge that adheres to vaginal walls
        (2) **pH > 4.5** (usually 5.0–5.5)
        (3) Presence of **clue cells** (i.e., epithelial cells studded with bacteria so that the cell borders are obscured)
        (4) **Fishy** (amine) **odor** when 10% potassium hydroxide solution is added
        (5) Paucity of lactobacilli
        (6) Relative absence of **white blood cells** (WBCs)

    d. **Management**

        (1) **Goal.** The goal is **restoration of a normal ecosystem.** This is achieved by eradicating the pathogens, restoring lactobacilli, and avoiding overgrowth of other potentially harmful microorganisms.
        (2) **Treatment** is recommended for the following patient groups:
            (a) Symptomatic gynecologic patients

(b) Selected asymptomatic gynecologic patients (e.g., before invasive vaginal or abdominal procedures)

(c) Symptomatic obstetric patients (after the first trimester, if possible)

(d) Selected asymptomatic obstetric patients (e.g., those with spontaneous rupture of membranes or preterm labor)

(3) Medications [Centers for Disease Control and Prevention (CDC), 1998]

(a) Oral agents include **metronidazole** 500 mg bid for 7 days; 2-g single dose or **clindamycin** 300 mg bid for 7 days.

(b) Vaginal agents include **metronidazole gel** (0.75%) bid for 5 days or **clindamycin cream** (2%) qid for 7 days.

(c) Side effects of metronidazole include a metallic taste and an Antabuse-like reaction to alcohol (i.e., nausea and vomiting).

(4) No treatment of the sexual partner is needed, because treatment does not decrease the rate of recurrence.

6. Candida vaginitis

a. Epidemiology. *Candida* vaginitis, most frequently with *Candida albicans,* is the second most common cause of vaginal complaints. Non-*albicans* species include *Candida tropicalis* and *Candida glabrata.*

b. Risk factors include:

(1) Factors altering the immune response include human immunodeficiency virus (HIV) infection, especially with a low CD4 count; immunosuppressive agents (e.g., corticosteroids); pregnancy; and oral contraceptive agents.

(2) Factors that increase glucose levels [e.g., uncontrolled diabetes mellitus (DM)]

(3) Factors that eradicate lactobacillus (e.g., broad-spectrum antibiotics)

c. Diagnosis

(1) Chief complaint: intense itching and burning

(2) Clinical findings include the following:

(a) Vulvar erythema and edema

(b) Whitish discharge varying from thin to curd-like consistency

(c) Vaginal pH usually normal (< 4.5)

(3) A wet-mount KOH prep is a low-cost office procedure that is 100% specific if branching **pseudohyphae** are present.

d. Management (CDC, 1998)

(1) Vaginal antifungal creams or suppositories such as butaconazole, clotrimazole, miconazole, terconazole, or ticonazole for 7–14 days

(2) Oral antifungal agents such as fluconazole in a single 150-mg tablet

(3) No treatment of the sexual partner is necessary, because treatment does not reduce the rate of recurrence.

7. *Trichomonas vaginalis* vaginitis

a. Epidemiology. Humans are the only host of *T. vaginalis,* a sexually transmitted protozoal parasite with four flagella. Most commonly, this parasite resides asymptomatically in male seminal fluid. *T. vagi-nalis* is the **most common cause of vaginitis worldwide.** Both patients and their partners require treatment.

    b. Diagnosis

      (1) Clinical findings include:

        (a) Vulvar erythema and edema

        (b) A profuse, malodorous, frothy, yellow-green discharge

        (c) *Trichomonas* cervicitis with red, punctate lesions (i.e., "strawberry patches")

        (d) Vaginal pH > 4.5

      (2) Wet-mount saline preparation is a low-cost office procedure that is 100% specific if motile organisms are present. However, it detects only 70% of infections.

      (3) Culture is the most sensitive diagnostic method.

    c. Management (CDC, 1998) involves treatment with **metronidazole.** The **patient** should receive 500 mg PO bid for 7 days or a single 2-g dose stat. Her **partner** should receive an immediate dose. Treatment during the first trimester of pregnancy should be avoided. **Side effects** include a metallic taste and an Antabuse-like reaction to alcohol (i.e., nausea and vomiting).

  8. Treatment options for other diagnoses of vaginal discharge include the following:

    a. Chlamydia infections should be treated with tetracycline, erythromycin, or doxycycline (see Chapter 9 II A).

    b. Gonorrhea should be treated with ceftriaxone, spectinomycin, or ciprofloxacin (see Chapter 9 II C).

    c. The severity and duration of **herpes virus lesions** may be decreased with acyclovir, famciclovir, or valacyclovir (see Chapter 9 I C).

    d. Chemical vaginitis is managed by identification and avoidance of the chemical agent.

    e. Physiologic discharge (from extensive exocervical columnar epithelium that produces increased mid-cycle cervical mucus) is managed by patient reassurance (further treatment is unnecessary).

V. VULVAR LESIONS

  A. Vulvar anatomy and physiology

    1. Anatomic components include the mons, labia majora/minora, clitoris, and vestibule, as well as Skene's and Bartholin's glands.

    2. Histologic features can be described as follows:

      a. Vulvar skin is keratinized stratified squamous epithelium with sebaceous glands.

      b. Vulvar structures *with* associated hair follicles and sweat glands include the mons pubis and the labia majora.

      c. Vulvar structures *without* hair follicles and sweat glands include the labia minora, clitoris, and vestibule.

3. **Nerve supply** is via the perineal, genitofemoral, and ilioinguinal nerves.

4. **Lymphatic drainage** is via superficial inguinal lymphatics.

B. **Pathophysiology**

1. **Range of pathology.** The vulva is susceptible to diseases that are common to skin generally as well as to specific genital diseases.

2. **Factors predisposing to vulvar symptoms** include sexual habits, recent systemic infections, use of antibiotics, and history of diabetes.

C. **Clinical issues**

1. **Classification of vulvar lesions**

   a. **Inflammatory dermatoses** include the following conditions:

   (1) **Intertrigo** occurs primarily on moist surfaces and is associated with a secondary fungal infection.

   (2) **Irritative vulvitis** is a localized reaction to chemicals (e.g., sprays, soaps) or aggravation from clothing (e.g., latex, nylon).

   (3) **Hidradenitis suppurativa,** a chronic, difficult-to-treat condition, arises from blockage or infection of the apocrine glands.

   (4) **Diabetic vulvitis** is associated with a secondary candidal infection. The vulva develops a beefy, red, inflammatory appearance.

   b. **Vulvar dystrophies** (Table 8-5) represent a spectrum of **hyperplastic** (squamous hyperplasia) and/or **atrophic** (lichen sclerosis) lesions.

   (1) **Cause.** Vulvar dystrophies are caused by a wide range of stimuli, resulting in both diffuse as well as localized **white lesions** of the vulva.

   (2) **Epidemiology.** White women **over 65 years** old are most commonly afflicted.

   (3) **Chief complaint** is frequently **itching** leading to secondary changes from prolonged scratching.

   (4) **Palpation** of squamous hyperplasia reveals a **white, firm, cartilaginous** lesion, whereas palpation of lichen sclerosis reveals a **thin, parchment-like** lesion.

   (5) **Biopsy is imperative** because areas of dysplasia or invasive cancer may mimic or coexist with vulvar dystrophies.

   (6) **Treatment** of squamous hyperplasia is **fluorinated corticosteroids** and that of lichen sclerosis is **testosterone cream.**

   c. **Benign tumors** include Bartholin's gland cysts or sebaceous gland cysts, as well as hidradenomas, nevi, fibromas, and hemangiomas.

2. **Diagnosis.** Physical examination or colposcopy cannot rule out vulvar dysplasia or carcinoma. **Vulvar biopsy must be performed for a definitive diagnosis.** With multiple lesions, the worst lesion should be selected for biopsy. With one large lesion, the biopsy should be taken from the margin of normal skin.

3. **VIN**

   a. **Definitions.** VIN refers to vulvar cellular atypia that is **limited to the epithelium** and has not penetrated the basement membrane. It includes a **spectrum** ranging from mild dysplasia (VIN I) to CIS (VIN III).

Table 8-5. Vulval Dystrophies

	Squamous Hyperplasia	Lichen Sclerosis	Mixed Dystrophy
Gross Appearance	White/grayish white, focal or diffuse	Small bluish-white papules that coalesce into white plaques	Combination of both
Symptoms	Pruritus	Pruritus; dyspareunia	Combination of both
Feel on Palpation	Firm cartilaginous	Thin, parchment-like	Combination of both
Histology	Thickened keratin with proliferative epithelium	Moderate hyperkeratosis with epithelial thinning	Combination of both
Patho-physiology	Reactive phenomena from irritation	Unknown	N/A
Method of Diagnosis	Biopsy	Biopsy	Biopsy
Treatment	Fluorinated corticosteroids	Testosterone cream	Combination of both

      (1) **Vulvar dysplasia** is marked by atypical cellular maturation that does not involve full epithelial thickness.

      (2) **Vulvar CIS** is marked by full-thickness atypical cellular maturation.

    b. **Epidemiology**

      (1) **VIN** is often found in association with **CIN,** and both conditions are frequently associated with **HPV types 16** and **18.** They have a similar histologic appearance, but with vulvar disease, progression to invasive carcinoma occurs much less than with cervical disease.

      (2) **VIN** is frequently multifocal in nature and often involves areas contiguous to the vulva with the most common sites being the anus and clitoris.

    c. **Differential diagnosis.** Viral diseases and early invasive carcinoma may produce histologic patterns that are indistinguishable from VIN.

    d. **Treatment.** Management of VIN involves **surgical excision** or **skinning vulvectomy** (removing only vulvar epithelium leaving subcutaneous tissue) or **laser ablation.** Topical chemotherapy is not usually successful.

    e. **Follow-up evaluations** should be scheduled every 4 months for 2 years, then every 6 months for the next 3 years.

  4. **Paget's disease,** which is generally seen in postmenopausal women, appears grossly as a diffuse **erythematous eczematoid lesion.** The fiery red background is mottled with white hyperkeratotic islands.

    a. **Epidemiology.** The disease is frequently **associated with other invasive carcinomas** [e.g., cervix, vulva, Bartholin's gland, breast,

    b. Histology. Large, pale apocrine cells involve the entire epithelium, and 90% of lesions are intraepithelial.

    c. Treatment. Management involves **wide excision** or **simple vulvectomy** (which removes epithelium and superficial subcutaneous tissue) to rule out invasion and node dissection, if there is invasive disease. Because the chance of recurrence is high, patients require careful follow-up.

5. Invasive vulvar carcinoma

    a. Epidemiology

        (1) Vulvar carcinoma is the **fourth most** common female reproductive tract malignancy, and it is responsible for 5% of gynecologic cancers.

        (2) The most common tumor type is **squamous cell** carcinoma (90%).

        (3) Average age at diagnosis is **65 years.**

        (4) Risk factors include obesity, hypertension, and **HPV 16** and **18.**

    b. Clinical findings and diagnosis

        (1) Pruritus is the **most common symptom,** but most early stage I disease is **asymptomatic.**

        (2) Definitive diagnosis requires a biopsy.

        (3) Primary spread is by local extension.

        (4) Lymphatic spread usually occurs in a sequential manner from the **superficial** inguinal lymph nodes to the **deep** inguinal lymph nodes.

    c. Staging. Staging is **surgical** using the tumor, nodes, metastasis (TNM) system (Table 8-6).

    d. Management. The overall 5-year survival rate is 70%. Treatment options include the following:

        (1) Basic treatment is **radical vulvectomy,** which removes tissue en bloc, including the mons pubis, clitoris, labia minora, labia majora, urethra, and perineal body, and **regional lymphadenectomy,** which is dissection of superficial and deep inguinal nodes.

Table 8-6. Surgical Staging System for Vulvar Carcinoma (FIGO*, 1989)

Stage	Description
0	Carcinoma-in-situ; carcinoma confined to epithelium
I	Tumor confined to vulva; ≤ 2 cm; negative nodes
II	Tumor confined to vulva; > 2 cm; negative nodes
III	Tumor any size with spread to lower urethra, vagina, anus; unilateral inguinal nodes
IVA	Tumor invades upper urethra, mucosa of bladder/rectum, pelvic bone; bilateral nodes
IVB	Any distant metastasis including pelvic nodes

*FIGO = International Federation of Gynecologists and Obstetricians.

(2) Radiation therapy and chemotherapy are adjunctive.

(3) **Cloquet's node** (i.e., the highest deep inguinal node beneath the inguinal ligament) is **predictive of distant metastases.**

VI. PELVIC RELAXATION

A. **Pelvic prolapse.** Disorders of pelvic support are described according to the organ primarily affected or displaced. They result from weakness in the pelvic diaphragm and specifically in the levator ani muscle (see Chapter 1 I H). Disorders of pelvic support affect one-third of parous women, but most are asymptomatic.

1. **Uterine prolapse.** Although uterine prolapse may occur as an isolated finding, it is more often found in association with one or more herniation defects of the vaginal walls.

   a. **Symptoms** include heaviness or fullness in pelvis, a feeling of "something falling out," low backache, and difficulty walking.

   b. **Degrees of uterine prolapse**

      (1) **First degree.** The cervix is in the vagina.

      (2) **Second degree.** The cervix is beyond the introitus.

      (3) **Third degree.** The entire uterus is outside the vagina (i.e., **procidentia**) because of failure of all genital supports, which results in purulent discharge, decubitus ulceration, and bleeding.

2. **Cystocele** (upper anterior vaginal wall herniation)

   a. **Symptoms**

      (1) Urinary frequency and urgency

      (2) Urinary incontinence

      (3) Urinary retention

   b. **Nature of prolapse.** The **bladder** is within the cystocele.

3. **Enterocele** (upper posterior vaginal wall herniation)

   a. **Symptoms** (often vague in presentation)

      (1) Backache or a pulling sensation when standing that is relieved by lying down

      (2) Uncomfortable pressure with a falling-out sensation in the vagina

   b. **Nature of prolapse.** The **pouch of Douglas** is herniated and the vagina contains loops of small bowel.

4. **Rectocele** (lower posterior vaginal wall herniation)

   a. **Symptoms**

      (1) The patient has difficulty emptying her rectum.

      (2) Digital help splinting the posterior vaginal wall is necessary.

   b. **Nature of prolapse.** The **rectum** is within the vagina.

B. **Predisposing factors**

1. Stretching of the pelvic supports by pregnancy

2. Genetic predisposition

3. Pelvic connective tissue weakness

4. Chronically increased intra-abdominal pressure as a result of chronic cough, ascites, heavy lifting, or constipation

C. Appropriate management

1. Nonsurgical approaches

a. Kegel exercises strengthen the pelvic diaphragm and levator ani muscles. The patient tightens the pubococcygeal muscle as if to stop the flow of urine.

b. Pessaries are objects inserted into the vagina that elevate the pelvic structures into a more normal anatomic position.

   (1) Indications include patients who are medically unfit for surgery, are pregnant, are postpartum, or require healing of a decubitus ulcer before surgery.

   (2) Side effects may include vaginal infection or discharge.

c. Estrogen replacement therapy (ERT) may improve tissue tone and connective tissue support in postmenopausal women.

4. Surgery is the definitive treatment of genital prolapse.

a. Anterior colporrhaphy, which plicates the pubocervical fascia

b. Posterior colporrhaphy, which plicates the endopelvic fascia

c. Enterocele repair, which plicates the uterosacral ligaments/levator ani muscles

d. Le Fort's partial colpocleisis, which partially occludes the vagina to support the uterus

e. Complete colpocleisis, which completely occludes the vagina to provide uterine support

VII. URINARY INCONTINENCE, the involuntary loss of urine (Table 8-7)

A. Prevalence. Incidence of urinary incontinence increases with age and parity.

1. Approximately 10% of women have regular urinary incontinence.

2. Approximately 50% of women have occasional urinary incontinence.

B. Normal micturition (urination) physiology. Continence of urine requires intravesical pressure to be lower than urethral sphincter pressure. This is achieved by a relaxed detrusor muscle combined with a contracted bladder neck and urethra. **Micturition** occurs when intravesical pressure exceeds urethral sphincter pressure. This is achieved by contracting the destrusor muscle and relaxing the urethral sphincter.

1. Urethral length. The longer the urethra, the easier continence is maintained. Because the female urethra is only 5 cm long (compared with 12 cm in the male), incontinence is much more common in females than males.

2. Pubourethral ligaments. The urethra is supported by the pubourethral ligaments of the pelvic diaphragm. Loss of support of these ligaments can lead to incontinence.

3. Innervation of the lower urinary tract

   a. Parasympathetic fibers from S2–S4 stimulate detrusor contractions that promote **micturition.** Uncontrolled cholinergic stimula-

Table 8-7. Female Urinary Incontinence

	Irritative	Stress	Urge	Overflow	Bypass
Amount	Small	Small	Large	Small	Small
Description	Complete emptying	In spurts	Complete emptying	Dribbling	Dribbling
Duration	Moderate, over several seconds	Brief, with stress	Moderate, over several seconds	Continuous	Continuous
Associated symptoms	Urgency, frequency, dysuria	None	Urgency and nocturia	Fullness and pressure	None
Position	Any	Upright and sitting but not supine or asleep	Any	Any	Any
Associated event	Coughing, exercise, bladder filling	Coughing, laughing; sneezing; physical activity	Coughing exercise; running water; touch; cold	None	None
Cause	Cystitis Bladder tumor Bladder foreign object	Intraabominal pressure increase transmitted more to bladder and less to urethra	Loss of voluntary bladder inhibition	Lower motor neuron lesions Systemic medications Urethral obstruction	Fistula, Urethral diverticulum
Residual volume	Normal	Normal	Normal	Increased	Normal
Sensation of fullness	Decreased volume	Normal volume	Decreased volume	Increased volume	Normal volume
Treatment	Antibiotics Resect tumor Remove foreign object	Kegel exercises Estrogen Urethropexy Collagen injections	Anticholinergics β = Adrenergic agonists Behavior modification Surgical denervation	Intermittent catheterization Cholinergic α-adrenergic blockers Discontinue medications Relieve obstruction	Surgical repair

tion, found with acute cystitis and radiation injury, leads to incontinence. Cholinergic stimulation is inhibited by perineal and anal stimulation.

     b. **Sympathetic fibers from T10–T12 and L1–L2** enhance the following responses that promote urinary **continence.**

         (1) **α-Adrenergics** contract the bladder neck and urethra.

         (2) **β-Adrenergics** relax the detrusor muscle of the bladder.

   4. Bladder muscle dynamics

     a. **Detrusor muscle** fibers have the unique intrinsic ability to relax in response to increasing bladder volume. Therefore the bladder can fill without concomitant increase in intraluminal pressure.

    b. Voluntary suppression of detrusor contractions, when the bladder is filled, normally allows control of micturition.

  5. Normal cystometric measurements (Box 8-2)

C. Urinary incontinence in pregnant women

  1. Intermittent urinary incontinence may be a normal third-trimester finding. The bladder becomes compressed by the enlarging fetus, and descent of the presenting part encroaches on the bladder.

  2. Infectious etiologies can cause urinary incontinence during pregnancy. It is important to differentiate upper and lower urinary tract disease as well as local and systemic processes (e.g., by fever, right or left flank tenderness).

    a. Asymptomatic bacteriuria criteria include the following:

      (1) Midstream, clean-catch specimen

      (2) Colony count of $> 100,000/ml$ on culture

      (3) Isolation of a single organism (not including lactobacillus, which is probably a vaginal contaminant)

    b. Urinary tract anomalies (i.e., urethral diverticulum, duplicated ureter) predispose to symptomatic or asymptomatic bacteriuria.

    c. Obstetric complications. Bladder inflammation irritates the underlying myometrium and may cause uterine contractions that may progress to preterm labor.

D. Urinary incontinence in nonpregnant women (see Table 8-7) may result from a number of causes. A **voiding diary,** kept by the patient, documents the temporal relationships of when urine loss occurs.

  1. Sensory irritative incontinence should be ruled out as the first step in a workup. A variety of irritative lower urinary tract conditions can result in involuntary loss of urine.

    a. Causes may include:

      (1) Infection (e.g., cystitis)

      (2) Neoplastic process (e.g., bladder tumor)

      (3) Foreign body in the urinary bladder

    b. Symptoms may include urinary urgency, frequency, and dysuria.

    c. Physical examination findings include the following:

      (1) Urinary leakage with urgency

Box 8–2. Normal cystometric measurements

Bladder residual volume	< 50 ml
Sensation-of-fullness volume	150–200 ml
Urge-to-void volume	400–500 ml

(2) Stable bladder without anatomic defect

(3) Normal neurologic examination

  d. Diagnostic workup includes the following:

    (1) WBCs and **bacteria** on **urinalysis** suggest an infectious etiology. A positive **urine culture** confirms the diagnosis.

    (2) Red blood cells (RBCs) on **urinalysis** suggest a tumor or foreign body. **Cystourethroscopy** confirms the diagnosis.

    (3) Normal **cystometric examination**

  e. Management is directed at the specific cause (e.g., **antibiotics** for cystitis, **resection** of tumor, or **removal** of foreign body).

2. Genuine stress incontinence occurs when intra-abdominal pressure increases are transmitted less to the urethra than to the bladder.

  a. Mechanisms

    (1) Weakness of the pelvic diaphragm leads to loss of bladder support, which results in anatomic descent of the proximal urethra so that it lies below the pelvic floor rather than being intra-abdominal.

    (2) Changes in the urethrovesical angle result in stressful activities producing a greater increase in intravesical pressure than in urethral pressure.

      (a) Urine loss occurs **only in spurts** during the brief time that the intravesical pressure exceeds the urethral pressure.

      (b) Detrusor muscle contractions do *not* **occur** so the bladder does not empty completely.

  b. Clinical findings

    (1) History of sporadic loss of small amounts of urine caused by coughing, laughing, sneezing, and physical activity

    (2) No loss when patients are supine or asleep (unique to stress incontinence)

    (3) Cystocele or urethrocele, with evidence of anterior vaginal wall relaxation, on physical examination (perhaps)

  c. Diagnosis is not based on any single test but includes **all of the following:**

    (1) A urine culture rules out an infection.

    (2) Neurologic examination is normal.

    (3) Cystometrogram is normal (i.e., normal residual volume, normal bladder capacity, normal sensation, no involuntary detrusor contractions).

    (4) Demonstrable urinary leakage is seen with voluntary stress.

    (5) Positive cotton-tipped applicator test **(Q-tip or Bonney test)** shows poor anatomic support. The angle of a lubricated Q-tip, when placed in the urethra, changes more than 30 degrees when intra-abdominal pressure is increased.

  d. Management may include either medical or surgical measures.

    (1) Medical approaches

      (a) Kegel exercises can strengthen the pelvic floor musculature.

      (b) ERT therapy in postmenopausal women dilates the periurethral venous plexus, thus elevating resting urethral pressure.

(2) Surgical approaches

(a) Elevation of the urethrovesical angle (urethropexy) is the only **definitive treatment** to restore the normal anatomic relationships. The proximal urethra and bladder neck become intra-abdominal structures and receive equal pressure transmission as the bladder with coughing and sneezing. The abdominal approaches have higher success rates (approaching 90%) than vaginal approaches.

(b) Collagen injections can compress the urethral mucosa, thus elevating resting urethral pressure.

3. **Motor urge incontinence,** the second most common cause of female urinary incontinence, increases in prevalence with advancing age. It results from detrusor instability. Other synonyms are detrusor dyssynergia/hyperreflexia, hypertonic bladder, and uninhibited/unstable bladder.

a. **Mechanisms** can be described as follows:

(1) Involuntary uninhibited detrusor muscle contractions occur. **This is the only cause of urinary incontinence in which detrusor contractions take place.**

(2) Contractions of the unstable bladder may occur spontaneously or on provocation by coughing, exercising, feeling cold, or hearing running water. This results in contractions of the detrusor muscle that **completely empty the bladder.**

b. **Symptoms** include the following:

(1) Urinary urgency and frequency, which occur even at rest or at night

(2) Unpredictable loss of large volumes

c. **Physical examination** may be normal and rarely provides strong supportive evidence of detrusor instability.

d. **Diagnosis** is confirmed by **all** of the following cystometric findings:

(1) Involuntary bladder contractions that are associated with urinary leakage

(2) Normal residual volume and sensation

(3) Decreased urge-to-void volume

e. **Management** is medical only (i.e., nonsurgical) and includes the following:

(1) Anticholinergic medications [e.g., oxybutynin (Ditropan), propantheline (Probanthine)] to suppress parasympathetic stimulation, leading to decreased detrusor muscle tone

(2) β-adrenergic agonists [e.g., flavoxate (Urispas)] to relax the detrusor muscle

(3) Nonsteroidal anti-inflammatory drugs (NSAIDs) [e.g., ibuprofen] to inhibit bladder contractions

(3) Bladder retraining to help patients regain cortical control of the voiding reflex that has been lost

4. **Overflow incontinence** results when intravesical pressure from an overdistended bladder exceeds urethral pressure. Urine leakage continues only until pressure in the bladder falls below the urethral pressure. **The bladder never empties. Detrusor contractions do not occur.**

a. **Underlying mechanisms** may include the following:

   (1) **Detrusor areflexia/hypotonia,** which can result from the following:

      (a) **Denervated bladder,** which can be caused by DM or lower motor neuron disorders

      (b) **Systemic medications** such as ganglionic blockers, anticholinergic medications, α-adrenergic agonists, and epidural or spinal anesthetics

   (2) **Urethral obstructive disorders** such as urethral kinking or pelvic masses

b. **Cystometric findings** include the following:

   (1) Increased residual volume

   (2) Increased bladder capacity (> 1000 ml)

   (3) Decreased sensation

   (4) Poor detrusor contractility

c. **Management** is only medical (i.e., nonsurgical) and includes the following:

   (1) Intermittent self-catheterization

   (2) **Cholinergic agents** [e.g., bethanechol (Urecholine)] to stimulate detrusor tone and contractility

   (3) **α-Adrenergic blockers** [e.g. phenoxybenzamine (Dibenzyline)] to decrease bladder outlet resistance

   (4) Discontinuation of causative systemic medications

5. **Bypass incontinence** results when the normal urethral sphincteric mechanism is bypassed, usually with a fistula.

   a. **Mechanisms**

      (1) **Formation of a fistula,** which is an abnormal passageway between two body areas that are normally separated by a tissue barrier

         (a) The location is usually ureterovaginal, vesicovaginal, or urethrovaginal.

         (b) Approximately 95% of fistulas result from extensive pelvic surgery or pelvic radiation.

      (2) **Urethral diverticulum,** which is a sac-like outpouching from the urethral lumen that creates a reservoir of urine that can empty unpredictably

   b. **Symptoms**

      (1) **Fistula:** constant urinary drainage after pelvic surgery or pelvic radiation

      (2) **Urethral diverticulum:** postvoid urinary incontinence, urgency, and frequency

   c. **Diagnosis**

      (1) **IVP** with contrast allows inspection for radiologic evidence of contrast leakage.

      (2) **IV indigo carmine dye injection** allows inspection for dye leakage into a fresh tampon inserted in the vagina.

      (3) **Urethroscopy** allows inspection for a diverticulum.

   d. **Management.** Surgery is the only definitive treatment, with a success rate higher than 90%.

Review Test

Directions: Each of the numbered items or incomplete statements in this section is followed by answers or by completions of the statement. Select the ONE lettered answer or completion that is BEST in each case.

1. What is the natural progression of most mild dysplasias of the cervix diagnosed in pregnancy?

(A) Undergoing metaplasia to adenosis
(B) Progressing slowly over the next 20 years
(C) Progressing rapidly over the next 5 years to invasive carcinoma
(D) Spontaneously regressing without treatment
(E) Remaining static without progression

2. Which one of the following statements is the presumptive explanation when a cervical biopsy is less severe than would be expected from the Papanicolaou (Pap) smear?

(A) The lesion has undergone spontaneous involution since the biopsy was taken
(B) The processing of biopsy specimens caused an artifact in the histologic appearance
(C) The Pap smear was overread by the cytologist or pathologist
(D) The less severe biopsy specimen was actually from another patient
(E) The biopsy was taken from a site other than the one from which cells were harvested for a Pap smear

3. Which one of the following stages is the International Federation of Gynecology and Obstetrics (FIGO) clinical staging for cervical carcinoma when the pelvic sidewall is not involved, but the lower one-third of the vagina is involved?

(A) Stage IIA
(B) Stage IIB
(C) Stage IIIA
(D) Stage IIIB
(E) Stage IV

4. Which one of the following effects of parasympathetic stimulation on the lower urinary tract is true?

(A) Detrusor contractions enhanced
(B) Detrusor contractions inhibited
(C) Urethral contraction
(D) Urethral relaxation

Directions: Each of the numbered items or incomplete statements in this section is negatively phrased, as indicated by a capitalized word such as NOT, LEAST, or EXCEPT. Select the ONE lettered answer or completion that is best in each case.

5. All of the following conditions are indications for cervical cone biopsy EXCEPT

(A) the cervical lesion(s) cannot be fully visualized
(B) a history of cervical dysplasia
(C) the endocervical curettage (ECC) is positive
(D) the biopsy reveals microinvasive squamous cell carcinoma
(E) the biopsy reveals adenocarcinoma in situ

6. All of the following are characteristics of a normal vaginal ecosystem EXCEPT

(A) the dominant microflora is lactobacillus
(B) high progesterone levels
(C) low vaginal pH
(D) glycogen metabolized into lactic acid
(E) a low concentration of anaerobic streptococcus

Directions: The set of matching questions in this section consists of a list of four to twenty-six lettered options (some of which may be in figures) followed by several numbered items. For each numbered item, select the ONE lettered option that is most closely associated with it. To avoid spending too much time on matching sets with large sets of options, it is generally advisable to begin each set by reading the list of options. Then, for each item in the set, try to generate the correct answer and locate it in the option list, rather than evaluating each option individually. Each lettered option may be selected once, more than once, or not at all.

Questions 7–11

For each of the following risk factors or etiologies, select the correct type of female urinary incontinence.
(A) Sensory irritation incontinence
(B) Motor urge incontinence
(C) Overflow incontinence
(D) Total incontinence
(E) Genuine stress incontinence

7. Diabetes

8. Bladder tumor

9. Pelvic radiation

10. Epidural anesthetic

11. Cystitis

Answers and Explanations

1. The answer is D [III F 1].

Spontaneous regression without treatment postpartum is found in 75% of patients with cervical dysplasia, which is a continuum of intraepithelial neoplastic transformation in which abnormal, immature, disorganized cells replace normal cells. The sequence of progression from minimal involvement to full-thickness change does not always occur. Undergoing metaplasia to adenosis is incorrect because the sequence is reversed with adenosis (columnar epithelium) undergoing metaplasia to squamous type. The remaining options are possible scenarios but are less likely in pregnancy.

2. The answer is E [III H].

The Papanicolaou (Pap) smear is a screening test, and the colposcopically directed cervical biopsy is the confirmatory test for detecting the true identity of the abnormal epithelium. A biopsy that does not agree with the cytology causes concern because a more advanced lesion may not have been identified. If an early invasive cervical cancer is present, but the treatment was for only an intraepithelial lesion, the missed cancer might spread. It is possible, but unlikely, that the lesion could undergo spontaneous involution. Artifacts created during processing of the biopsy should be apparent to the pathologist. Pap smear overreading is a rare occurrence, and mistakes in labeling specimens are more infrequent.

3. The answer is C [Table 8-4].

Stage IIIA assesses the degree to which the cervical cancer has spread from the cervix. Cervical carcinoma staging is clinically based and is the only female reproductive tract cancer that is not surgically staged. Stage IIA and stage IIB are incorrect because involvement of the lower one-third of the vagina excludes stage II. Stage IIIB does involve the pelvic sidewall or the kidney. Stage IV is incorrect because there is no invasion beyond the true pelvis or bladder or rectal mucosa.

4. The answer is A [VII B 3].

Enhancement of detrusor contractility is by parasympathetic stimulation. Innervation of the lower urinary tract involves the detrusor muscle, the bladder neck, and the urethra. Parasympathetic fibers largely control the detrusor muscle, and sympathetic fibers innervate the bladder neck and urethra. Detrusor inhibition is the result of parasympathetic suppression. Urethral contraction occurs from α-adrenergic stimulation, whereas urethral relaxation results from β-adrenergic stimulation.

5. The answer is B [III H 7].

A previous history of cervical dysplasia is the correct answer (but the statement is incorrect) because when the dysplasia is adequately treated with ablative therapy and follow-up confirms normal cytology, cone biopsy is not indicated. Lack of visualization of the cervical lesion(s), a positive endocervical curettage (ECC), and biopsy specimens showing either microinvasive carcinoma or adenocarcinoma in situ are all appropriate indications for cone biopsy.

6. The answer is B [IV A].

A healthy vagina is fostered by high estrogen levels, not high progesterone levels. A healthy vagina is the result of many factors maintained in a delicate physiologic balance. A change in any of these factors could result in an altered state of pathology. Characteristics of a normal environment are lactobacillus as the dominant organism, an acidic pH as the result of lactobacilli metabolizing glycogen to lactic acid, and low concentrations of anaerobic organisms.

7–11. The answers are: 10-C [VII D 3], 11-A [VII D 2], 12-D [VII D 1], 13-C [VII], 14-A [VII D 1].

Bladder denervation caused by diabetes results in overflow incontinence. The irritation of a bladder tumor can lead to sensory irritation incontinence. The development of a bladder fistula secondary to pelvic radiation results in total incontinence. Epidural anesthesia may lead to a detrusor hypotonia characterized by overflow incontinence. The irritation of cystitis can lead to sensory irritation incontinence.

9

Sexually Transmitted Diseases

I. SEXUALLY TRANSMITTED DISEASES (STDs) WITH GENITAL ULCERS

A. Chancroid

1. **Epidemiology.** *Haemophilus ducreyi,* a small, gram-negative, non-motile facultative anaerobic bacterium, is the causative agent of this **uncommon STD. Chancroid is rare in the United States** but common in developing countries. The **male:female ratio is 5:1.** Although this condition is highly contagious, it cannot penetrate and invade normal skin but requires tissue trauma and excoriation.

2. **Signs.** The initial lesion is a small papule, which becomes a pustule that ulcerates in 48–72 hours. The vulvar ulcer is soft and **painful** with a characteristic ragged edge. The exudate is dirty, gray, and necrotic without induration. Within 2 weeks, 50% of infected women develop a pseudobubo (acutely tender, unilateral inguinal adenopathy).

3. **Diagnosis** involves identifying the organism on Gram strain or culture of ulcer discharge or node aspirate.

4. **Management.** The Centers for Disease Control and Prevention (CDC) [1998] recommends oral **erythromycin** base (500 mg qid) for 7 days. A single dose of intramuscular (IM) ceftriaxone 250 mg or oral azithromycin 1 g is also effective. Fluctuant nodes should be aspirated to prevent abscess rupture. Sexual partner(s) should always be treated.

B. Granuloma inguinale (donovanosis)

1. **Epidemiology.** *Calymmatobacterium granulomatis,* a gram-negative, nonmotile, encapsulated rod-shaped bacterium, is the causative agent. **This infection is rare in the United States** but common in the tropics. It can be spread by both **sexual and nonsexual contact.** Infectivity is low.

2. **Signs.** A symptomatic nodule forms at the site of infection, leading to skin ulceration and formation of a **painless** beefy red ulcer of granulation tissue. Multiple nodules or ulcers may coalesce. Secondary infection

can develop. Inguinal adenopathy is minimal. The chronic form may lead to scarring, lymphatic obstruction, and vulvar edema.

3. **Diagnosis** involves identifying the characteristic **Donovan bodies** in smears or biopsies from the ulcer.

4. **Differential diagnosis** includes lymphogranuloma venereum (LGV), chancroid, syphilis, herpes, and vulvar carcinoma.

5. **Management.** The CDC (1998) recommends oral **trimethoprim-sulfamethoxazole** bid or oral **doxycycline** 100 mg bid for 3 weeks. An initial response is seen within 1 week, but complete resolution may take up to 1 month.

C. **Herpes simplex virus (HSV)** [see Chapter 5 V and Table 5-1]

1. **Epidemiology** (see Chapter 5 V A)

2. **Clinical findings** (see Chapter 5 V B 1)

3. **Diagnosis** (see Chapter 5 V B 2)

4. **Management.** There is no effective cure.

   a. **Abstinence** from sexual contact until complete lesion reepithelialization occurs

   b. **Symptomatic relief** from hot sitz baths and use of diluted Burow's solution

   c. **Antiviral agents,** which include **acyclovir, famciclovir,** or **valacyclovir** (CDC, 1998)

      (1) Primary infections are treated by intravenous (IV) or oral routes (depending on disease severity) for 7–10 days.

      (2) Recurrent infections are treated by oral medications for 5 days.

      (3) Suppression of recurrences may be treated by continuous twice-daily oral medications. Recurrences are not prevented, but their frequency and severity may be decreased. **Suppression of recurrence may not decrease risk of sexual transmission.**

D. **Lymphogranuloma venereum (LGV)** is an uncommon STD that affects men six times more frequently than women. Although LGV occurs primarily in Africa and Asia, the causative organism can also be found in the southeastern United States.

1. **Risk factors** (same as those for chlamydia infections) [see II A 2]

2. **Pathophysiology**

   a. **Causative organism:** one of the aggressive L serotypes (1, 2, and 3) of *Chlamydia trachomatis*

   b. **Sexual transmission**

      (1) **Women.** The organisms are carried by lymphatic drainage from the genital lesion to the perirectal and pelvic lymph nodes predominantly. Rectal involvement, which is common in women, occurs by contiguous spread from the perirectal nodes, leading to proctocolitis and rectal strictures.

      (2) **Men.** Drainage is primarily to the inguinal nodes where the classic **bubo** (i.e., purplish, indurated, tender, inguinal mass) is found. The bubo is found less often in women.

   3. **Diagnosis.** Determination of LGV is based on clinical examina-

tion and is extremely difficult until the late stages of the disease. Subclinical infections are common.

   a. Clinical findings. The lesions start as a **painless** vesicopustular eruption that spontaneously disappears. After a few weeks, the sequelae of lymphatic spread appear with few systemic manifestations.

   b. Laboratory findings

     (1) The **Frei test** is based on a delayed skin hypersensitivity to the antigen.

     (2) The **complement fixation test** is more sensitive for LGV than the Frei test, but neither test can distinguish between current or past disease.

     (3) False-positive serologic tests for syphilis may occur.

  4. Complications. Problems are largely related to scar tissue formation.

   a. Proctitis may progress to **colitis** with perirectal strictures.

   b. Severe stricture formation may lead to **intestinal obstruction** requiring colostomy.

   c. Rectovaginal fistulas are often found in patients with strictures.

   d. Vulvar carcinoma has been implicated as a complication of LGV.

  5. Management. The CDC recommends **doxycycline** 100 mg PO bid for 21 days. Tetracycline, erythromycin, or sulfisoxazole 500 mg PO qid for 3–6 weeks is also effective. Surgical therapy is required for strictures or fistulas.

E. Syphilis is an STD caused by the motile spirochete ***Treponema pallidum*** (see Chapter 5 VI and Table 5-1). **Transmission** is by contact with either intact mucous membranes or contact with broken skin. In women, the **most frequent entry sites** are the vulva, vagina, and cervix.

  1. Clinical findings and diagnosis (see Chapter 5 VI B 2 a)

   a. Clinical findings with untreated disease include primary, secondary, latent, and tertiary syphilis.

   b. Laboratory tests (see Chapter 5 VI B 2 b)

   c. Screening serology tests are associated with up to 15% false-positive rates (see Chapter 5 VI B 2 c).

  2. Management

   a. Benzathine penicillin 2.4 million units IM once is the treatment of choice. With penicillin allergy, erythromycin or tetracycline 500 mg PO qid is administered for 14 days.

   b. Jarisch-Herxheimer reaction is an acute febrile reaction occurring within the first 24 hours after any therapy for syphilis. **Clinical findings** include headache, myalgia, uterine contractions, and late decelerations. It occurs in all women with primary syphilis and half of women with secondary syphilis.

   c. Venereal Disease Research Laboratory (VDRL) titers should decrease fourfold in 3 months and become negative in 12 months after treatment. A spinal tap should be performed to rule out neurosyphilis if titers remain positive after 1 year.

   d. Sexual partners of infected patients should be treated.

II. SEXUALLY TRANSMITTED DISEASE (STDs) WITHOUT GENITAL ULCERS

A. Chlamydia infection (see Chapter 13 IV; pelvic inflammatory disease)

1. **Epidemiology.** This condition is the **most common** sexually transmitted genital infection in women. *C. trachomatis* is the causative organism.

2. **Risk factors** include sexual activity at age less than 20 years, multiple sexual partners, new sexual partner within the previous 3 months, low socioeconomic status, and history of other STDs.

3. **Protection.** Use of barrier contraception may help prevent infection.

4. **Pathophysiology.** *C. trachomatis,* an **obligate intracellular microorganism,** attaches only to **columnar epithelial cells** without invading deep tissues. Adverse outcomes result from chronic inflammation and fibrosis.

5. **Diagnosis**

   a. **Clinical findings.** Patients are **frequently asymptomatic,** even when salpingitis is present. Physical findings include mucopurulent cervical discharge; hypertrophic, friable cervical inflammation; and acute urethral syndrome.

   b. **Laboratory findings.** Positive laboratory identification is the only way to make a definitive diagnosis.

      (1) **Cell culture** is the "gold standard," with 100% specificity. However, it may take up to 7 days for the culture to be read, and the test can be expensive.

      (2) **Direct-smear fluorescent antibody testing** has higher than 95% specificity and higher than 90% sensitivity. It is rapid, and results can be obtained in less than 1 hour.

6. **Complications**

   a. Complications **from salpingitis** arise from postinflammatory scar tissue and include:

      (1) **Infertility** caused by fimbrial agglutination or occlusion (see Chapter 16 III B)

      (2) **Ectopic** pregnancy from intraluminal tubal adhesions (see Chapter 13 V)

      (3) **Pelvic pain** from fibrosis of peritoneal surfaces leading to a "frozen pelvis"

      (4) **Dyspareunia** from pelvic visceral adhesions (see Table 14-2)

   b. **Neonatal infection** may occur as a result of delivery through an infected birth canal and may lead to inclusion conjunctivitis and otitis media.

   c. **Obstetric problems** that may occur from chlamydia infection coexistent with pregnancy include preterm delivery and postpartum endometritis.

7. **Management**

   a. **Tetracycline (contraindicated in pregnancy):** 500 mg PO qid for 7 days

   b. **Doxycycline (contraindicated in pregnancy):** 100 mg PO bid for 7 days

    c. Erythromycin: 500 mg PO bid for 7 days

    d. Amoxicillin: 500 mg PO tid for 7 days

    e. Ofloxacin (contraindicated in pregnancy): 300 mg PO bid for 7 days

B. Condyloma acuminatum

  1. Epidemiology. Human papilloma virus (HPV) is the causative agent, with 20 subtypes (of 70 identified) causing genital infections.

    a. Types 6 and 11 are associated with euploid, benign lesions.

    b. Types 16 and 18 are associated with aneuploid, premalignant, and malignant lesions of the cervix, vagina, vulva, and anus.

    c. Simultaneous infection can occur with multiple HPV types.

    d. Transmission is by sexual contact between mucous membranes, with peak incidence between ages 15 and 25.

      (1) Chance of acquiring the infection from an infected sexual partner is more than 50%.

      (2) Risk factors include immunosuppression, diabetes, pregnancy, and perineal trauma.

  2. Signs

    a. Most HPV infections are asymptomatic, subclinical, or unrecognized. In addition, most clinical lesions are asymptomatic.

    b. The initial lesions are pedunculated, soft papules 2–3 mm in diameter and 10–20 mm in length that may occur singly or in clusters. The lesions, which may coalesce into cauliflower-like masses, can be painful, friable, or pruritic.

    c. Clinical lesions are most commonly located in the following anatomic sites: cervix (70%), vulva (25%), anus (20%), and vagina (10%).

    d. Secondary infections may occur, leading to pain, odor, and bleeding.

  3. Diagnosis of clinical lesions is generally by gross inspection. Suspicious lesions should be biopsied. They demonstrate the characteristic histology.

  4. Management. The primary goal of treating visible HPV lesions is removal of symptomatic warts. Current treatments probably do not significantly affect the natural history of HPV infection or prevent the development of cervical carcinoma.

    a. Only clinical lesions are managed with local treatment. Therapeutic modality chosen depends on the location, size, and extent of the lesions(s), as well as the presence of pregnancy.

    b. No present therapy eliminates subclinical infection. The recurrence rate with all therapies is disappointing.

    c. Methods of treatment include the following:

      (1) Topical therapy is used for small lesions and includes **podofilox, podophyllin, trichloroacetic acid,** and **5-fluorouracil.** An immune response modifier, **imiquimod,** a new HPV topical therapy, may induce cytokines, including interferon-α (IFN-α).

      (2) Destructive, ablative procedures are used for larger lesions and include cryotherapy, electrodesiccation, laser vaporization, and surgical excision.

      (3) Immunotherapy with IFN may be intralesional or systemic.

C. Gonorrhea

1. **Epidemiology**

   a. *Neisseria gonorrhoeae,* a gram-negative diplococcal bacteria, is the causative organism.

      (1) **Bactericidal agents** include most disinfectants, as well as drying, sunlight, and heat.

      (2) **Sites of recovery** include the urethra, cervix, anal canal, and pharynx.

      (3) **Principal sites of invasion** are the following:

         (a) Columnar epithelium of the genital tract

         (b) Transitional epithelium of the urinary tract

   b. The **infection rate** after exposure to an infected sexual partner is as follows:

      (1) 35% in men

      (2) 75% in women

         (a) Approximately 15% develop salpingitis if untreated.

         (b) Approximately 30% develop a coexistent chlamydia infection.

2. **Diagnosis**

   a. **Early clinical findings**

      (1) **Asymptomatic** infections may be found in the pharynx, cervix, or rectum.

      (2) **Vulvovaginal/perineal infection** may result in inflammation, discharge, itching, and burning.

      (3) **Other findings** include cervical purulent discharge, urinary frequency/dysuria, and rectal discomfort.

   b. **Late clinical findings**

      (1) **Bartholinitis** is an inflammation of Bartholin's gland, which may develop into an abscess. With resolution, an asymptomatic fluid-filled cyst forms because of occlusion of Bartholin's duct.

      (2) **Disseminated infection** may develop from asymptomatic infection.

         (a) **Triad of common symptoms:** polyarthralgia, tenosynovitis, and dermatitis

         (b) **Additional findings** may include purulent arthritis as well as dermatitis, pericarditis, endocarditis, and meningitis.

      (3) **Ophthalmic infections may occur.**

         (a) **Conjunctivitis** (adults) as a result of autoinoculation

         (b) **Ophthalmia neonatorum** (newborns) as a result of delivery through an infected birth canal

      (4) **Vulvovaginitis may occur.** The invasion of nonkeratinized stratified squamous epithelium develops in **prepubertal** children and **postmenopausal** women because of low estrogen levels. In adults, keratinized membranes are resistant to gonorrhea, but when estrogen levels are low, the lack of keratinization increases vulnerability to vulvovaginitis.

   c. **Laboratory findings**

      (1) **Presumptive.** Gram stain of intracellular gram-negative diplococci may indicate gonorrhea.

(2) **Definitive.** A positive culture on **Thayer-Martin media** definitely indicates gonorrhea.

3. **Complications**

    a. **Acute salpingitis–peritonitis** (see Chapter 13 IV) is diagnosed by the presence of:

        (1) **All of the following criteria:**

            (a) Bilateral lower abdominal-pelvic pain usually following menses

            (b) Abdominal, uterine, adnexal, and cervical motion tenderness

            (c) Vaginal discharge

        (2) **Plus one or more of the following:**

            (a) Temperature $\geq$ 100.4°F (38°C)

            (b) WBC count > 10,000/mm^3

            (c) Inflammatory pelvic mass

            (d) Elevated sedimentation rate or C-reactive protein

            (e) Gram-negative intracellular diplococci in cervical secretions

    b. Untreated or inadequately treated infections can lead to **pelvic abscesses** such as:

        (1) **Pyosalpinx,** which is an occluded oviduct distended by pus

        (2) **Tubo-ovarian abscess,** which is an inflammatory mass involving the oviduct, ovary, and broad ligament

        (3) **Cul-de-sac abscess,** which is a collection of pus in the pouch of Douglas

    c. **Fimbrial agglutination or adnexal destruction** may lead to infertility.

    d. **Adhesion formation** in the pelvis can cause intestinal obstruction and pelvic pain.

4. **Management.** Treatment options (CDC, 1998) for women with gonorrhea involve outpatient therapy plus treatment of all male partners.

    a. **Cefoxitin** 2 g IM plus **probenecid** 1 g PO, followed by 14 days of

        (1) **Doxycycline:** 100 mg PO bid, **or**

        (2) **Tetracycline** 500 mg PO qid

    b. **Ceftriaxone** 250 mg IM plus **probenecid** 1 g PO, followed by 14 days of

        (1) **Doxycycline:** 100 mg PO bid, **or**

        (2) **Tetracycline:** 500 mg PO qid

    c. **Ofloxacin** 400 mg PO bid, followed by 14 days of

        (1) **Clindamycin:** 450 mg PO qid, **or**

        (2) **Metronidazole:** 500 mg PO bid

D. **Hepatitis B virus (HBV)** [see Chapter 5 VII and Table 5-1]

    1. **Epidemiology** (see Chapter 5 VII A 1)

    2. **Immunologic markers for HBV** (see Chapter 5 VII C)

    3. **Diagnosis** (see Chapter 5 VII D 2)

    4. **Management** (see Chapter 5 VII D 3)

    5. **Prevention**

        a. Hepatitis B surface antigen (HbsAg)–negative women at high risk for

HBV should receive **passive immunization** with hepatitis B immune globulin and **active immunization** with hepatitis B vaccine.

b. All adolescents should receive active immunization against HBV, because HBV is the only STD that can be prevented by immunization (CDC, 1998).

E. Human immunodeficiency virus (HIV) [see Chapter 5 VIII and Table 5-1]

1. **Likelihood of sexual transmission** from an infected partner (see Chapter 5 VIII A 2 a). Transmission may also occur via other body fluids (e.g., blood, oral secretions, breast milk).

2. **Microbiology** (see Chapter 5 VIII A 3)

3. **Course of disease** (see Chapter 5 VIII B 1). Antiviral agents, particularly multidrug regimens, may prolong life expectancy.

4. **Diagnosis of acquired immune deficiency syndrome (AIDS)** [see Chapter 5 VIII B 2]

5. **Prevention of HIV and AIDS** (see Chapter 5 VIII B 3)

6. **HIV testing** (see Chapter 5 VIII B 4)

7. **Screening recommendations** (see Chapter 5 VIII B 5)

8. **Initial evaluation of HIV-positive women**

   a. Evaluation for other STDs, including gonorrhea (culture), chlamydia (culture), syphilis (VDRL or RPR), HBV (HbsAg), and HPV [cervical Papanicolaou (Pap) smear]

   b. Assessment for susceptibility to toxoplasmosis (toxoplasmosis antibody) and tuberculosis [purified protein derivative (PPD) skin test and chest x-ray]

   c. Quantitative CD4 T-lymphocyte analysis and HIV plasma RNA level (HIV viral load)

9. **Management using antiretroviral agents**

   a. Asymptomatic individuals with CD4 T-cell counts below $500/mm^3$ should be offered therapy.

   b. All patients with advanced or symptomatic HIV disease should receive aggressive antiretroviral therapy.

   c. Decisions regarding initiating or changing antiretroviral therapy are guided by monitoring the quantitative **HIV RNA viral load** and **CD4 T-cell count** as well as the patient's condition. The goal is to reduce the viral load to undetectable levels with minimal medication side effects.

   d. Current recommendations include a three-drug regimen with two **nucleoside reverse transcriptase inhibitors** and one **protease inhibitor.** However, knowledge in this field is evolving so rapidly that recommendations change rapidly.

F. Toxic shock syndrome (TSS)

1. **Epidemiology**

   a. This acute febrile illness, which has a mortality rate of 5%, is produced by a **bacterial endotoxin.**

   b. Blood cultures are seldom positive, but in 90% of cases, *Staphylococcus aureus* is isolated.

    c. **Menses** and **tampon use** are associated in 50% of cases.

2. **Signs**

    a. A high fever abruptly begins on day 2–4 of menses. It is associated with headache, myalgias, sore throat, vomiting, diarrhea, and hypotension.

    b. An classic intense **sunburn-like rash** lasts for 48 hours. The skin then becomes macular within a few days.

    c. Desquamation of the face and trunk occurs within 1–2 weeks. The skin of the palms and soles may completely slough.

    d. Many cases are less severe "formes frustes."

3. **Management**

    a. Treatment is largely supportive, involving intensive care, monitoring, and support.

    b. Cultures for *S. aureus* (cervical, vaginal, blood) should be obtained.

    c. Endotoxin from the vagina should be irrigated with saline or dilute iodine solution.

    d. Treatment involves beta-lactamase–resistant penicillin for 10–14 days.

4. **Prevention.** Recurrences are markedly decreased with antibiotic treatment. Tampons should be changed every 4–6 hours, and superabsorbent tampons should be avoided.

Review Test

Directions: Each of the numbered items or incomplete statements in this section is followed by answers or by completions of the statement. Select the ONE lettered answer or completion that is BEST in each case.

1. Which one of the following infections is the most common sexually transmitted disease (STD) in females?

(A) Human immunodeficiency virus (HIV)
(B) Genital herpes
(C) Hepatitis B virus (HBV)
(D) Gonorrhea
(E) Chlamydia

2. Which one of the following regions is the most common site of gonococcal infection in sexually active adult females?

(A) Lower genital tract
(B) Gastrointestinal (GI) tract
(C) Upper urinary tract
(D) The eye
(E) Upper genital tract

3. A 23-year-old woman complains of headache, myalgia, and diarrhea of 1 day's duration. Her last menstrual period began 2 days ago, and she is using vaginal tampons. She recently ate Chinese food at a restaurant and spent a weekend in Mexico 1 week ago. On examination, her temperature is 102°F (38.9°C), and she has a sunburn-like rash. Which one of the following conditions is the most likely diagnosis?

(A) *Escherichia coli* food poisoning
(B) Toxic shock syndrome (TSS)
(C) Erythema multiforme
(D) Allergic pollen reaction
(E) Acute rubella syndrome

4. Which one of the following sexually transmitted diseases (STDs) is the only one that can be prevented by immunization?

(A) Genital herpes
(B) Chlamydia
(C) Gonorrhea
(D) Hepatitis B
(E) Lymphogranuloma venereum (LGV)

5. A 26-year-old woman requests screening for sexually transmitted diseases (STDs). She says that her boyfriend has been treated for an STD. On examination you find a painless vulvar ulcer. Which of the following STDs is the most likely diagnosis?

(A) Human immunodeficiency virus (HIV)
(B) Gonorrhea
(C) Human papilloma virus (HPV)
(D) Chlamydia
(E) Syphilis

6. A 35-year-old woman has been treated for perineal condyloma with a variety of therapies. No gross lesions are now visible. However, a cervical DNA probe was once positive for human papilloma virus (HPV). Which one of the following therapies is appropriate at this time?

(A) Topical podophyllin
(B) 5-fluorouracil
(C) Imiquimod
(D) Interferon-α (IFN-α)
(E) No therapy is indicated

Directions: Each of the numbered items or incomplete statements in this section is negatively phrased, as indicated by a capitalized word such as NOT, LEAST, or EXCEPT. Select the ONE lettered answer or completion that is best in each case.

7. All of the following are risk factors for chlamydia infection EXCEPT

(A) multiple sexual partners
(B) sexual activity before age 20 years
(C) history of other sexually transmitted disease (STDs)
(D) lower socioeconomic status
(E) use of barrier contraception

264

Answers and Explanations

1. The answer is E [II A].

Chlamydia trachomatis involves an obligate intracellular microorganism that attaches only to columnar epithelial cells without deep tissue invasion. Chronic inflammation and fibrosis leading to chronic pain and infertility may occur if chlamydia is untreated. Human immunodeficiency virus (HIV), genital herpes, hepatitis B virus (HBV), and gonorrhea are all significant sexually transmitted diseases (STDs) in females, but they are not as prevalent as chlamydia.

2. The answer is A [II C 1 a].

The cervix, along with Bartholin's and Skene's glands of the adult female lower genital tract, is the most frequent site of gonococcal infection. The upper genital tract is the second most common site of gonorrhea in sexually active adult females. The gastrointestinal (GI) tract and upper urinary tract are unlikely sites in the adult female. Eye infections are more likely in untreated neonates born to mothers with infected genital tracts.

3. The answer is B [II F].

Toxic shock syndrome (TSS) should be the first consideration when fever and a classic sunburn-like rash are seen during menses. TSS is a potentially life-threatening illness produced by a bacterial endotoxin from *Staphylococcus aureus*. The high fever differentiates this case from food poisoning, erythema multiforme, and an allergic pollen reaction. The rash of acute rubella does not look like sunburn.

4. The answer is D [II D 5].

Sexually transmitted diseases (STDs) involve both bacterial and viral organisms. Development of vaccines against viruses has tended to be more successful than against bacteria. Hepatitis B is the only viral disease of the five STDs listed that can be prevented by both active and passive immunization. The Centers for Disease Control and Prevention (CDC) recommends that all adolescents receive active immunization against hepatitis B.

5. The answer is E [I E (Chapter 5 VI B 2 a)].

Because this patient has a genital ulcer, the sexually transmitted disease (STD) syphilis is the answer. The STDs can be divided into two groups: those with ulcers and those without ulcers. The first four options name STDs without ulcers; only option E, syphilis, is characterized by genital ulcers. Genital ulcers may be painful or painless. Painful ulcers are manifestations of the STDs chancroid and herpes. Painless ulcers are characteristic of syphilis and other STDs, including granuloma inguinale and lymphogranuloma venereum (LGV).

6. The answer is E [II B 4].

No present therapy for human papilloma virus (HPV) eliminates subclinical infection. Current treatment does not significantly affect the natural history of subclinical infection. In this scenario, the patient has no observable clinical disease. The first four options presented are appropriately used for clinical disease.

7. The answer is E [II A 2].

Use of barrier contraception is the correct answer because it provides protection rather than being a risk factor for chlamydial infections. Multiple sexual partners, early age of onset of coitus, history of sexually transmitted disease (STDs), and lower socioeconomic status are all risk factors for chlamydia.

10

Fertility Control

I. CONTRACEPTION

A. Categories of contraceptive effectiveness

1. **Theoretical effectiveness** describes when a device or substance is used perfectly, consistently, reliably, and predictably. It is never lower than the use effectiveness.

2. **Use effectiveness** takes into account **human frailties** and reflects the impact of passions of the moment, forgetfulness, running out of supplies, and improper use. It can never exceed theoretical effectiveness.

B. Ideal contraceptive characteristics. (An ideal method has yet to be described.)

1. Inexpensive
2. Easy and simple to use
3. Use unrelated to the time of intercourse
4. Freely reversible effect (Figure 10-1)
5. Free of side effects
6. Readily available
7. Free of cultural barriers

C. Contraceptive methods: categories

1. **"Folk" methods** intuitively seem helpful, but they actually have a poor degree of reliability and effectiveness.

   a. **Coitus interruptus,** which is the withdrawal of the penis from the vagina prior to ejaculation

      (1) **Advantage.** The method is inexpensive and readily available.
      (2) **Disadvantage.** The method demands a high degree of discipline.
      (3) **Limitation.** Semen can escape into the vagina and cervical mucus prior to ejaculation.

   b. **Postcoital douche**

      (1) **Theoretical basis.** Water, vinegar, or other products theoreti-

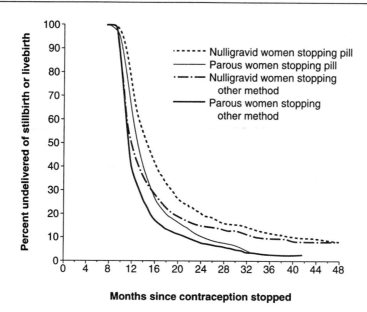

Figure 10-1. Fertility in women who have terminated contraception so that they could conceive. (Reprinted with permission from Scott JR, DiSaia PJ, Hammond CB, et al (eds): *Danforth's Obstetrics and Gynecology,* 6th ed. Philadelphia, J.B. Lippincott Co., 1990, p 720.)

cally flush semen out of the vagina. The liquid is thought to possess spermicidal properties.

(2) **Limitation.** Sperm may enter cervical mucus within 90 seconds of ejaculation.

c. **Prolongation of lactation**

(1) **Theoretical basis.** A delay in ovulation is assumed during breastfeeding because of increased prolactin levels.

(2) **Advantage.** Epidemiologically, there is a statistical delay in preventing conception.

(3) **Disadvantage.** Individual women differ in their length of ovulation delay, which makes the method unreliable.

(4) **Limitation.** Approximately 6% of lactating women ovulate before their first postpartum menstrual cycle.

2. **Barrier and spermicidal methods** vary, but each may result in method failure (Table 10-1).

a. The **male condom** is a sheath that is placed on the erect penis, preventing sperm deposition into the vagina. It is the **most widely used** mechanical contraceptive in the world, and its use is second only to oral contraceptive pills in the United States.

(1) **Advantages**

(a) Condoms are inexpensive, readily available, and convenient.

(b) Condoms provide major protection against sexually transmitted diseases (STDs).

(c) One size fits all.

(2) **Disadvantages**

(a) Use is linked directly to the act of intercourse.

Table 10-1. Barrier and Spermicidal Contraception

	Condom	Diaphragm	Female Condom	Cervical Cap	Sponge	Spermicide
Description	Sheath on erect penis prevents sperm deposition in vagina	Mechanical and spermicidal barrier to sperm between vagina and cervical canal	Vaginal pouch with inner ring fitting over cervix and outer ring outside the vagina	Cup-like diaphragm placed tightly over cervix without spermicide	Spermicidal sponge placed in proximal vagina	Foams and tablets with spermicidal activity
Advantages	Widely available	Place up to 2 hours before coitus	STD protection Female-controlled	May leave in place for weeks	Place up to 24 hours before coitus	Prevents some common STDs Female-controlled
Individual fitting needed?	No	Yes	No	Yes	No	No
Female controlled?	No	Yes	Yes	Yes	Yes	Yes
Decreases STDs?	Yes	Yes	Yes	No	Yes	Yes
Disadvantages	Reduction of penile sensation	Spermicidal re-application may be needed	Expensive, bulky	Woman may not feel her own cervix	Off the market in the United States	Dispersion of agent may not occur
Genital skin irritation	No	No	No	No	Yes	Yes
Coitus related?	Yes	No	Yes	No	No	Yes
Problems with method failures?	Yes	Yes	Yes	Yes	Yes	Yes
Failure rate	10%–15%	15%–20%	15%–20%	15%–20%	15%–20%	15%–20%

STD = sexually transmitted disease

   (b) There is a reduction of penile sensation.
   (c) Sexual spontaneity is lost.
   (d) Breakage is possible.
   (e) Use is male-controlled.
  b. The **female condom** consists of a polyurethane pouch with two flexible rings. The blind pouch end fits over the cervix, and the open end rests outside the vagina on the vulva (Figure 10-2).
   (1) **Advantages**
    (a) Female condoms provide protection against STDs.
    (b) Use is female-controlled.
   (2) **Disadvantages**
    (a) Use is linked directly to the act of intercourse.
    (b) Bulkiness and awkwardness are present.
    (c) The method is relatively expensive.
  c. The **vaginal diaphragm** is a mechanical and spermicidal barrier that is placed between the posterior vaginal fornix and the pubic symphysis, holding spermicidal jelly against the external cervical os.

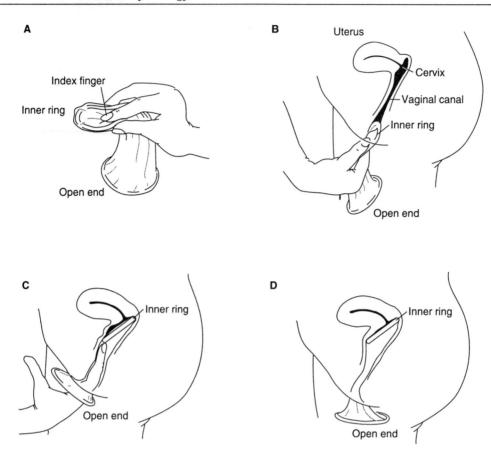

Figure 10-2. Insertion and positioning of the female condom (reality). (*A*) The inner ring is squeezed for insertion. (*B*) The sheath is inserted in a manner similar to inserting a diaphragm. (*C*) The inner ring is pushed up with the index finger as far as it will go. (*D*) The vaginal pouch is in place. (Reprinted with permission from Cunningham FG, MacDonald PC, Gant NF, et al: *Williams' Obstetrics,* 19th ed. Norwalk, Connecticut. Appleton & Lange, 1993, p 1348.)

      (1) Advantages
          (a) Placement may occur up to 2 hours before ejaculation.
          (b) Removal may be delayed for at least 6 hours after ejaculation.
          (c) Use may prevent some STDs (e.g., chlamydia, gonorrhea).
          (d) Use is female-controlled.
      (2) Disadvantages
          (a) Individual fitting by a trained person is required.
          (b) Placement must occur before penile insertion.
          (c) Use is linked directly to the act of intercourse.
          (d) The risk of urinary tract infection (UTI) or bladder infection is present.
          (e) Reapplication of spermicide is required for repeated intercourse.
    d. The **cervical cap** is a cup-like diaphragm that is placed tightly over the cervix without spermicide.
      (1) Advantages

    (a) Insertion may occur from 30 minutes to 48 hours before intercourse.

    (b) It may be left in place for a prolonged period.

    (c) Use may prevent some STDs (e.g., chlamydia, gonorrhea).

    (d) Use is female-controlled.

  (2) Disadvantages

    (a) Individual fitting by a trained person is required.

    (b) Many women cannot feel their own cervix.

e. The **vaginal contraceptive sponge** is a spermicide-impregnated polyurethane disk that is placed in the proximal vagina. The spermicide nonoxynol 9 is released when the sponge is moistened and by the action of intercourse.

  (1) Advantages

    (a) Insertion may occur up to 24 hours before intercourse.

    (b) Use may prevent some common STDs (e.g., chlamydia, gonorrhea).

    (c) There is no need to reapply spermicide for repeated intercourse.

    (d) Use is female-controlled.

    (e) One size fits all.

  (2) Disadvantage. Nonoxynol 9, the active ingredient, attacks lipid membranes and may cause epithelial irritation.

f. **Spermicidal preparations** consist of vaginal foams, suppositories, and tablets with spermicidal activity.

  (1) Advantages

    (a) Use may prevent some common STDs (e.g., chlamydia, gonorrhea).

    (b) Use is female-controlled.

  (2) Disadvantages

    (a) Thirty minutes are needed for a tablet to foam or for a suppository to melt and disperse.

    (b) Nonoxynol 9 may cause epithelial irritation.

    (c) Teratogenesis of nonoxynol 9 has not been proven.

3. Steroid hormone–based methods

  a. Oral agents are the **most commonly used** methods of reversible contraception in the United States, where they are second only to sterilization in popularity as a method of family planning. They are available in both estrogen–progestin combinations and progestin-only forms (mini-pill).

  (1) Advantages

    (a) Contraceptive protection is continuous when taken correctly.

    (b) The contraceptive effect is readily reversible when the pills are discontinued (see Figure 10-1).

    (c) Noncontraceptive health benefits, summarized in Table 10-2, are the result of either suppressed ovulation or decreased menstrual flow.

  (2) Disadvantages

    (a) Oral contraceptives must be remembered and taken daily.

Table 10-2. Noncontraceptive Health Benefits of Estrogen–Progestin Contraceptive Agents

Organ	Decreased Incidence of	Mechanism
Ovary	• Functional ovarian cysts • Epithelial ovarian carcinoma	• Suppression of gonadotropins eliminates formation of follicular and corpus luteum cysts • Ovarian epithelial capsule is not broken with ovulation
Uterus	• Primary and secondary dysmenorrhea • Dysfunctional uterine bleeding • Endometrial carcinoma	• Decreased strength of menstrual contractions from prostaglandin suppression • Eliminates unopposed estrogen state • Decreased duration of unopposed estrogen stimulation
Oviduct	• Pelvic inflammatory disease • Ectopic pregnancy	• Progesterone-induced hostile cervical mucus inhibits sperm migration • Decreased PID and decreased pregnancy overall
Breast	Benign breast disease	Decreased hormonal stimulation
Blood	Microcytic anemia	Decreased amount and duration of menstrual flow
Other	Endometriosis	Decreased amount and duration of menstrual flow

PID = pelvic inflammatory disease

        (b) Intermenstrual bleeding and headaches may be noted in the first few months of use.

        (c) Weight gain may be noted in patients taking higher dosage formulations.

    b. Intramuscular (IM) agents use the slow release of depomedroxy-progesterone acetate (DMPA), which is a progestin-only formulation.

      (1) Advantages

        (a) DMPA is highly effective, with a failure rate less than 1%.

        (b) Use is independent of the act of intercourse.

        (c) Administration of the agent can be performed with ease.

      (2) Disadvantages

        (a) IM injections (150 mg) must be repeated **every 3 months.**

        (b) Return of regular ovulation and normal menses may be delayed up to 12 months after discontinuing DMPA.

        (c) Side effects include **irregular bleeding** (the most common reason for discontinuation), fluid retention, and weight gain (from fluid retention).

    c. Subcutaneous depot methods agent (e.g., Norplant) use another progestin, L-norgestrel, which is contained in six Silastic capsules. Each capsule implanted beneath the upper arm skin contains 36 mg of L-norgestrel.

      (1) Advantages

        (a) Contraception is highly effective, with a failure rate of less than 1%.

        (b) Capsules need to be replaced only **every 5 years.**

        (c) Fertility returns rapidly after the subcutaneous rods are removed.

    (2) Disadvantages

        (a) Placement and removal of the subcutaneous capsules must be performed by a trained health care professional.

        (b) Capsule removal can be difficult because of scar tissue formation.

        (c) Side effects include **irregular bleeding** (the most common reason for discontinuation), fluid retention, and weight gain (from fluid retention).

  d. Mechanisms of action for steroid hormone–based methods

    (1) Suppression of gonadotropins leads to anovulation. This effect is more predictable and reliable with combination estrogen–progestin preparations, but it also occurs with progestin-only agents.

    (2) Cervical mucus is altered by the progestin, which renders the mucus hostile to sperm penetration and migration.

    (3) Endometrial atrophy is a progestin effect that makes the uterine lining unfavorable for blastocyst implantation.

  e. Contraindications for steroid contraceptive agents, which are summarized in Table 10-3, can be absolute (never to be used) or relative (benefits must be weighed against the risks). The majority of these are related to the estrogen component of steroid contraceptives.

  f. Drugs that decrease the effectiveness of oral contraceptives can be categorized by their mechanism of action.

    (1) Drugs that increase liver metabolism of contraceptive steroids include the following:

        (a) Anticonvulsant agents such as phenytoin, phenobarbital, primidone, and carbamazepine

Table 10-3. Contraindications for Combination Steroid Contraception

Absolute	Relative
Pregnancy	**Systemic disease**
	Diabetes mellitus
Cardiovascular	Sickle cell disease
Venous thrombosis	Chronic hypertension
Pulmonary embolism	Hyperlipidemia
Cerebrovascular accident	
Coronary heart disease	**Neurologic**
	Vascular headache
Malignancy	Depression
Breast	
Endometrium	Poor lifestyle habits (e.g.,
Melanoma	smoker > 35 years age)
Hepatic	
Liver tumor	
Abnormal liver function tests	

(b) Antifungal agents such as griseofulvin

(c) Antituberculosis agents such as rifampin

(2) Drugs that change the enterohepatic circulation of contraceptive steroids because they alter intestinal flora include **antibacterial agents** (e.g., ampicillin, tetracycline, erythromycin, metronidazole). However, the data supporting this are controversial.

MATE

4. **Intrauterine devices (IUDs)**

a. **Types.** IUDs may be either medicated or nonmedicated (not available in the United States).

(1) **Progesterone-impregnated IUDs** (e.g., Progestasert), which release the medication rapidly, must be replaced every year.

(2) **Copper IUDs** [e.g., Paraguard (Copper T-380A)], which release the copper slowly, must be replaced every 10 years.

b. **Mechanisms.** These are not well defined. No data suggest that the major action of IUDs is as an abortifacient. Probable mechanisms of action include the following:

(1) **Altered tubal motility,** for both sperm and egg transport, from altered ciliary action

(2) **Endometrial inflammatory response** from foreign body mobilization of leukocytes

(3) **Altered implantation** from disruption of endometrial maturation

c. **Advantages**

(1) Use is independent of the act of intercourse.

(2) Contraception is highly effective, with a failure rate of only 2%.

(3) There are no systemic side effects.

(4) Minimal patient compliance is required.

d. **Disadvantages**

(1) Insertion requires a trained clinician.

(2) The initial expense of insertion is high.

(3) Menstrual duration, blood loss, and pain are increased depending on the degree of endometrial compression and myometrial distention.

e. **Complications**

(1) Uterine perforation, which is highest with a retroverted uterus, occurs mostly at the time of insertion.

(2) Risk of septic abortion is 50% if the IUD is left in place after a pregnancy occurs.

(3) Risk of salpingitis is increased in the first 2 months after insertion.

(4) *Actinomyces israelii* organisms may be noted on Papanicolaou (Pap) smears but do not appear to be associated with increased pelvic infections.

f. **Absolute contraindications**

(1) Pregnancy

(2) Undiagnosed uterine bleeding

(3) Acute cervical, uterine, or tubal infection

(4) History of salpingitis

(5) Suspected gynecologic malignancy

g. **Relative contraindications**
   (1) Nulliparity or desired future pregnancies
   (2) Prior ectopic pregnancy
   (3) History of STDs or multiple sexual partners
   (4) Moderate or severe dysmenorrhea
   (5) Abnormal uterine cavity
   (6) Chronic menometrorrhagia
   (7) Iron-deficiency anemia

5. **Natural family planning**
   a. **Mechanisms**
      (1) **Avoidance of intercourse** during the periovulatory fertile period of the woman's menstrual cycle
      (2) **Prediction of ovulation** by a variety of methods including the following:
          (a) Keeping a calendar
          (b) Basal body temperature (BBT) chart noting the mid-cycle postovulatory increase (0.5°F) caused by increasing progesterone levels
          (c) Cervical mucus changing from thin and watery to thick and sticky at mid-cycle, which is caused by the effect of progesterone
          (d) Preovulatory symptoms (e.g., mittelschmerz)
   b. **Advantages**
      (1) Wide religious and cultural acceptance
      (2) No dependence on hormones or chemicals
   c. **Disadvantages**
      (1) Requirement of discipline and self-control
      (2) Low effectiveness rate
      (3) Possibility of variable cycles
      (4) Hyperthermia arising from nonovulatory causes

II. STERILIZATION

A. **Description of procedures**

   1. **Men.** Worldwide, **vasectomy** is performed as frequently on men as **tubal ligation** is performed on women. However, in the United States, tubal ligation is the more common method of sterilization (Figure 10-3). Objective criteria for a successful vasectomy is **azospermia** on a semen collection after 12 ejaculations.

   2. **Women.** The **most common method** of prevention of pregnancy in the United States for women is **surgical sterilization.** No objective criteria exist for a successful female sterilization. Procedures include the following:

      a. **Abdominal surgery**
         (1) Postpartum abdominal infraumbilical curvilinear incision
         (2) Laparoscopic infraumbilical with intraperitoneal CO_2 insufflation
         (3) Interval minilaparotomy abdominal with suprapubic incision
         (4) Interval vaginal with colpotomy

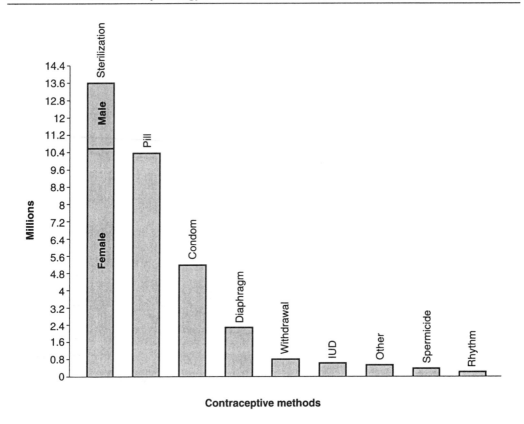

Figure 10-3. Types and users (in millions) of contraceptive methods used by women in the United States aged 15 to 44 years. (Reprinted with permission from Cunningham FG, MacDonald PC, Gant NF, et al: *Williams' Obstetrics,* 19th ed. Norwalk, Connecticut. Appleton & Lange, 1993, p 1322.)

    b. Laparoscopy

        (1) Electrocautery destroys a segment of the oviduct by fulguration or thermal injury.

        (2) The **falope ring** causes necrosis of the loop of oviduct distal to the Silastic ring.

        (3) The **Hulka or Filshie clip** causes necrosis of the oviduct at the site of the clip.

    c. Laparotomy or minilaparotomy (Figure 10-4)

        (1) The **Pomeroy method** consists of elevating a loop of the oviduct, placing a ligature around it, and excising the distal loop.

        (2) The **Irving method** consists of incising the mid-oviduct, ligating the distal end, and burying the proximal end in the myometrium.

        (3) The **Parkland method** places two suture ligatures, 3 cm apart, encircling the mid-oviduct through the mesosalpinx. The intervening segment of tube is removed by cauterizing the mesosalpinx.

        (4) The **Kroener fimbriectomy** involves ligating the tube across the ampulla. The distal portion of the ampulla, including all of the fimbriae, is resected.

    d. Posterior colpotomy. This method consists of a vaginal approach to the oviducts through the posterior fornix into the cul-de-sac.

A. Pomeroy

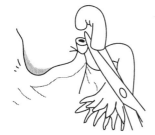

B. Irving

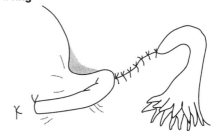

C. Parkland

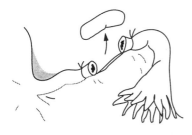

D. Kroener fimbriectomy

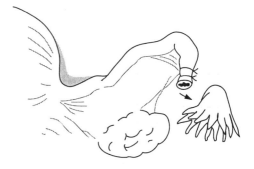

Figure 10-4. Various techniques for tubal sterilization. (Reprinted with permission from Cunningham FG, MacDonald PC, Gant NF, et al: *Williams' Obstetrics,* 19th ed. Norwalk, Connecticut. Appleton & Lange, 1993, p 1354.)

    e. Hysteroscopy. This method uses a plug, cautery, or a chemical to block or scar the tubal ostia.

   3. Female chemical procedure consists of a transcervical injection of a sclerosing chemical agent into the uterus. The objective is to scar the tubal ostia. The procedure is considered experimental.

B. Risks

   1. Surgical procedure risks are as follows:

    a. Bleeding or hematoma at the entry incision, from the perforation of great vessels, or at the ligation site on the mesosalpinx

    b. Infection of the entry incision or at the ligation site on the mesosalpinx

    c. Visceral trauma from inadvertent cutting or cautery, which may develop in the bowel and bladder or on other viscera

   2. Risks of procedure failure (resulting in pregnancy) occur at an overall rate of 0.5% after 1 year but rise to 1.5% cumulatively after 10 years. Most occur in women under 30 years of age and are caused by spontaneous fistula formation.

    a. Lowest failure rates are found after unipolar coagulation and postpartum partial salpingectomy (0.7% after 10 years).

    b. Highest failure rates are found after bipolar coagulation and spring clip application (up to 3% after 10 years).

3. **Increased menstrual bleeding** (post-tubal ligation syndrome) is presumed to be an ovarian follicle dysfunction caused by interruption of ovarian blood supply as a result of mesosalpinx injury from the sterilization procedure. There is no consensus that such an entity exists. Heavier bleeding may simply be a return of normal menstrual periods after discontinuing oral contraceptives.

C. **Benefits.** Avoiding the medical risks of reversible contraceptive methods and gaining psychological relief from concern regarding undesired pregnancy are possible benefits.

D. **Historical risk factors for complications**

1. **Bleeding history** may be indicative.
   a. Personal history of easy bruising
   b. Personal history of prolonged bleeding after cuts or dental extractions
   c. Family history of bleeding disorders passed from generation to generation

2. **Surgical history** of previous pelvic or abdominal surgery, including ectopic tubal pregnancy, tubal reconstructive procedures, cesarean deliveries, or appendectomy

3. **Medical history** of adhesion formation caused by a previously ruptured appendix, previous pelvic inflammatory disease (PID), or previous intraperitoneal radioactive phosphorus chemotherapy

E. **Contraindications**

1. **Medical conditions** that put patients in physical jeopardy include the following:
   a. Morbid obesity
   b. Cardiovascular arrhythmias, thrombophlebitis, embolic predisposition, and structural heart disease (e.g., Eisenmenger's syndrome)
   c. High anesthesia risk
   d. Pulmonary conditions such as severe asthma or obstructive/restrictive lung disease
   e. Coagulation complications caused by anticoagulation medications (e.g., warfarin, heparin) or by an inherited defect (e.g., hemophilia)
   f. Metabolic immunosuppression from any cause

2. **Emotional conditions,** including life events that cause psychic upheaval such as divorce, death, or loss of employment

3. **Ethical concerns** regarding morality and freedom of choice include the following:
   a. Coercion from spouse or family
   b. Planning a procedure secretly without the knowledge of one's spouse
   c. Using a procedure to manipulate another person

4. **Developmental conditions,** including incompetence, lack of experience, immaturity, or mental retardation

5. **Surgical conditions** that place the patient in physical jeopardy, including diffuse intraperitoneal adhesions as a result of previous surgery or previous radiation therapy

F. Possible regret. Factors associated with regret after a sterilization procedure include:

  1. Age < 30 years

  2. Medically indicated sterilization

  3. Recent emotional trauma (e.g., divorce, death, sickness)

  4. Coercion from spouse or family

III. INDUCED ABORTION. The deliberate termination of a pregnancy in a manner that ensures the death of the embryo or fetus is known as induced abortion.

  A. Epidemiology. Worldwide statistics indicate the following:

   1. **Abortion** is the most common method of reproductive limitation, with one of every four pregnancies ending in abortion.

   2. The **legal status** internationally regarding abortion rights indicates that:

      a. One-third of the world's women live under nonrestrictive laws.

      b. One-third of the world's women live under some legal restrictions.

      c. One-third of the world's women live where abortion is illegal.

  B. General risks of abortion

   1. **Uterine perforation** is unique to those methods during which intrauterine instrumentation occurs [e.g., dilation and curettage (D&C), dilation and evacuation (D&E)].

   2. **Cervical trauma** can follow excessively rapid cervical dilation, resulting in an incompetent cervix in subsequent pregnancies. These occur mostly in second-trimester abortions from the following causes:

      a. Overly aggressive use of metal cervical dilators

      b. Tumultuous uterine contractions from excessive doses of uterotonic agents

      c. Laminaria tents (Figure 10-5). These can prevent injury by bringing about gradual cervical dilation. Laminaria are hydrophilic rods placed in the cervical canal 6 hours before the abortion procedure. They absorb cervical fluid and enlarge to many times their original volume, thus dilating the cervix.

   3. **Bleeding and hemorrhage** usually occur from the placental site before uterine contractions can close the vessels.

   4. **Infection** arises from normal genital flora and results in lymphatic-mediated endomyoparametritis.

   5. **Aspiration pneumonitis** is more likely to occur when **general anesthetics,** rather than local anesthetics, are used.

   6. **Psychological sequelae** tend to be related to the **degree of ambivalence** of the woman regarding the decision to abort.

  C. Factors associated with abortion hazards

   1. **Risks** are increased with **advancing gestational age,** use of **general versus local anesthesia,** and maternal **systemic medical diseases.**

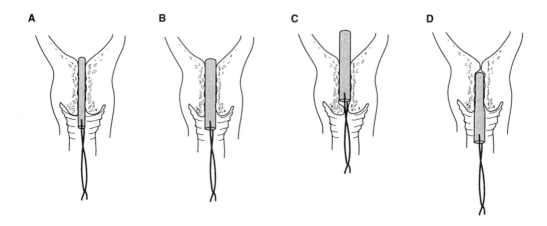

Figure 10-5. Insertion of laminaria before dilation and curettage (D&C). (*A*) Laminaria immediately after being appropriately placed with its upper end just through the internal os. (*B*) The swollen laminaria and dilated, softened cervix several hours later. (*C*) Laminaria inserted too far through the internal os; the laminaria may rupture the membranes. (*D*) Laminaria not inserted far enough to dilate the internal os. (Reprinted with permission from Cunningham FG, MacDonald PC, Gant NF, et al: *Williams' Obstetrics,* 19th ed. Norwalk, Connecticut. Appleton & Lange, 1993, p 681.)

  2. Risk is generally not increased with advancing maternal age.

D. Medical methods of induced abortion (Table 10-4)

  1. Mefipristone (RU-486) is a progesterone antagonist that was developed and used initially in France for first-trimester abortions. It is now in clinical trials in the United States. Mefipristone is an oral preparation used with a prostaglandin agent to induce contractions. When administered before 10 weeks' gestation, 95% of pregnancies are interrupted.

  2. Methotrexate is a folic acid antimetabolite used widely in cancer chemotherapy. Currently, it is not widely used as an abortifacient. However, when administered orally during the first trimester, a high rate of pregnancies are interrupted with a mechanism of action similar to mefipristone.

E. First-trimester surgical abortion methods (see Table 10-4)

  1. Menstrual extraction is an obsolete method from a time before pregnancy tests were readily available. It was performed within 14 days after the missed menstrual period. In an office procedure, the uterine cavity was aspirated transcervically using low-pressure suction. Because a narrow-gauge cannula was used, no cervical dilation or anesthesia was necessary.

  2. Suction curettage is performed at a gestational age of less than 12 weeks. This is the **most commonly performed** abortion procedure.

  a. Procedure. The anesthesia used is either a local paracervical block or an intravenous (IV) sedation. The cervix is dilated with either laminaria tents (see Figure 10-5) or metal dilators. Strong vacuum pressure is used to aspirate the uterine contents.

  b. Morbidity. In up to 2% of cases, morbidity is primarily caused by hemorrhage resulting from uterine atony, uterine perforation, and infection.

Table 10-4. Methods of Induced Abortion

Method	Weeks Gestation	Procedure	Cervical Dilation	Anesthesia	Risks and Complications	Maternal Mortality
Medical Mefipristone (RU-486)	< 10 weeks	Progesterone-antagonist pills induce contraction	None	None	Retained tissues; failed abortion (< 3%) if used with prostaglandin	Negligible
Surgical **First trimester** **Suction curettage**	< 12 weeks	Vacuum aspiration	Laminaria or dilators	Local or sedation	Bleeding, uterine perforation, infection	1/100,000
Sharp curettage	< 12 weeks	Sharp scraping	Laminaria or dilators	Local or sedation	Bleeding, uterine perforation, infection, Asherman syndrome	1/100,000
Second trimester **Dilation and evacuation (D & E)**	14–20 weeks	Morcellation of fetus and extraction of body parts	Laminaria or dilators	Paracervical block, intravenous sedation	Cervical laceration, uterine perforation, hemorrhage, infection, emotional stress	4/100,000
Labor induction	> 14 weeks	Amniotic infusion (e.g., hypertonic saline, hyperosmolar urea, prostaglandin $F_{2\alpha}$) or vaginal suppository (i.e., prostaglandin E_2)	Laminaria	Regional or narcotics	Retained placenta, cervical laceration, hemorrhage, emotional stress	8/100,000
Hysterotomy	> 14 weeks	Mini-cesarean section	N/A	General	Anesthesia, hemorrhage, visceral injury, infection	25/100,000
Hysterectomy	Any gestational age	Removal of pregnant uterus	N/A	General	Anesthesia, hemorrhage, visceral injury, infection	25/100,000

    c. Mortality. The rate of mortality is **1 per 100,000** procedures, which is the **lowest of all abortion methods.**

  3. Sharp curettage was also performed at a gestational age of less than 12 weeks. Widely used before the availability of the suction method, it is seldom performed today.

    a. Procedure. Anesthesia and cervical dilation is the same as in the suction curettage procedure. However, the uterine contents are scraped out the same as in a standard D&C.

    b. Morbidity. Causes of morbidity are similar to suction curettage, except increased rates of hemorrhage, uterine perforation, and cervical injury are found. Intrauterine synechiae **(Asherman's syndrome)** is a unique complication of this procedure.

    c. Mortality. The rate of mortality is **1 per 100,000** procedures.

  F. Second-trimester abortion methods (see Table 10-4)

1. **D&E** is performed between 14 and 20 weeks' gestation. It is the **safest** second-trimester procedure.
   a. **Procedure.** The anesthesia used is either local paracervical block or IV sedation. The cervix is dilated to 15 mm or more by serial placement of laminaria tents or metal dilators. The fetus is morcellated, and the body parts are systematically extracted from the uterus.
   b. **Morbidity** causes are similar to those occurring with suction curettage (i.e., hemorrhage from uterine atony, uterine perforation, and infection), but the incidence is higher. Retained placental or fetal tissue can occur. Staff may experience significant emotional stress.
   c. **Mortality** rate is **4 per 100,000** procedures.

2. **Labor induction by intra-amniotic infusion** is performed between 14 and 20 weeks' gestation. This method is seldom performed today.
   a. **Procedure**
      (1) Amniocentesis is used to aspirate as much amniotic fluid as possible, followed by instillation of hypertonic **saline,** hyperosmolar **urea,** or **prostaglandin** F_{2a} to stimulate uterine contractions.
      (2) Progressive cervical dilation generally ensues with expulsion of the fetus and placenta within 24 hours.
      (3) **Laminaria** tents decrease the induction-to-delivery interval and reduce cervical trauma.
      (4) Methods of analgesia include regional anesthetics or narcotic sedatives.
   b. **Morbidity**
      (1) Retained placenta, cervical lacerations, and hemorrhage may occur in up to 20% of cases.
      (2) A **liveborn fetus** may be delivered with hyperosmolar urea or prostaglandin F_{2a}. Hypertonic saline usually results in **fetal death.**
      (3) **Hypernatremia** and **coagulopathy** may result from use of hypertonic saline.
      (4) Both the patient and staff may experience significant emotional stress.
      (5) Infection risk is increased with prolonged induction-to-delivery intervals.
   c. **Mortality** rate is **8 per 100,000** procedures, which is the same rate as an uncomplicated term vaginal delivery.

3. **Labor induction by vaginal prostaglandin** is performed between 14 and 20 weeks' gestation.
   a. **Procedure**
      (1) Vaginal suppositories of prostaglandin E_2 are used to stimulate uterine contractions.
      (2) Progressive cervical dilation generally ensues with expulsion of the fetus and placenta occurring within 24 hours.
      (3) Laminaria tents reduce the induction-to-delivery interval and decrease cervical trauma.
      (4) Methods of analgesia include regional anesthetics or narcotic sedatives.

      b. Morbidity is similar to that with intra-amniotic prostaglandin F_{2a}. However, **fever,** nausea, vomiting, and diarrhea can occur uniquely with the use of vaginal prostaglandins.

      c. Mortality rate is **8 per 100,000** procedures, which is the same rate as an uncomplicated term vaginal delivery.

G. Hysterotomy and hysterectomy (see Table 10-4). These are major surgical procedures, but they can be performed at any gestational age. These procedures should not be used as primary abortion methods because of the associated high morbidity and mortality rates.

  1. Procedure

      a. Hysterotomy is the opening of the uterine cavity with a classical incision to remove the uterine contents. The only appropriate use is to manage a failed mid-trimester procedure or its complications.

      b. Hysterectomy is the removal of the entire pregnant uterus. The indications for this procedure are management of invasive cervical carcinoma or uncontrollable bleeding.

  2. Morbidity includes infection, hemorrhage, visceral injury, and complications from anesthesia, and it is similar to the morbidity associated with a cesarean section or hysterectomy procedure.

  3. Mortality rate is **25 per 100,000** procedures, which is the **highest of all abortion methods.**

Review Test

Directions: Each of the numbered items or incomplete statements in this section is followed by answers or by completions of the statement. Select the ONE lettered answer or completion that is BEST in each case.

1. Which of the following statements correctly describes the mechanism of action of mefipristone (RU-486)?

(A) It is a gonadotropin-releasing hormone agonist
(B) It is a progesterone antagonist
(C) It is a prostaglandin synthetase inhibitor
(D) It is a progesterone agonist
(E) It is an estrogen antagonist

2. Which one of the following contraceptive methods is almost identical in its use effectiveness rating as well as its theoretical effectiveness rating?

(A) Condom
(B) Diaphragm
(C) L-Norgestrel (Norplant)
(D) Cervical cap
(E) Spermicide

3. Which one of the following contraceptive methods results in the lowest percentage of pregnancies within the first year of use?

(A) Condom
(B) Diaphragm
(C) Oral contraceptive pill
(D) Intrauterine device (IUD)
(E) Depomedroxyprogesterone acetate (DMPA)

4. Which one of the following complications is the most common cause of tubal ligation failure?

(A) Preoperative adhesions
(B) Human error
(C) Spontaneous fistula formation
(D) Mistaking the round ligament for the oviduct on the part of the physician
(E) Use of permanent suture materials

5. Which one of the following abortion procedures that is appropriate at 17 weeks' gestation has the lowest maternal mortality rate?

(A) Hysterotomy
(B) Labor induction by intra-amniotic infusion
(C) Hysterectomy
(D) Labor induction by vaginal suppository
(E) Dilation and evacuation (D&E)

Directions: Each of the numbered items or incomplete statements in this section is negatively phrased, as indicated by a capitalized word such as NOT, LEAST, or EXCEPT. Select the ONE lettered answer or completion that is BEST in each case.

6. All of the following devices protect against sexually transmitted diseases (STDs) EXCEPT

(A) Condoms
(B) Diaphragms
(C) Contraceptive sponges
(D) Intrauterine devices (IUDs)
(E) Spermicides

Answers and Explanations

1. The answer is B [III D 1].

Mefipristone (RU-486) is a progesterone antagonist (not agonist) that has been associated with medical abortions, although it has many other potential uses. It is highly effective when used in conjunction with a prostaglandin to terminate pregnancies of less than 10 weeks' gestation.

2. The answer is C [I C 3 c].

L-Norgestrel (Norplant), which is subcutaneous progestin-impregnated rods, requires no user involvement after the rods have been placed. Theoretical effectiveness takes into consideration the forgetfulness, passions, and human frailties of the user. Use effectiveness expresses how well a contraceptive method works when used consistently and reliably. The less human involvement required of a contraceptive method, the closer the two kinds of effectiveness. Condoms, diaphragms, cervical caps, and spermicides all have a significant human element, which reduces their use effectiveness.

3. The answer is E [I C 3 b].

Depomedroxyprogesterone acetate (DMPA) results in conception in less than 1% of users in the first year of use. All contraceptive methods are imperfect, with each one having offsetting advantages and disadvantages. The overall use effectiveness is a significant characteristic to compare. The rate of conception during the first year of use is 10%–15% with condoms, 15%–20% with diaphragms, 2%–3% with oral contraceptives, and 1%–2% with intrauterine devices (IUDs).

4. The answer is C [II A 2 c, B].

Tubal ligation failures occur at a rate of 1 in 200 procedures for the first year. Studies show that most failures are a consequence of fistula formation in the healing process. Although preoperative adhesions, human error, mistaking the round ligament for the oviduct, and use of permanent suture materials may each play a role in some failures, they are responsible for fewer failures than spontaneously developing fistulas.

5. The answer is E [III F 1].

Second-trimester terminations have higher maternal morbidity and mortality rates than first-trimester procedures. Dilation and evacuation (D&E) has the lowest rate of complications. Hysterotomy, labor induction by intra-amniotic infusion, hysterectomy, and labor induction by vaginal suppository are all available for second-trimester abortions, but each has a higher maternal mortality rate than the D&E procedure.

6. The answer is D [I C 4 e].

The intrauterine device (IUD) is the correct answer because the IUD may increase the risk of pelvic inflammatory disease (PID) rather than protect against it. Protection against sexually transmitted diseases (STDs) can be provided by a condom or a cervical cap as a mechanical barrier, by a spermicidal/bacterial agent such as a diaphragm, or by a contraceptive sponge with spermicide.

11

Menstrual and Endocrine Disorders

I. PRECOCIOUS PUBERTY

A. **Normal puberty is described as follows** (Figure 11-1):

1. **Pubertal changes** are mediated for both genders through sex steroids that are normally produced by the gonads in response to maturation of the hypothalamic-pituitary-gonadal axis. **Developmental endocrinologic events** leading to puberty are shown in Table 11-1.

2. **Ovarian estrogens** are the normally dominant sex steroids in **females,** and **testicular androgens** are the normally dominant sex steroids in **males.**

3. The **lower age limits** of normal puberty are 8 years in girls and 9 years in boys. **Age of puberty onset** in females may depend on attainment of a critical mean body weight or a critical percentage of body fat. This coincides with a decreasing sensitivity of the gonadotropin-releasing hormone (GnRH) receptors to the negative feedback from the low levels of circulating estrogens. The low estrogen levels are not enough to suppress GnRH. The resultant rising GnRH stimulates anterior pituitary follicle-stimulating hormone (FSH), which acts on the gonads to produce sex steroids.

4. **Sequential changes** of normal female puberty involve changes in the rate of growth and the development of secondary sexual characteristics as shown in Table 11-2 (see Figure 11-1).

B. **Precocious puberty** occurs when pubertal changes occur prior to the expected age. The female:male ratio of precocious puberty is 5:1.

1. **Incomplete precocity** occurs when **only one sign** of pubertal development is present (e.g., thelarche or adrenarche).

   a. The **diagnosis** is one of exclusion. Incomplete precocity is most likely caused by transient hormone elevations (estrogens or androgens) or unusual end-organ sensitivity (breast or pubic regions).

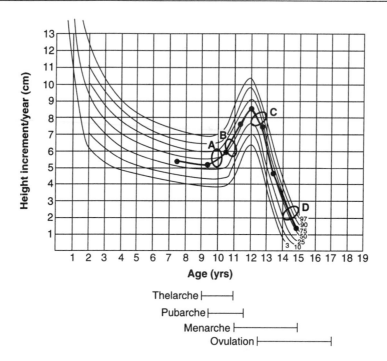

Figure 11-1. Pubertal development chart for the normally developing females. *A* = thelarche; *B* = pubarche; *C* = menarche; *D* = onset of ovulation. (Reprinted with permission from Reindollar RH, Mcdonough PG: Delayed sexual development: Common causes and basic clinical approach. *Pediatr Ann* 10:178, 1981.)

    b. Management is conservative with no significant sequelae noted.

  2. **Complete precocity** occurs when **all signs** of pubertal development are present (e.g., thelarche, adrenarche, menarche).

    a. Hazards of precocious puberty consist of **premature closure** of long bone epiphysis with resultant **short stature.**

    b. There is no impact on sexual function or fertility.

C. Isosexual complete precocity occurs when girls experience breast development and develop normal female body contours. Isosexual maturation is always mediated by an **increase in circulating estrogens.** The origin of the increased estrogens may be caused by premature activation of normal mechanisms [hypothalamic-pituitary-ovarian (HPO) axis] or by pathologic mechanisms (Table 11-3).

  1. **GnRH-dependent causes** are mediated through **estrogen** from activation of the HPO axis.

    a. Approximately 90% of patients with isosexual precocity are girls older than 4 years who have **idiopathic** premature activation of normal mechanisms. These patients have a good prognosis with appropriate treatment.

    b. Approximately 10% of patients have central nervous system (CNS) lesions, which are associated with a poor prognosis. These lesions usually cause the isosexual precocity found in girls younger than 4 years.

    c. Treatment of idiopathic precocious puberty utilizes GnRH agonists administered in a nonpulsatile fashion, initially stimulating but

Table 11-1. Developmental Endocrinologic Changes

	Sex Steroid Levels	**Gonadostat* Function**	**Gonadotropin Levels**
Fetus < 20 weeks	**ESTROGENS HIGH** from maternal-placental sources	Negative feedback becoming functional	**RAPIDLY RISING** for 20 weeks to adult levels
Fetus > 20 weeks	**ESTROGENS HIGH** from maternal-placental sources	**NEGATIVE FEEDBACK HIGH** from maternal estrogens	**GRADUALLY FALL** until term
Newborn	**ESTROGENS FALL RAPIDLY** in first week after delivery to low basal level	**NEGATIVE FEEDBACK LOST** due to low estrogen levels	**RAPIDLY RISE** with a peak at 3 months of age
Early childhood	**ESTROGENS AT LOW BASAL LEVELS** from ovarian follicles	**GONADOSTAT SENSITIVITY GRAD-UALLY INCREASES** resulting in maximal suppression even with low estrogen levels	**GRADUALLY FALL** to low basal levels by age 4 years
Late childhood	**ESTROGENS AT LOW BASAL LEVELS** from ovarian follicles	**GONADOSTAT SENSITIVITY HIGH**	**REMAIN AT LOW LEVELS**
Prepuberty	**ADRENAL ANDRO-GENS RISE GRADUALLY** (adrenarche) between ages 6 and 9 years	**ADRENARCHE INDEPENDENT OF GONADOSTAT**	**REMAIN AT LOW LEVELS**
Puberty	**ESTROGENS RISE GRADUALLY** from ovarian follicle stimulation	**GONADOSTAT SENSITIVITY GRADUALLY DECLINES,** allowing increasing stimulation of follicles	**GRADUALLY RISE** from sleep-associated increases in GnRH

*Functional concept, not anatomic location.

Table 11-2. Normal Development of Secondary Sexual Characteristics

Age (Years)	Pubertal Change
8–9 years	Slowest growth rate
9–10 years	Thelarche: Breast budding
10–11 years	Adrenarch: Pubic and axillary hair
11–12 years	Maximal growth rate
12–13 years	Menarche: Onset of menses
13–14 years	Adult pubic hair
14–15 years	Ovulation

Table 11-3. Comparison of Types of Sexual Precocity

Type	Specific Etiology	Proposed Mechanism	Treatment
Isosexual (Estrogen mediated) **True** (central: gonadotropin GnRH dependent)	**Idiopathic** (75%)	Premature activation of normal hypothalamic-pituitary–ovarian axis	GnRH agonists suppress ovarian follicle stimulation of estrogen
	CNS lesion (10%) • Obstruction (e.g., hydrocephalus) • Infection (e.g., meninigitis, sarcoid, tuberculosis) • Tumor (e.g., glioma, astrocytome)	Unknown	Directed at the specific lesion identified
	Prolonged hypo-thyroidism (rare)	THS mimics GnRH to stimulate gonadotropin release	Thyroid hormone replacement
Pseudo (peripheral, GnRH independent)	**McCune-Albright syndrome (5%)**	Autonomous premature ovarian estrogen production	Aromatase enzyme inhibitor
	Tumor (rare) • Granulosa Cell • Fibrothecoma	Autonomos estrogen production by a hormonally active tumor	Surgical removal of the tumor
	Exogenous (rare) • Combination oral contraceptive pill • Estrogen creams	Medication effect	Discontinue offending medication
Heterosexual (Androgen-medicated)	**Tumor (rare)** • Sertoli-Leydig cell • Hilar cell	Autonomous androgen production by a hormonally active tumor	Surgical removal of the tumor
	Congenital adrenal hyperplasia (rare)	Excessive androgens produced because of enzyme deficiency	Corticosteroid replacement
	Exogenous (rare) • Anabolic steroids • Androgen creams	Medication effect	Discontinue the offending medication

CNS = central nervous system; GnRH = gonadotropin-releasing hormone; TSH = thyroid-stimulating hormone.

then downregulating the GnRH receptors. When an appropriate height or developmental age has been reached, the medication is discontinued, and normal mechanisms resume.

2. GnRH-independent causes are mediated through autonomous estrogen production without HPO axis involvement. The resultant conditions are rare.

   a. The **most frequent cause is McCune-Albright syndrome,** characterized by polyostotic fibrous dysplasia and café au lait skin spots, in which ovarian follicles autonomously start producing estrogens. Management involves aromatase enzyme inhibitors.

   b. **Estrogen-producing ovarian tumors** (e.g., granulosa cell or fibrothecoma) can also occur. A pelvic mass is identifiable. Management involves surgical removal of the tumor.

D. **Heterosexual complete precocity** occurs when girls experience virilization changes (e.g., facial hair, clitoromegaly, male body contours). Heterosexual maturation in females is always mediated by an **increase in circulating androgens** and is always pathological. The **most common cause** is **congenital adrenal hyperplasia (CAH).**

II. AMENORRHEA

A. The **sequence of normal menstrual physiology** is as follows:

   1. **Hypothalamus.** GnRH is released in pulses from the GnRH neurons within the **arcuate nucleus** into the hypophyseal portal circulation.

   2. **Pituitary gland.** The anterior pituitary **gonadotroph cells** respond to the stimulation of the GnRH pulses and release FSH and luteinizing hormone (LH) into the general circulation.

   3. **Ovarian follicle.** The primary follicles respond to FSH stimulation progressing in development through the preantral and antral phases to the preovulatory follicle. The **granulosa cells** of the follicles produce increasing levels of **estrogen,** which stimulates a thickening of the uterine endometrium into the proliferative phase.

   4. **Corpus luteum.** The increasing estrogen level suppresses FSH but leads to the midcycle LH surge that induces ovulation. At the ovulatory site, the luteinized granulosa cells of the corpus luteum produce **progesterone,** which ripens the endometrium to the secretory phase.

   5. **Endometrium.** If conception does not occur, the corpus luteum rapidly degenerates, after a lifespan of 14 days, resulting in a decrease in progesterone levels. The progesterone withdrawal results in endometrial **spiral arteriolar spasm,** ischemic tissue disorganization, and breakdown shedding.

   6. **Outflow tract.** The menstrual flow makes its way through the cervical canal into the vagina, through which it is ultimately released from the body.

B. **Causes of amenorrhea** are numerous and can arise from abnormalities at each of the six steps in the process of normal menses. The causes can be organized into anatomic levels, which can be further classified into three groups based on the gonadotropin levels (Table 11-4).

   1. **Low** levels (**hypogonadotropic** amenorrhea) suggest a **hypothalamic-pituitary** etiology.

Table 11-4. Amenorrhea Etiology by Anatomic Site

Anatomic Level	Anatomic Site	Type of Pathology	Gonadotropin Level	Diagnostic Methods
1	**Hypothalamus**	• Tumors • Anorexia nervosa • Severe weight loss, stress, and exercise	**Low**	• History • Magnetic resonance imaging (MRI) • Computed tomography (CT scan)
2	**Pituitary** (anterior)	• Sheehans syndrome • Panhypopituitarism	**Low**	• History • Gonadotropin-releasing hormone stimulation test
3	**Ovarian follicle**	• Gonadal dysgenesis • Ovarian failure • Vanishing testes • Steroidogenic enzyme defects • Postradiation, infection or chemotherapy	**High**	• History • Karyotyping • Gonadal biopsy
4	**Corpus luteum** (anovulation)	• Polycystic ovary syndrome • Hyperprolactinemia (tumors, drugs, chest wall stimulation) • Weight loss, stress, exercise	**Normal**	• History • Progesterone challenge test • MRI, CT scan
5	**Uterus or endometrium**	• [Pregnancy] • Androgen insensitivity • Müllerian agenesis • Asherman syndrome	**Normal**	• History • Testosterone level • Karyotyping • Hysteroscopy
6	**Outflow tract**	• Imperforate hymen • Vaginal agenesis • Cervical stenosis	**Normal**	• Pelvic examination

2. **High** levels (**hypergonadotropic** amenorrhea) suggest an **ovarian follicle** etiology.

3. **Normal** levels (**eugonadotropic** amenorrhea) suggest **anovulation** or **outflow tract** etiology.

C. **Primary amenorrhea** has an incidence of 2%–3%.

1. **Diagnostic criteria** include the following:

a. No menses by age **14 years,** and **absence** of secondary sex characteristics

b. No menses by age **16 years,** with **presence** of secondary sex characteristics

2. One **clinical approach** uses four categories based on whether breasts and a uterus are absent or present. The presumptions and distinguishing tests for each type of patient are summarized in Table 11-5.

3. The three **most common causes** of primary amenorrhea and the percentages of cases that they account for include:

   a. **Gonadal dysgenesis (30%),** which is also known as **Turner's syndrome** or **monosomy X.** Breasts are absent but a uterus is present.

      (1) **Examination** reveals short stature, web-shaped neck, no secondary sexual characteristics (including breasts absent), but a uterus present.

      (2) **Diagnosis** is confirmed by high FSH and 45,X karyotype.

      (3) **Management** includes estrogen therapy to induce secondary sex characteristics along with cyclic progestin to prevent unopposed estrogen-induced endometrial hyperplasia.

   b. **Müllerian agenesis (20%),** which is also known as **Rokitansky-Küster-Hauser** syndrome. Breasts are present but a uterus is absent. As an accident of development, müllerian duct derivatives (oviducts, uterus, cervix, proximal vagina) have failed to develop. Otherwise, patients are phenotypically and endocrinologically normally functioning females.

      (1) **Examination** reveals normal female phenotype with secondary sex characteristics (including breasts, pubic and axillary hair) and a short blind vaginal pouch but no müllerian duct derivatives.

      (2) **Diagnosis** is confirmed by normal female testosterone level and normal female 46, XX karyotype.

      (3) **Management.** A neovagina can be developed through progressive dilation of the vaginal pouch or surgically created (McIndoe procedure) through a split-thickness skin graft placed between the bladder and the rectum. Although an affected woman is unable to carry a pregnancy, she can produce her own biologic children with follicle aspiration, in-vitro fertilization, and embryo transfer into a surrogate mother.

   c. **Androgen insensitivity (10%),** which is also known as male **pseudohermaphroditism:** the genitalia are opposite of the gonads. Breasts are present but a uterus is absent. Such individuals have a 46,XY karyotype with a body (in complete forms) that lacks androgen receptors. Müllerian inhibitory factor, produced by the testes, results in involution of the müllerian duct and its derivatives. Wolffian duct differentiation, external genitalia development, and axillary/pubic terminal hair growth is dependent on androgen stimulation. Because no androgens are recognized by the body, the wolffian duct also involutes, the external genitalia differentiate in a female direction, and no terminal hair develops in the axillary/pubic areas. Female breast development does occur in response to estrogen normally produced by male testes.

      (1) **Examination** reveals a normal female phenotype (with female body contours and breasts), but no pubic/axillary hair, a short blind vaginal pouch, and no müllerian duct derivatives (oviducts, uterus, cervix, and proximal vagina). Undescended testes are palpable in the inguinal canal.

Table 11-5. Primary Amenorrhea

Patient Type	Assumptions	Differential Diagnosis	Evaluation
Breasts absent uterus present	**Absence of breasts: no estrogen is being produced by the gonads** because of: • lack of two functional X chromosomes • nonfunctional hypothalamic-pituitary axis • absence of ovarian follicles **Presence of uterus:** normal müllerian development AND absence of a Y chromosome	• **Gonadal dysgenesis (30%)** • Hypothalamic-pituitary failure	• FSH level • Gonadotropin-releasing hormone stimulation test • Karyotype
Breasts present; uterus absent	**Presence of breasts: estrogen was or is being produced by the gonads,** and the following conditions must be present: • two functional X chromosomes • normal hypothalamic-pituitary axis • former or current response of ovarian follicles **Absence of uterus:** no development of müllerian system OR presence of Y chromosome	• **Congenital absence of uterus (20%)** • **Androgen insensitivity (10%)**	• Serum testoterone • Karyotype
Breasts absent; uterus absent	**Absence of breasts: no estrogen is being produced by the gonads** because of: • lack of two functional X chromosomes • nonfunctional hypothalamic-pituitary axis • absence of ovarian follicles **Absence of uterus:** no development of müllerian system OR presence of Y chromosome	• Vanishing testes (agonadism) • Enzyme deficiency (17, 20–desmolase deficiency; 17-hydroxylase deficiency)	• Karyotype • Gonadal biopsy • Human chorionic gonadotropin stimulation of testoterone
Breasts present; uterus present	**Presence of breasts: estrogen was or is being produced by the gonads,** and the following conditions must be present: • two functional X chromosomes • normal hypothalamic-pituitary axis • former or current response of ovarian follicles **Presence of uterus:** normal müllerian development AND absence of a Y chromosome	• Outflow tract anomaly • Anovulation • Current hypothalamic-pituitary failure	• Pelvic examination • Serum prolactin • Progesterone challenge: -if LH is positive, look for PCO -if FSH is negative, look for hypothalamic-pituitary failure

FSH = follicle-stimulating hormone; LH = luteinizing hormone; PCO = polycystic ovarian syndrome

(2) Diagnosis is confirmed by normal male testosterone levels and a normal male 46, XY karyotype.

(3) Management. A neovagina can be created as described in II C 3 b (3). To prevent malignant transformation, the gonads should be removed from the inguinal canal. Estrogen replacement therapy (ERT) should then be administered.

D. Secondary amenorrhea can be described as follows:

1. **Diagnostic criteria** include the following:
   a. No menses for **3 months,** if previous menses were **regular**
   b. No menses for **6 months,** if previous menses were **irregular**

2. **At the time of the last normal menses,** the following conditions must have been satisfied.
   a. The müllerian system was functional.
   b. The ovaries had responsive follicles.
   c. The hypothalamic-pituitary axis was functional.

3. **Since the last normal menses,** changes in one or more of the following have resulted in amenorrhea.
   a. **Müllerian system** changes, which may include the following:
      (1) Pregnancy, the most common cause of secondary amenorrhea
      (2) Intrauterine adhesions (**Asherman's syndrome**) that have scarred the endometrium
      (3) Cervical stenosis from cone biopsy or cryotherapy
   b. **Ovarian follicles** may have been exhausted from the following:
      (1) Radiation, infection, or chemotherapy
      (2) Autoimmune disease
      (3) Idiopathic primary ovarian failure
   c. **Hypothalamic-pituitary axis changes from the following:**
      (1) Anovulation may have resulted from elevated prolactin due to anterior pituitary or CNS tumor, hypothyroidism, medication effect, or chest wall–mediated stimulation. Galactorrhea is frequently noted with these disorders (Table 11-6; Figure 11-2).
      (2) Pituitary necrosis may result from obstetrical hemorrhage, causing Sheehan's syndrome (see Chapter 7 II A 3 c).

E. Clinical workup of amenorrhea involves the following steps:

1. A **β-human chorionic gonadotropin (β-hCG) test** should be obtained to identify or rule out pregnancy.

2. The **progesterone challenge test** should be obtained to assess the level of **endogenous estrogen** and the competence of the **outflow tract.** Parenteral progesterone in oil (150 mg) or oral medroxyprogesterone acetate (10 mg for 5 days) is administered.
   a. A **positive withdrawal response** is diagnosed if there is bleeding within 2–7 days in any amount beyond a few drops. **The patient can be considered anovulatory.**
      (1) Evaluate if the patient has a serious but correctable cause of anovulation.

Table 11-6. Amenorrhea and Galactorrhea

Type	Mechanism	Specific Causes	Diagnosis
Hyperprolactinemia associated with galactorrhea	**Prolactin-producing tumor**	Pituitary prolactinoma	Physical examination Prolactin level CNS imaging
	CNS tumor that interferes with portal circulation, cutting off dopamine inhibition of prolactin	Craniophyaryngioma	Physical examination Prolactin level CNS imaging
	Dopamine antagonist agents decrease dopamine inhibition of prolactin	Phenothiazines Tricyclic antidepressants Narcotics	Physical examination Prolactin level history
	Estrogen stimulates pituitary lactotrophs	Combination oral contraceptives	Physical examination Prolactin level History
	Prolonged TRH levels stimulate pituitary lactotrophs	Hypothyroidism	THS level
	False transmitter agents	α-Methyldopa	Physical examination Prolactin level History
	Catecholamine-depleting agents	Reserpine	Physical examination Prolactin level History
Chest wall-mediated stimulation	**Peripheral neural stimulation**	Chest or breast surgery Herpes zoster Burns	History Examination
	Nipple stimulation	Stimulation of nipple Chronic nipple irritation	History Examination
Other causes	**Tonically elevated LH**	Polycystic ovary syndrome	History Examination
	Central suppression of GnRH	Weight loss Stress Exercise	History Examination

CNS = central nervous system, *GnRH* = gonadotropin-releasing hormone, *LH* = luteinizing hormone, *TSH* = thyroid-stimulating hormone, *TRH* = thyrotropin-releasing hormone.

(a) **Hypothyroidism.** If the **thyroid-stimulating hormone (TSH) level** is high, the patient should receive treatment with appropriate thyroid hormone replacement.

(b) **Pituitary prolactinoma.** If the **fasting serum prolactin**

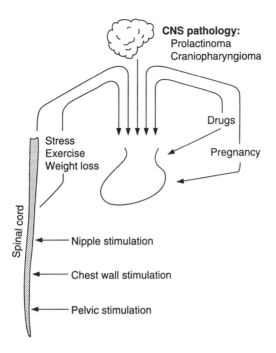

Figure 11-2. Causes of hyperprolactinemia. (Reprinted with permission from Scott JR, DiSaia PJ, Hammond CB, et al (eds): *Danforth's Obstetrics and Gynecology,* 6th ed. Philadelphia, JB Lippincott, 1990, p 765.)

level is elevated (> 50 ng/ml) or if galactorrhea is present, CNS imaging studies [cone view of the sella turcica or magnetic resonance imaging (MRI)] is essential to rule out a tumor.

(2) The patient requires **periodic progestin** withdrawal cycling to prevent **endometrial hyperplasia** from unopposed estrogen stimulation.

(3) Progestin cycling does not return the patient to an ovulatory condition. She may require **ovulation induction** to become pregnant.

b. A **negative withdrawal response** is diagnosed if no flow occurs. Possible explanations include the following:

(1) **Inadequate estrogen priming** of the endometrium, which is unable to respond to the exogenous progestin

(2) **Inoperative outflow tract** due to an obstruction (e.g., cervical stenosis), or intrauterine adhesions (e.g., Asherman's syndrome)

3. A **combined estrogen and progestin challenge test** assesses if the problem is inadequate estrogen stimulation. Oral conjugated estrogens (1.25 mg for 21 days) combined with oral medroxyprogesterone acetate (10 mg for the last 5 days) are administered.

a. A **negative response** is diagnosed if no flow occurs. The cause is either an outflow tract obstruction or a defect in the endometrium. Diagnosis is by hysteroscopy and/or hysterosalpingogram. Management is based on the specific diagnoses identified.

b. A **positive response** is diagnosed if there is withdrawal flow within

2–7 days. It can be assumed that the problem is one of inadequate estrogen production. The possible explanations of a positive response include:

(1) The ovaries do not contain adequate functional follicles.

(2) Follicles are present but there is inadequate pituitary gonadotropic stimulation.

4. **FSH levels** determine whether the lack of estrogen is due to a deficiency of ovarian follicles or in the CNS–pituitary axis. Regardless of the cause, appropriate estrogen replacement (and cyclic progestin) should be instituted to prevent the sequelae of estrogen deficiency (see Chapter 12).

   a. **High levels of FSH** are presumptive of **ovarian failure,** and the patient can be considered sterile.

      (1) If the patient is older than 30 years, premature menopause is diagnosed.

      (2) If the patient is younger than 30 years, a karyotype should be performed to identify possible **mosaicism with a Y chromosome.** This would put her at risk for malignant tumor formation in any testicular component within the gonads. Autoimmune ovarian failure can also occur, which is often associated with autoimmune thyroid disease.

   b. **Low levels of FSH** indicate that the patient's problem involves the CNS–pituitary axis. It is important to perform **CNS imaging,** using either computed tomography (CT) scan with contrast or MRI, to evaluate the sella turcica for signs of abnormal change. If no tumor is found, a presumptive diagnosis is made of **hypothalamic amenorrhea,** which is the result of suppression of pulsatile GnRH secretion below its critical range.

III. DYSMENORRHEA. The presence of painful menstrual periods is known as dysmenorrhea. Prevalence is estimated at 50% of menstruating women, with 10% having severe symptoms.

A. **Classification of dysmenorrhea**

   1. **Primary dysmenorrhea** occurs in young women in their early reproductive years within 2 years of menarche at the onset of ovulatory cycles (Figure 11-3 and Table 11-7). Familial predisposition occurs.

      a. **Pathophysiology** is excessive myometrial contractions (mediated by prostaglandins) as a result of progesterone withdrawal resulting in uterine ischemia. The ischemic pain results in a "uterine attack."

      b. **Examination** reveals absence of specific pelvic pathology.

      c. **Management** is suppression of prostaglandin release by nonsteroidal anti-inflammatory drugs (NSAIDs) or combination oral contraceptives.

   2. **Secondary dysmenorrhea** occurs usually after ovulatory cycles are well established and is associated with specific pelvic pathology (see Table 11-7).

      a. **Differential diagnosis** includes **endometriosis, pelvic inflam-**

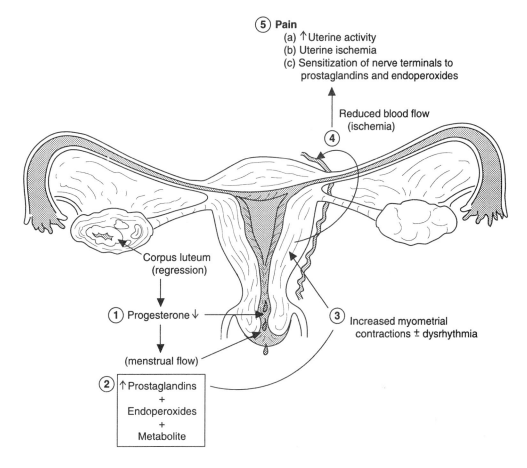

Figure 11-3. Postulated mechanism in the generation of pain in patients with primary dysmenorrhea. Factors affecting central nervous system (CNS) perception of pain are not depicted. (Reprinted with permission from Hacker NF, Moore JG (eds): *Essentials of Obstetrics and Gynecology,* 2nd ed. Philadelphia, WB Saunders, 1992, p 334.)

matory disease **(PID),** cervical stenosis, adenomysosis, uterine leiomyomas, pelvic congestion syndrome, and cervical stenosis.

  b. Examination often is abnormal with findings variable depending on the specific cause.

  c. Management depends on the diagnosis identified.

B. Causes of secondary dysmenorrhea

  1. Endometriosis is a benign condition in which the endometrial glands and stroma are present outside the uterine cavity (Figure 11-4). It is estimated to occur in 15% of women, and it is the most common gynecologic diagnosis responsible for hospitalization of women in the reproductive years.

    a. Pathogenesis theories, although not clearly established, include the following:

      (1) Retrograde menstruation occurring with viable endometrial fragments being shed through the patent oviducts into the peritoneal cavity

      (2) Lymphatic and vascular drainage from the uterus transporting endometrial tissues to distal sites

Table 11-7. Dysmenorrhea

	Primary	Secondary
Onset	Within 2 years of menarche; just prior to or at menses, lasting 48–72 hours	20–30 years of age. May extend pre- or postmenstrually
Description	**Cramping** located in lower abdomen, radiating to lower back, inner thighs	Variable but often **dull, aching**
Associated symptoms	Nausea and vomiting Fatigue Diarrhea Headache	Dyspareunia (painful intercourse) Infertility Abnormal bleeding
Pelvic examination	Normal	Variable, depending on cause
Etiology	Excessive myometrial contractions Decreased uterine blood flow Uterine ischemia Excessive endometrial prostaglandin production ($PGF_{2\alpha}$, PGE_2)	Endometriosis Pelvic inflammation Adenomyosis Leiomyomata Pelvic congestion syndrome Ovarian cysts
Management	Reassurance, explanation NSAIDs Oral contraceptive agents Psychotherapy Surgical procedures (e.g., D&C presacral neurectomy, uterosacral ligament transection) should be avoided	Directed at primary cause

D&C = dilation and curretage; *NSAIDs* = nonsteroidal anti-inflammatory drugs.

    (3) Metaplastic transformation of peritoneal mesothelium into endometrial tissue

  b. Most frequent sites of occurrence in decreasing order are the ovary, cul-de-sac, uterosacral ligaments, broad ligaments, and fallopian tubes (see Figure 11-4).

  c. Pathological appearance can vary from small, red petechial implants on the peritoneal surface to thickened, scarred "powder-burn" implants of various sizes. **Endometriomas** of the ovary result from accumulation of old blood, forming "chocolate cysts."

  d. Degree of symptomatology may be unrelated to the gross extent of the disease (i.e., minimal disease may be associated with severe pain, and extensive disease may be asymptomatic). Characteristic symptoms of endometriosis, in addition to dysmenorrhea, include:

    (1) Painful intercourse **(dyspareunia),** particularly with deep penetration as a result of posterior vaginal fornix involvement

    (2) Painful defecation **(dyschezia)** from rectosigmoid involvement

    (3) Infertility, which may be present with minimal gross findings

  e. The **diagnosis** can be strongly suspected on the basis of a careful

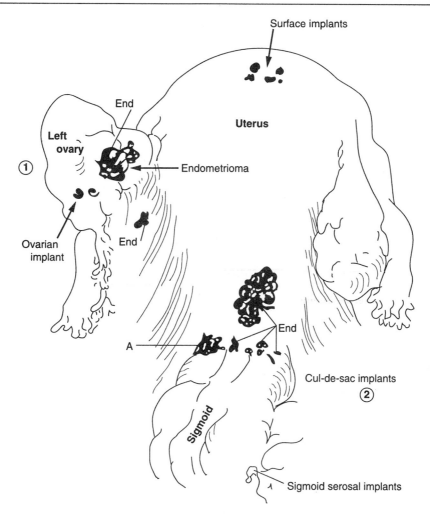

Figure 11-4. Clinical features of endometriosis. *A* = uterosacral implants; *End* = endometriosis. (Reprinted with permission from Beckmann CR, Ling FW, Barzansky BM, et al: *Obstetrics and Gynecology,* 2nd ed. Baltimore, Williams & Wilkins, 1995, p 345.)

history and physical examination. **Confirmation** of the diagnosis should await direct surgical visualization of lesions by **laparoscopy.**

f. **Management** can be medical or surgical, depending on the patient's circumstances.

    (1) **Medical management** attempts to induce atrophy of the endometrial tissue. Appropriate patients are those with symptomatic disease who desire fertility preservation. Approaches used include:

        (a) **Pseudopregnancy,** using continuous progestins or combination oral contraceptives

        (b) **Pseudomenopause,** using danazol (an antiestrogen); or a GnRH agonist (e.g., leuprolide), which initially stimulates, but with sustained levels blocks the GnRH receptors and suppresses gonadotropins

    (2) **Surgical management** may be conservative or radical. **Con-**

servative surgery (e.g., excision, cauterization, or ablation) is used to lyse adhesions to enhance fertility. **Radical** surgery (e.g., total abdominal hysterectomy, bilateral salpingo-oophorectomy, and excision of remaining adhesions) is reserved for those with severe disease who have completed fertility.

2. **Cervical stenosis,** if severe, can impede menstrual flow, causing an increase in intrauterine pressure. Retrograde menstrual flow can occur associated with endometriosis. Etiology may be congenital or result from cervical injury from infection, scarring, or operative trauma. Diagnosis is confirmed by failure to pass a thin probe into the uterus or by hysterosalpingography. Management involves cervical dilation under anesthesia.

3. **Pelvic congestion syndrome** results from vascular engorgement of the uterus and the vessels of the broad ligament. The pain is chronic and described as pelvic burning or throbbing. It is exacerbated by prolonged standing and is worse at night. Pathophysiology appears to be stress-related with psychosomatic features. Diagnosis is confirmed by laparoscopic visualization of pelvic engorgement. Management involves stress reduction and counseling.

4. **Ovarian cysts** (see Chapter 13 I)

5. **Uterine leiomyomas** (see Chapter 13 III B)

6. **Adenomyosis** (see Chapter 13 III C)

7. **PID** (see Chapter 13 IV)

IV. ABNORMAL MENSTRUAL BLEEDING

A. **Characteristics of the normal menstrual cycle** are described as follows:

1. Cycle **length** can vary between 21 days and 35 days.

2. Cycle **duration** can vary from 2 days to 7 days.

3. **Volume** of menstrual blood loss in one cycle is up to 80 ml.

4. Cycles generally are **regular** and **predictable** from month to month.

B. **Ovulatory cycles** resulting from estrogen–progesterone withdrawal bleeding are **self-limited** for the following reasons:

1. Menstrual changes occur simultaneously in **all segments** of the endometrium.

2. Endometrium that has responded to estrogen proliferation followed by **progesterone** is **structurally stable** and is not prone to random breakdown.

3. **With progesterone withdrawal,** the ischemic disintegration of the endometrium leading to tissue collapse is **orderly and progressive.**

4. Prolonged **vasoconstriction** enables clotting factors to seal off the exposed bleeding sites.

C. **Anovulatory bleeding,** resulting from estrogen stimulation (without progesterone withdrawal), is **not self-limited** for the following reasons:

1. Menstrual changes occur at **random sites** and times in various segments of the endometrium.

2. Endometrium that has been stimulated by **unopposed estrogen** proliferation is structurally **unstable** and is prone to random breakdown.

3. **Without progesterone withdrawal,** bleeding occurs from **spontaneous, random breakdown** of hyperproliferative endometrium without stromal structural support.

4. There is no orderly tissue collapse to induce stasis because of the **lack of vasoconstriction** of the endometrial spiral arterioles.

D. **Traditional classification** of abnormal uterine bleeding is based on cycle regularity, cycle length, volume, and duration of flow (Table 11-8).

E. **Differential diagnosis** of abnormal uterine bleeding by genital site is described as follows:

    1. **Vagina and vulva.** Atrophy, trauma, infections, and malignancy are possible causes.

    2. **Cervix.** Eversion, inflammation, polyps, and malignancy are possible causes.

    3. **Uterus.** First-trimester bleeding, molar pregnancy, endometritus, polyps, submucous leiomyomas, adenomyosis, hyperplasia, and malignancy are possible causes.

    4. **Oviducts.** Salpingitis, ectopic pregnancy, and malignancy are possible causes.

    5. **Ovaries.** Estrogen-producing tumors and malignancy are possible causes.

F. **Clinical workup** of abnormal menstrual bleeding is described as follows:

    1. **Cycle characteristics** should meet one or more of the following criteria:

        a. Cycle length < 21 days or > 35 days

        b. Bleeding of > 7 days' duration

        c. Volume of menstrual flow > 80 ml per cycle

        d. Occurrence of intermenstrual bleeding

    2. **β-hCG test** should be performed to identify or rule out pregnancy.

    3. **Evaluation of cycles** should be performed to determine whether they are ovulatory or anovulatory. Usually a history is adequate to make the diagnosis.

        a. Characteristics of **ovulatory cycles** include the following:

           (1) **Cycle predictability and regularity, which should be retained**

           (2) Basal body temperature (BBT) chart showing midcycle elevation

           (3) Serum progesterone level > 500 ng/dl

           (4) Endometrial biopsy indicating secretory changes

        b. Characteristics of **anovulatory cycles** include the following:

           (1) **Loss of cycle predictability and regularity**

           (2) Monophasic BBT and progesterone as well as biopsy evidence of ovulation

Table 11-8. Menstrual Bleeding

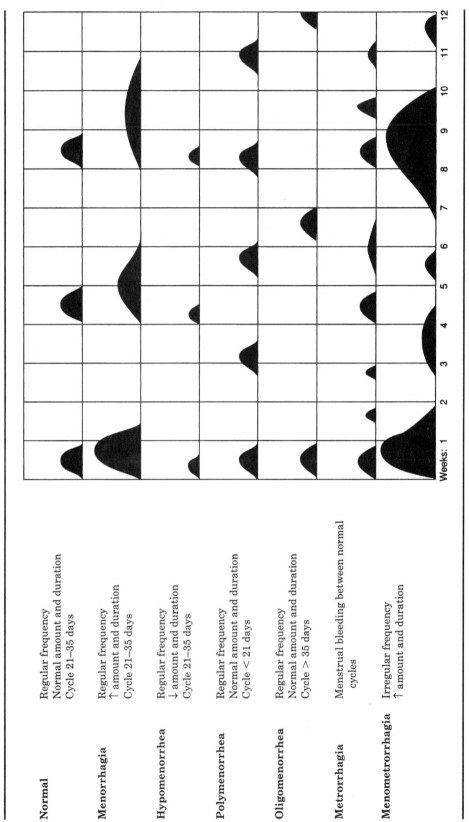

Normal	Regular frequency Normal amount and duration Cycle 21–35 days
Menorrhagia	Regular frequency ↑ amount and duration Cycle 21–35 days
Hypomenorrhea	Regular frequency ↓ amount and duration Cycle 21–35 days
Polymenorrhea	Regular frequency Normal amount and duration Cycle < 21 days
Oligomenorrhea	Regular frequency Normal amount and duration Cycle > 35 days
Metrorrhagia	Menstrual bleeding between normal cycles
Menometrorrhagia	Irregular frequency ↑ amount and duration

4. Anovulatory bleeding is often referred to as **dysfunctional uterine bleeding (DUB).** Most women affected with DUB are in the extremes of the reproductive years.

   a. **Adolescent women** may experience DUB in the first few years after menarche, before the establishment of regular ovulation.

      (1) Endometrial biopsy is **not necessary,** because malignancy is rarely present.

      (2) Cyclic progestin therapy is used in **chronic** bleeding and results in maturing of the endometrium that allows predictable cycles.

      (3) Parenteral estrogen is useful for stopping the **acute** hemorrhaging that results from DUB. The mechanism of action is stimulation of rapid endometrial proliferation. Immediate follow-up with cyclic progestin therapy is essential.

   b. **Reproductive-age women** may experience DUB as a result of chronic anovulation syndromes.

      (1) **Endometrial biopsy** should be performed only in selected patients at high risk for endometrial hyperplasia or cancer (e.g., patients who are > 35 years, obese, chronically hypertensive, or diabetic).

      (2) Medical management with cyclic **progestins** usually secures normal cycles.

      (3) **Endometrial ablation** (by iatrogenic thermal injury to the endometrium) or hysterectomy is indicated only if hormonal management fails.

   c. **Perimenopausal women** experience increasingly frequent anovulatory cycles and therefore DUB.

      (1) **Endometrial biopsy** should be performed to rule out complex hyperplasia.

      (2) **Management** is based on histologic findings. If unopposed estrogen effect is noted, cyclic progestin therapy is imperative.

   d. **Postmenopausal women** can never experience DUB because they have exhausted their ovarian follicles. **Malignancy must always be ruled out by endometrial histologic evaluation.**

5. **If cycles appear to be anovulatory,** the missing hormone, progesterone, should be added. A progestin trial should be initiated.

   a. **Medroxyprogesterone acetate** (10 mg) should be administered orally for 10 days.

   b. The following changes in menses should be anticipated **if the cycles are definitely anovulatory:**

      (1) Bleeding should **stop within 48 hours** of starting the progestin trial.

      (2) Bleeding should **remain stopped** until the progestin course is completed.

      (3) **Normal withdrawal bleeding** should occur after the progestin is completed.

   c. **If anovulation is confirmed,** the following steps should be taken:

      (1) A fasting serum prolactin to rule out a pituitary prolactinoma

      (2) A TSH level to rule out hypothyroidism

      (3) Periodic progestin cycling to prevent endometrial hyperplasia

6. **If cycles appear to be ovulatory** (or a progestin trial does not normalize cycles), the existence of a structural abnormality within the uterus should be investigated.

    a. **Hysterosonography,** which is performed by instilling saline into the uterine cavity through a transcervical catheter, to allow visualization of endometrial thickness, endometrial polyps, and uterine submucous leiomyomas

    b. **Hysteroscopy with dilation and curettage (D&C)** to visualize endometrial pathology (e.g., endometrial polyps, submucous leiomyomas)

    c. **Cervical cytology** is unreliable for assessing pathology of the endometrium.

G. **Polycystic ovarian (PCO) syndrome** is an endocrinologic disorder characterized by excessive androgen production and chronic anovulation. Hypersecretion of LH and hyperinsulinism are common.

1. **Symptoms:** anovulation, DUB, infertility, and excess male-pattern body hair

2. **Signs:** mild bilateral ovarian enlargement (all patients); obesity and hirsutism (one-half of cases); acanthosis nigricans, diabetes, and hypertension

3. **Hormonal profile:** noncyclic levels of estradiol (high normal), FSH level (low normal), LH (high normal), androgens (mild elevation), sex hormone–binding protein (SHBG) [decreased]

4. **Diagnosis:** high normal estradiol, elevated LH:FSH ratio (> 3), and sonographic evidence of > 10 follicles in both mildly enlarged ovaries

5. **Management** depends on which aspect of the disorder is of greatest concern.

    a. **Hirsutism.** Combination **oral contraceptives** decrease androgens in the following ways:

        (1) Suppression of LH stimulation of androgen production by ovarian stroma

        (2) Increased SHBG, thus binding testosterone and decreasing free testosterone levels

    b. **DUB.** Combination **oral contraceptives** are effective in the **following ways:**

        (1) Offset the hyperproliferative effect of prolonged unopposed estrogen

        (2) Ensure cyclic shedding of the endometrium

    c. **Infertility. Clomiphene** can be utilized for ovulation induction when pregnancy is desired.

V. PREMENSTRUAL SYNDROME.

A psychoneuroendocrine disorder with biological, psychological, and social parameters is known as premenstrual syndrome (PMS). Up to 90% of women experience some degree of premenstrual symptomatology. The highest incidence is found in women between the ages of 25 and 35 years.

A. The **definition** of PMS generally includes the following temporal criteria:

1. Symptoms are present only in the **second half** of the menstrual cycle.

2. The **first week** of the cycle is symptom free.

3. Symptoms are **recurrent,** being present through a minimum of three consecutive cycles.

4. Symptoms are **severe** enough to interfere with normal functioning, thereby requiring treatment.

B. **Symptoms** vary, with more than 150 attributed to PMS. Table 11-9 lists four different symptom clusters: fluid retention, autonomic symptoms, emotional symptoms, and musculoskeletal complaints.

    1. Each patient has a unique symptom constellation that must be determined.

    2. The specific symptoms are less important than their predictable recurrence in relation to the menstrual cycles.

C. **Theories of pathogenesis** abound, but currently there is no unified explanation. Suggested etiologies include estrogen–progesterone imbalance, fluid retention caused by renin–angiotensin–aldosterone activity, endogenous endorphin deficiency, prostaglandin excess, vitamin deficiencies, and serotonin deficiency.

D. **Diagnosis** is based on history alone and is confirmed by a **menstrual diary.** The patient keeps a daily record in which she identifies the day of her

Table 11-9. Premenstrual Syndrome

Symptom Clusters	Treatment Options
Fluid retention • Breast tenderness • Extremity edema • Weight gain • Bloating	**Medications** • **SSRIs** • Progesterone suppositories • Spironolactone • Pyridoxine (vitamin B_6)
Autonomic • Heart pounding • Confusion • Dizziness • Insomnia • Fatigue	**Lifestyle** • Relaxation techniques • Regular exercise • Support groups
Emotional • Nervous tension • Forgetfulness • Mood swings • Depression • Irritability • Anxiety • Crying	**Nutritional** • Balanced diet • Decrease caffeine • Decrease sugar • Decrease salt
Musculoskeletal • Muscle aches • Joint aches • Headache • Cramps	

SSRI = selective serotonin-reuptake inhibitors

cycle, the specific symptoms she experiences, and the intensity of her symptoms. A symptom-free follicular phase and a symptom-present luteal phase confirm the diagnosis.

E. Management

1. The patient should be assured that her condition is real and that it is taken seriously. Assurance of clinician support is vital.

2. The patient and her family should be educated regarding what is known about PMS and the realistic expectations associated with therapeutic modalities.

3. The constellation of symptoms should be examined to determine if a specific symptom cluster predominates. Treatment should address the symptom clusters that are identified (see Table 11-9).

   a. **Nutrition.** Balanced diet, decreased caffeine/sugar/salt, and multivitamins are of benefit for all patients.

   b. **Lifestyle.** Stress reduction, relaxation techniques, support groups, and regular exercise can be recommended safely for all patients.

   c. **Medication**

      (1) **Fluoxetine (Prozac)** or other selective serotonin reuptake inhibitors **(SSRIs)** are the **only treatment that has been shown to improve PMS in randomized prospective studies.**

      (2) **Spironolactone,** a potassium-sparing diuretic, may be helpful for complaints of bloating and fluid retention.

      (3) **NSAIDs** may be useful for musculoskeletal complaints.

      (4) **Bromocriptine** may be helpful for treatment of breast tenderness.

      (5) **Progesterone** has not been shown to be more effective than placebo in randomized prospective studies.

VI. HIRSUTISM

A. Terminology

1. **Hypertrichosis** is the excess growth of nonsexual hair (e.g., eyebrows, eyelashes, forearms, lower legs).

2. **Hirsutism** is the excess growth of male-pattern, pigmented, terminal hairs on the body midline (e.g., face, upper lip, chin, chest, abdomen, back, inner thighs).

3. **Defeminization** is the early stage of virilization (e.g., decreased breast size, loss of vaginal lubrication).

4. **Virilization,** always a pathologic condition, is an excess of male-pattern hair in addition to the following conditions:

   a. Increased muscle mass

   b. Clitoromegaly

   c. Temporal balding

   d. Deepening voice

B. Physiology

1. A **pilosebaceous unit** consists of a hair follicle and its sebaceous glands, which are extremely sensitive to the effects of sex hormones.

2. **Phases of hair activity** occur asynchronously but recurrently, with each follicle maintaining an independent rhythm of growth and rest.
    a. **Anagen** is the phase of active hair growth, during which there is proliferation of the hair shaft from the follicle bulb.
    b. **Catagen** is the phase of involution, during which mitoses cease, and the follicle regresses.
    c. **Telogen** is the resting phase, during which the hair is loosely attached to the follicle and is easily shed.

3. **Hair length** is determined by the anatomic location of the follicle.
    a. **Short hair** is found on the extremities, eyebrows, and eyelashes as a result of a short anagen phase, with a longer telogen.
    b. **Long hair** is found on the scalp and is the result of an extended anagen phase followed by a short telogen.

4. **Hair types** are classified as follows:
    a. **Vellus hair** is finely textured, short, and lightly pigmented. All hair on the fetus is of this type and is called **lanugo**.
    b. **Terminal hair** is coarse, longer, and darkly pigmented. It is characteristically found on the scalp, eyebrows, eyelashes, and sites of secondary sexual hair distribution.

C. **Mechanism**

1. **Number and location of hair follicles** are determined genetically in utero. Mediterranean whites have the most follicles, followed by northern European whites, then blacks, with Asians having the fewest follicles.

2. **At the time of puberty,** with the development of secondary sexual characteristics, sex steroids from gonadal and adrenal sources convert certain vellus hair to terminal hair. This occurs in very specific anatomic sites, which vary as to the level of circulating androgens required for hair conversion.
    a. **Low levels of androgens,** which are normally present in both genders, cause this conversion in the axillae, lower pubic triangle, forearms, and legs.
    b. **High levels of androgens,** normally found only in males, are required for growth of terminal hair on the face, upper lip, chin, chest, upper abdomen, and back.

3. **Final hair growth** is determined by a combination of two factors: the **level of circulating androgens** and the **sensitivity of hair follicles** to androgens.
    a. The **free, unbound** form of circulating androgens is the **active moiety.** This is a product of total androgen production combined with the binding capacity of SHBG. Hirsute women tend to have increased levels of free testosterone and decreased levels of SHBG.
    b. The **active androgen** within the hair follicle is **dihydrotestosterone** (DHT), the product of 5α-reductase enzyme conversion of androstenedione and testosterone to DHT. Hirsute women tend to have increased androgen sensitivity of the hair follicles, as indicated by high levels of 5α-reductase activity.

D. Androgenic steroids (Table 11-10). The table includes the relative potencies of these steroids compared with **dehydroepiandrosterone sulfate (DHEAS)**. Note that **dehydroepiandrosterone (DHEA)** and DHEAS derive mostly from the adrenal glands, and DHT derives mostly from peripheral conversion.

E. Causes of hirsutism (Table 11-11) may arise from any of the following:

1. **Ovaries:** hormonally active tumor (Sertolic-Leydig cell tumor), PCO syndrome, luteoma of pregnancy

2. **Adrenals:** hormonally active tumor, late-onset CAH [overproduction of androgenic precursor (17-OH progesterone)], Cushing's syndrome

3. **Exogenous medications** (anabolic steroids, danazol)

4. **Hair follicle sensitivity**

F. Diagnostic workup

1. **A detailed history** should be obtained, including the following:

a. **Ethnic or racial origin and family history** of hirsutism or an idiopathic cause (e.g., hair follicle sensitivity)

b. **Age of onset,** rapidity of development, and duration of findings

(1) **Onset gradually after puberty** is suggestive of PCO syndrome, late-onset CAH, or an idiopathic cause.

(2) **Onset rapidly after age 25 years** suggests an androgen-producing tumor.

(3) **Onset during pregnancy** suggests a **luteoma** of pregnancy or **theca lutein cysts.**

c. **Defeminization and virilization symptoms** are always abnormal and suggest a tumor.

d. **Gynecologic history** of irregular menses suggests PCO syndrome.

e. **Medication history** may elicit ingestion of specific androgenic steroids, anticonvulsants, or antibiotics that cause excessive body hair (see Table 11-11).

Table 11-10. Types of Androgenic Steroids

Androgen	Potency*	Source		
		Ovary	Adrenal	Peripheral Conversion
DHEAS	1	0%	100%	0%
DHEA	3	10%	90%	0%
Androstenedione	10	45%	45%	10%
Testosterone	100	25%	25%	50%
DHT	200	2%	2%	96%

DHEAS = dehydroepiandrosterone sulfate; *DHEA* = dehydroepiandrosterone; *DHT* = dihydrotestosterone.
*Potency is expressed in a comparison to DHEAS with a given potency of 1.

Table 11-11.　Causes of Hirsutism

Cause	Mechanism	Diagnostic Information	Treatment
Ovarian androgens	**Androgen-producing tumor** (e.g., Sertoli-Leydig cell, Hilar cell)	• Rapid onset • High testosterone level • Pelvic mass noted • Clitorimegaly	• Remove tumor
	Polycystic ovarian syndrome	• Long-term duration • Mildly elevated testosterone • Elevated LH/FHS ratio • Anovulation, infertility, obesity	• Oral contraceptive pills
	Luteoma of pregnancy Theca lutein cysts	• Onset during pregnancy	• Conservative management
Adrenal androgens	**Androgen-producing tumor**	• Rapid onset • High DHEAS level • Abdominal mass noted • Clitorimegaly	• Remove tumor
	Congenital adrenal hyperplasia (late onset) • 21-hydroxylase deficiency	• Elevated serum 17-dhydroxy progesterone level	• Glucocorticoid replacement and suppression
	Cushing syndrome	• Elevated plasma cortisol	• Varies as to etiology
Exogenous androgens	**Hormonal medications**	• Methyltestosterone • Anabolic steroids • Danazol	• Discontinue offending medications
Hair follicle sensitivity	**Excessive conversion of androgens to DHT in the hair follicle**	• Long-term duration • Positive family history • Mediterranean origin	• Spironolactone • Depilatory creams • Electrolysis • Waxing • Shaving
Exogenous etiology of hypertrichosis (nonsexual hair)	Nonhormonal medications	• Phenytoin • Diazoxide • Minoxidil • Streptomycin • Penicillamine	• Discontinue offending medications

DHEAS = dihydroepiandrosterone sulfate; *DHT* = dihydrotestosterone;
FSH = follicle-stimulating hormone; *LH* = luteinizing hormone.

2. **A thorough physical examination** should be performed to identify the following (specifically):

   a. **Height-to-weight ratio,** body habitus, presence of acne

   b. **Hair distribution pattern** and anatomic location

   c. **Cushingoid findings,** including centripetal obesity, extremity wasting, abdominal striae, buffalo hump, and moon face

   d. **Clitoral enlargement,** which is found in patients with virilization

   e. **Adnexal masses,** which suggest an ovarian tumor

3. **Laboratory testing** may include the following:

   a. **Serum total testosterone** in the male range, which identifies an androgen-producing ovarian tumor

   b. **Serum DHEAS,** which suggests an androgen-producing adrenal tumor

   c. **Serum 17-OH progesterone,** which identifies CAH

   d. **Overnight dexamethasone suppression test,** which identifies Cushing's syndrome

   e. **Serum LH:FSH ratio > 3,** which suggests PCO syndrome

   f. **Serum 3α diol glucuronide** is a stable metabolic breakdown product of DHT, which correlates with peripheral conversion of androgens

G. Management

1. **Exogenous medications** associated with increased hair growth should be discontinued.

2. **Androgen-secreting tumors** should be surgically removed.

3. **Adrenal overproduction of androgens** caused by CAH should be suppressed with glucocorticoid replacement.

4. **Ovarian overproduction of androgens** caused by PCO should be suppressed with oral contraceptive agents.

5. **Peripheral conversion of androgens** to DHT in the hair follicle should be suppressed with **spironolactone** by blocking androgen receptors.

6. **Cosmetic measures** may be helpful by removing unwanted hair (e.g., electrolysis, waxing, depilatory creams) or making the hair less visible (e.g., shaving, bleaching).

Review Test

Directions: Each of the numbered items or incomplete statements in this section is followed by answers or completions of the statement. Select the ONE lettered answer or completion that is BEST in each case.

1. During what period of human female development does the hypothalamic-pituitary-gonadal axis first become completely functional?

(A) Fetal period
(B) Neonatal period
(C) Childhood
(D) Prepuberty
(E) Puberty

2. A 15-year-old female adolescent with pubic hair and developing breasts has not started to menstruate. Which one of the following terms provides the best explanation for her condition?

(A) Normal development
(B) Pituitary tumor
(C) Abnormal karyotype
(D) Imperforate hymen
(E) Müllerian agenesis

3. A 28-year-old woman has a history of increased facial and body hair since onset of puberty at age 13. Serum testosterone and dehydroepiandrosterone sulfate (DHEAS) are normal. Which one of the following medical treatments is most likely to be beneficial in this case?

(A) Estrogen
(B) Progesterone
(C) Luprolide
(D) Spironolactone
(E) Prednisone

4. A 32-year-old woman has a history of regular menses until 4 months ago. A qualitative serum β-human chorionic gonadotropin (β-hCG) test is negative. A progesterone challenge test 10 days ago has produced no withdrawal bleeding. Which one of the following hormone assays would best identify the cause of her secondary amenorrhea?

(A) Follicle-stimulating hormone (FSH)
(B) Estrogen
(C) Progesterone
(D) Gonadotropin-releasing hormone (GnRH)
(E) Prolactin

5. Beginning at the age of 7 years, a female patient undergoes a sequence of developmental changes, including thelarche, adrenarche, and menarche. Which of the following explanations is most likely the correct interpretation for this developmental process?

(A) Sarcoid-induced complete isosexual precocious puberty
(B) Constitutional complete isosexual precocious puberty
(C) Pseudoisosexual precocious puberty
(D) Incomplete isosexual precocious puberty
(E) Pseudoheterosexual precocious puberty

6. A 28-year-old woman has had predictable, regular menstrual cycles until 3 months ago. Two years ago, she had a copper intrauterine device placed for contraception. She has a 3-year-old son and a 5-year-old daughter. Which one of the following descriptions of a hormone level is the most likely finding in this patient?

(A) Decreased estrogen level
(B) Increased thyroid-stimulating hormone (TSH) level
(C) Increased β-human chorionic gonadotropin (β-hCG) level
(D) Decreased dopamine level
(E) Decreased prolactin level

7. Which one of the following substances is the most potent androgen?

(A) Dihydroepiandrosterone (DHEA)
(B) Dihydrotestosterone (DHT)
(C) Dihydroepiandrosterone sulfate (DHEAS)
(D) Testosterone
(E) Androstenedione

Directions: Each of the numbered items or incomplete statements in this section is negatively phrased, as indicated by a capitalized word such as NOT, LEAST, or EXCEPT. Select the ONE lettered answer or completion that is BEST in each case.

8. All of the following are characteristics of dysfunctional uterine bleeding (DUB) EXCEPT

(A) DUB lacks pelvic pathology
(B) DUB is associated with anovulation
(C) DUB is diagnosed by dilation and curettage (D&C)
(D) DUB reflects prolonged unopposed estrogen
(E) DUB can be found in postmenopausal women

9. Which one of the following types of abnormal menstrual bleeding is NOT associated with either anovulation or polyps?

(A) Menorrhagia
(B) Hypomenorrhea
(C) Metrorrhagia
(D) Menometrorrhagia
(E) Polymenorrhea

Answers and Explanations

1. The answer is A [I A; Tables 11-1, 11-2].

The hypothalamic-pituitary-gonadal axis is activated during fetal life. During prenatal life, the pituitary gland can produce adult levels of gonadotropins, but it characteristically produces low levels because of the negative feedback response to the high level of placental steroids. During the neonatal period, with loss of placental steroid, the levels of follicle-stimulating hormone (FSH) and luteinizing hormone (LH) rapidly increase then gradually decrease while developing increasing sensitivity to the low estrogen levels of childhood. During puberty, the loss of hypothalamic sensitivity to negative feedback of sex steroids causes the level of gonadotropin-releasing hormone (GnRH) to begin to increase.

2. The answer is A [II C 1].

A 15-year-old girl with pubic hair and developing breasts but no onset of menses is normal, although the mean age of the onset of menses is 12 years. Primary amenorrhea is diagnosed when no menses have occurred by age 16 years with the presence of secondary sexual characteristics or by age 14 years if no secondary sexual development is present. Although pituitary tumor, abnormal karyotype, imperforate hymen, and müllerian agenesis are possible underlying pathologies, they are not the most likely explanations.

3. The answer is D [VI G 5].

The scenario described is that of constitutional or familial hirsutism, caused by increased peripheral androgen metabolism. Treatment is optimally a medication that blocks androgen receptors at the hair follicles. Spironolactone blocks the conversion of testosterone to dihydrotestosterone (DHT) at the hair follicle. Estrogen and progesterone have no effect on hirsutism treatment. Luprolide is an effective gonadotropin-releasing hormone (GnRH) agonist that suppresses androgen secretion but does not block receptors at the hair follicle. Prednisone suppresses the adrenal gland but does not block androgen receptors at the hair follicle.

4. The answer is A [II E 2].

A negative progesterone challenge test indicates a serum level of estrogen that is inadequate to prime the endometrium (< 40 mg/ml). A low level of estrogen may mean that either the ovaries do not have follicles to produce estrogen or that the hypothalamus and pituitary gland are not stimulating the follicles that may be present. An elevated level of follicle-stimulating hormone (FSH) would suggest ovarian failure, whereas a normal or decreased level would suggest hypothalamic-pituitary failure. An assay for estrogen is incorrect because the negative progesterone challenge is an in vivo bioassay for low estrogen. An assay for progesterone is incorrect because measuring progesterone is absurd when it is administered as part of the challenge test. An assay for gonadotropin-releasing hormone (GnRH) would not be the best way to differentiate the cause of secondary amenorrhea. A prolactin assay would be appropriate if the progesterone challenge test was positive.

5. The answer is B [I C; Table 11-3].

Precocious puberty is diagnosed as the onset of secondary sexual development in a girl before the age of 8 years. In this case, constitutional complete isosexual precocious puberty is the best explanation. Although sarcoid can induce developmental changes that are similar to constitutional complete isosexual precocious puberty, the incidence is 10 times lower. Pseudoisosexual precocious puberty, although rare, has similar physical findings as constitutional complete isosexual precocious puberty. However, the mechanism of constitutional complete isosexual precocious puberty involves the pituitary gland and hypothalamus, and the mechanism of pseudoisosexual precocious puberty involves an estrogen-producing tumor. Incomplete isosexual precocious puberty means that not all pubertal changes are present, which is not the case with the patient described. Pseudoisosexual precocious puberty is a possible diagnosis in this case, but pseudo-heterosexual precocious puberty is not a clinical entity.

6. The answer is C [II D,E].

Secondary amenorrhea is defined as absence of menstrual periods for 3 months if menses were previously regular or absence for 6 months if they were previously irregular. An increased β-human chorionic gonadotropin (β-hCG) level is the most likely finding because the most common cause of secondary amenorrhea is pregnancy. The second most common cause of amenorrhea is anovulation. A decreased estrogen level is found in patients with ovarian failure or severe hypothalamic dysfunction. Decreased, not increased, thyroid-stimulating hormone (TSH), can cause anovulation. Decreased dopamine levels allow prolactin levels to increase, possibly causing amenorrhea and anovulation. Decreased prolactin levels are not associated with amenorrhea.

7. The answer is B [VI D; Table 11-10].

Androgens vary in relative potency. Dihydrotestosterone (DHT) has relative potency of 200 compared with a potency of 1 for dihydroepiandrosterone sulfate (DHEAS), which is the weakest androgen. The relative potencies of the other androgens are 1 for DHEA, 10 for androstenedione, and 100 for testosterone.

8. The answer is E [IV F 4 d].

Dysfunctional uterine bleeding (DUB) is a disorder of premenopausal or perimenopausal women because it requires the presence of ovarian follicles, which produce estrogen. Postmenopausal women have no functional ovarian follicles, and therefore E is the correct answer. Standard characteristics of DUB include the absence of pelvic pathology, the association with anovulation (i.e., estrogen-producing follicles are not released), the diagnosis made by dilation and curettage (D&C), and prolonged unopposed estrogen contributing to the cause.

9. The answer is B [IV D; Table 11-8].

Abnormal menstrual bleeding is generally caused either by abnormal patterns of hormonal stimulation or by alterations in normal anatomy. The most common abnormal pattern of hormonal stimulation is anovulation, in which the endometrium is exposed to prolonged unopposed estrogen. This is also known as dysfunctional uterine bleeding (DUB). Hypomenorrhea, diminished or lighter menses, is usually caused by oral contraception, cervical stenosis, or intrauterine adhesions (Asherman's syndrome). Menorrhagia, cyclic and regular bleeding of excessive amount or duration, may be anovulatory in origin. Metrorrhagia (intermenstrual bleeding) and menometrorrhagia (intermenstrual bleeding that is irregular in frequency and excessive in amount) are usually associated with ovulatory cycles and usually arise from anatomic pathology such as polyps or neoplasia. Polymenorrhea, cycles that occur fewer than 21 days apart, is often associated with anovulation.

12

Menopause

I. OVERVIEW. Table 12-1 and Figure 12-1 summarize the reproductive events leading up to menopause. Note that menopause is characterized by absence of ovarian functional follicles resulting in low estrogen levels and elevated gonadotropins.

   A. Definitions. The terminology used to describe menopause is based on differing etiologies and the age at which menopause occurs (Table 12-2).

   1. **Perimenopause** is a 3- to 5-year period with increasingly frequent irregular anovulatory bleeding, followed by episodes of amenorrhea gradually lengthening associated with intermittent menopausal symptoms. Perimenopause tends to be short if menopause is early and prolonged if menopause is late.

   2. **Menopause** is the point in time at which menstrual cycles permanently cease. The mean age of occurrence of menopause is 51 years. The diagnosis is retrospective; after 12 months of amenorrhea, a woman is classified as being menopausal.

   B. Risk factors

   1. **Smoking.** Women who smoke experience menopause an average of 2 years earlier than women who do not smoke. A dose-response relationship exists.

   2. **High-altitude residence.** Women who live at high altitudes tend to have early onset of menopause.

   C. Early effects of menopause

   1. **Symptoms** of menopause are largely related to decreased estrogen levels.

      a. **Cessation of menses is the most common symptom.** Normally, the amount and duration of flow decrease gradually. Abrupt cessation is rare.

      b. **Hot flashes** are the classic evidence of estrogen decrease; they are experienced by 75% of women. A sensation of heat begins in the face, neck, and chest followed by profuse sweating in the upper body that lasts an average of 4 minutes. The duration of this symptom is 1–5

Table 12-1. Reproductive Events Leading to Menopause

Reproductive Stage	Germ Cell Number	Ovulation Status	Menstrual Cycles	Estrogen Level	Gonadotropin Level
Fetal life	Rapid mitotic increase to 6–7 million oogonia by 20 weeks and then rapid depletion to 1.5 million at birth	NA	NA	↑ **levels** from maternal/ placental source	↑ **rapidly** to adult levels by 20 weeks then gradually falls to term
Childhood (Birth to 8 years)	Further gradual depletion of follicles	NA	NA	↓ **levels** from ovarian follicles	↓ to **low basal levels**
Puberty (9 to 14 years)	Follicle number has declined to 350,000	**Irregular ovulation** initially but becoming more regular	**Anovulatory** cycles initially but becoming ovulatory	**Gradually increasing** to adult levels	
Reproductive years (15 to 45 years)	For every follicle that ovulates, 1000 become atretic	**Regular ovulation** with each cycle	**Ovalatory** from regular follicle maturation	**Normal cyclic variation** with menstrual cycles	
Perimenopause (45 to 55 years)	Only a few thousand less responsive follicles remain	**Irregular ovulation** becomes increasing frequent	**Anovulatory** cycles becoming increasingly frequent followed by oligomenorrhea	**Fluctuating** as follicle sensitivity varies	
Menopause (Average age 51 years)	No functional follicles remain	**Ovulation ceases**	**Menstrual cycles cease**	↓ **levels** from peripheral aromatization of androgens	↑ **levels** from loss of estrogen feedback

years. Physiologically, there is cutaneous vasodilation, decreased body core temperature, and increased heart rate associated with pulses of luteinizing hormone (LH). Hot flashes adversely affect rapid eye movement (REM) sleep.

   c. **Reversal of premenstrual syndrome** complaints is observed, including decreases of breast tenderness, abdominal bloating, edema, headaches, and cyclic emotions.

   d. **Urinary symptoms** of urgency, frequency, and nocturia develop from urothelium atrophy.

   e. **Psychological changes** are noted by many women. Depression and irritability are common complaints, but wide variability in degree is found. The mechanism is thought to be decreased levels of central neurotransmitters and endogenous opioids.

2. **Physical findings** of menopause are related to decreased estrogen levels.

   a. **Reproductive tract**

     (1) **Vagina.** Vaginal changes include flattening of rugae and thinning

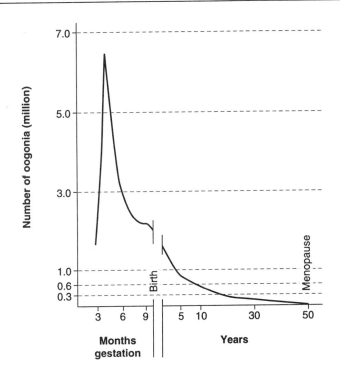

Figure 12-1. Changes in total population of germ cells in the human ovary with increasing age. (Reprinted with permission from Baker TG: *Am J Obstet Gynecol* 110:746, 1971.)

Table 12-2.   Menopause Terminology

Term	Age	Cause
Natural menopause	After 40 years	Time-related depletion of ovarian follicles
Premature menopause	Between 30 and 40 years	Mostly unknown but may occur after oophorectomy or ovarian follicle injury due to infection, radiation, or chemotherapy
Ovarian failure	Before 30 years	Autoimmune condition or caused by a mosaic karyotype that includes a Y chromosome

of the epithelium, as well as an increase in pH and a decrease in lubrication.

(2) **Cervix.** Cervical changes include a decrease in size, retreat of the squamocolumnar (SC) junction into the endocervical canal, and decreased cervical mucus.

(3) **Uterus.** Uterine changes include a decrease in overall size with shrinkage of myomas and atrophy of adenomyosis.

(4) **Ovaries.** Ovaries decrease in size; they usually become nonpalpable.

b. **Urinary tract.** Urothelium atrophy may lead to loss of urethral tone and development of urethral caruncle. The bladder may become hypertonic, leading to **detrusor instability** (see Chapter 8).

c. **Pelvic floor.** Loss of tissue tone can lead to pelvic relaxation, including uterine and vaginal prolapse (see Chapter 8).

d. **Breast.** Changes include a decrease in size of the breasts and fewer benign cysts than before menopause.

e. **Skin.** Collagen content and skin thickness decrease at 2% per year, resulting in generalized thinning, loss of elasticity, and wrinkling.

3. **Changes in hormone levels** during menopause are largely related to the loss of endocrine activity of ovarian follicles (estrogen and progesterone) with continued secretion of ovarian stroma (testosterone) [Table 12-3].

D. Late effects of menopause

1. **Osteoporosis** is a disorder of decreased bone density, which results from increased osteoclastic activity (resorption) and frequently unchanged osteoblastic (formation) activity. The loss of bone initially is asymptomatic but eventually leads to decreased skeletal strength and fractures.

a. **Physiology of bone loss.** Bone density peaks in one's 20s. After age 40, resorption exceeds formation by 0.5% per year. This negative balance increases after menopause to a loss of 5% of trabecular bone per year.

(1) **Vertebral crush fractures** are the most common occurrences. Untreated women can lose 2.5 inches in height.

(2) **Hip and wrist fractures** are the next most common sites.

b. **Types of osteoporosis**

(1) **Type I** affects **trabecular** bone primarily, with the vertebral bodies being most involved. Postmenopausal women are most often affected.

(2) **Type II** affects both **trabecular and cortical** bone, with the hip being the most involved bone. Both **men** and **women** are affected with advancing age.

Table 12-3. Changes in Hormonal Levels With Menopause

	Source of Estrogens	Source of Testosterone	Source of Androstenedione	Source of Progesterone	Gonadotropin Levels
Prior to menopause	Ovarian follicles stimulated by follicle-stimulating hormone	Ovarian stroma and peripheral conversion of androstenedione	Ovarian follicles and adrenal secretion	Corpus luteum secretion by ovary	Fluctuates with menstrual cycles
After menopause	Peripheral conversion of adrenal androstenedione	Ovarian stroma and peripheral conversion of adrenal androstenodione	Adrenal secretion only	Peripheral aromatization of adrenal steroids	Persistently elevated

   c. **Risk factors** (Table 12-4) include gender, body mass index, race, family history, lifestyle factors, and steroid medications.

   d. **Diagnosis.** Symptoms and bone fractures are late findings.

     (1) **Current bone density** is best assessed by dual-energy x-ray absorptiometry (DEXA) scanning. This assessment of bone densitometry can demonstrate if bone density is above or below the fracture threshold.

     (2) **Rate of bone loss** is best assessed by 24-hour urinary hydroxyproline or deoxypyridoline measurements. These are sensitive measures of changes in osteoclastic activity.

   e. **Prevention**

     (1) **Lifestyle**

       (a) Dietary calcium and supplements should equal 1500 mg/day.

       (b) Vitamin D supplements should equal 1500 mg/day.

       (c) Weight-bearing exercise should be performed regularly.

       (d) Cigarettes and alcohol should be eliminated.

     (2) **Medications**

       (a) **Estrogen** replacement therapy (ERT) is the mainstay of prevention and treatment (see I E).

       (b) **Alendronate** (Fosamax) is a biphosphonate that inhibits osteoclastic activity and has minimal side effects.

       (c) **Raloxifene** (Evista) is a selective estrogen receptor modulator (SERM) that belongs to the benzothiophene group. SERMs are molecules that bind with high affinity to estrogen receptors but have tissue-specific effects distinct from estradiol. Raloxifene has some estrogen-like effects [e.g., increasing bone density, decreasing low-density lipoprotein (LDL) cholesterol] but acts as an estrogen antagonist on endometrial and breast tissue. This agent results in the exacerbation of hot flashes.

       (d) **Calcitonin** inhibits osteoclastic activity and also has an analgesic effect.

       (e) **Fluoride** increases trabecular bone, but because the bones are made more brittle, fracture rates may be increased.

  2. **Cardiovascular disease** is the number one cause of death in women, causing almost 150 times more deaths in the United States than endometrial carcinoma.

Table 12-4. Risk Factors for Osteoporosis

Gender	Genetic	Lifestyle	Steroids
• Occurs more often in **women** (male-female ratio, 1:3)	Positive family history	• **Smoking**	• **Exogenous medications**
• Risk highest in **fair-skinned, slender, white** women	• Highest in **whites** • Moderate in Asians • Lowest in blacks	• ↑ **caffeine** intake • ↑ **alcohol** use • ↑ **protein** in diet • ↓ **vitamin D** intake • ↓ **calcium** intake	• **Cushing's syndrome**

a. **Epidemiology.** Before menopause, a woman's risk of a heart attack is one-third that of a man's. After menopause, the heart attack rate in women increases progressively until it is the same for both genders at age 70 years.

b. **Estrogen therapy** decreases the heart attack risk in women by 50%, with the oral and transdermal routes of administration **being equally effective. The mechanisms by which estrogen decreases cardiovascular risk are as follows:**

   (1) Estrogen increases the high-density lipoprotein (HDL) fraction while lowering the LDL fraction.

   (2) Estrogen decreases atherogenic plaque formation by direct action on vascular endothelium.

E. **Hormone replacement therapy**

1. **Benefits** of ERT are realized only as long as the therapy is continued. Once ERT is discontinued, the underlying pathophysiological process resumes.

   a. **Vagina.** Estrogen thickens and cornifies the epithelium, which decreases dyspareunia. It also produces an acidic pH, which decreases infectious vaginitis.

   b. **Urinary tract.** Estrogen decreases atrophy of the urothelium, thus enhancing normal bladder function.

   c. **Osteoporosis.** Loss of bone density can be halted with stabilization of trabecular bone formation. Fractures can be reduced by more than 50%.

   d. **Cardiovascular disease.** Estrogen can decrease the risk of a heart attack by 50%, mostly in women with high-risk factors (Figure 12-2).

   e. **Skin.** Estrogen may halt the loss of collagen, which stabilizes elasticity. The greatest benefit is in women with low natural levels of estrogen.

   f. **Alzheimer's disease** may be reduced 50%, with the benefit directly related to length of estrogen use.

   g. **Colon carcinoma** risk is reduced up to 50%, possibly due to reduction of colon bile salts.

2. **Confirmed risks** regarding ERT are endometrial carcinoma and gallbladder disease.

   a. **Endometrial carcinoma.** The risk of endometrial carcinoma increases (up to 10-fold) with increases in dosage and duration of therapy. The disease is usually localized and of low-grade malignancy. **Adding progestins to ERT eliminates the increased risk of endometrial cancer.** Progestins can be administered for 12 days of each 28-day cycle or daily in combination with ERT.

   b. **Gallbladder disease.** ERT increases plasma triglycerides and total cholesterol, thus increasing the risk of gallstone formation.

3. **Unconfirmed risks** regarding ERT are breast cancer, hypertension, and thromboembolic disease. At the estrogen dosages currently recommended, there are no replicated studies showing a persistent relation between ERT and the development of breast cancer, hypertension, or thromboembolic disease.

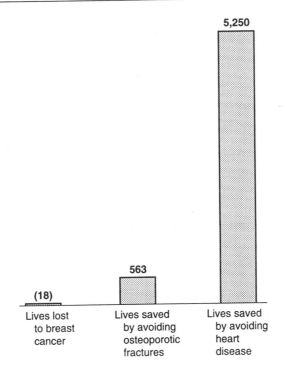

Figure 12-2. Lives saved or lost per 100,000 women between the ages of 50 and 75 years by taking 0.626 mg/day of oral conjugated estrogens. (Reprinted with permission from Henderson: *Am J Obstet Gynecol* 154:1181–1186, 1986.)

    4. Contraindications to ERT include the following:

        a. Undiagnosed vaginal bleeding

        b. Acute liver disease

        c. Chronic impaired liver function

        d. Acute vascular thrombosis

        e. Hormonally dependent carcinoma

    5. Hormone selection is based on presence or absence of a uterus.

        a. Estrogen should be administered **continuously** at a **physiologic** replacement dose (e.g., conjugated estrogen 0.625 mg PO, micronized estradiol 1 mg PO; 0.05 mg transdermally) to all patients.

        b. Progestin should be administered to all women **with a uterus** to prevent endometrial hyperplasia, but is unnecessary in those who have undergone hysterectomies. Medroxyprogesterone acetate 2.5 mg is given **continuously.** Within 3 months virtually all patients become amenorrheic. Progestins do not negate the beneficial estrogen effects on vasomotor symptoms or bone density, but may diminish the improved lipid profile response and adversely affect irritability and depression.

II. POSTMENOPAUSAL BLEEDING

    A. Endometrial cancer is a primary concern when vaginal bleeding occurs after 12 months of amenorrhea in middle-aged women who are not receiving hormone replacement therapy. With loss of functional ovarian follicles, bleeding from normal ovulatory cycles is impossible. Postmenopausal bleeding can never be "dysfunctional" or anovulatory in nature.

1. **Endometrial cancer is the most common gynecological malignancy.**

   a. The total number of **new cases** equals the combined number of new cases of ovarian and cervical cancer.

   b. The **mortality rate** from endometrial cancer has steadily decreased during the past 50 years.

2. **Endometrial neoplasia** can progress from simple hyperplasia to invasive cancer caused by unopposed estrogen (Table 12-5; Figure 12-3).

3. **The mechanism** for many endometrial carcinomas is prolonged estrogen stimulation of the endometrium unopposed by progesterone. The source of endometrial stimulation may be any of the following:

   a. Exogenous estrogen (e.g., ERT)

   b. Peripheral aromatization of androstenedione to estrone

   c. Estrogen-producing tumor

   d. Tamoxifen stimulation of the endometrium

4. **Risk factors** for endometrial carcinoma include no pregnancies; prolonged reproductive time; unopposed estrogen; and the triad of diabetes mellitus (DM), hypertension, and obesity (Table 12-6).

5. **Patterns of spread** of endometrial carcinoma are described as follows:

   a. **Direct extension** to adjacent structures is the most common route of spread. The cancer can invade the myometrium, extend downward to the cervix, or (rarely) involve the vagina, rectum, and bladder.

   b. **Transtubal migration** of malignant cells can lead to involvement of ovaries, peritoneum, and omentum.

   c. **Lymphatic spread** is mainly to the pelvic lymph nodes with pro-

Table 12-5. Endometrial Hyperplasia

Type of Endometrial Neoplasia	Findings on Histology	Progress to Cancer
Simple hyperplasia	Crowding of normal glands with normal stroma	< 1%
Complex hyperplasia without atypia	Complex crowded glands with little intervening stroma	5%
Simple hyperplasia with atypia	Glands lined by enlarged cells with increased nuclear to cytoplasmic ratio	10%
Complex hyperplasia with atypia	Glands lined by enlarged cells with increased nuclear to cytoplasmic ratio	30%
Endometrial carcinoma	Obvious glandular anaplasia, with stromal, myometrial, or vascular invasion	100%

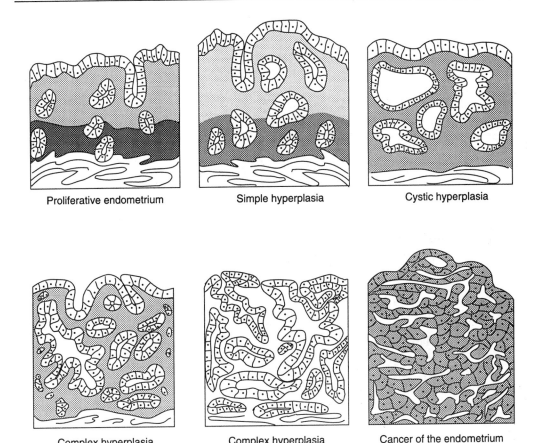

Proliferative endometrium   Simple hyperplasia   Cystic hyperplasia

Complex hyperplasia without atypia   Complex hyperplasia with atypia   Cancer of the endometrium

Figure 12-3. Endometrial histology: hyperplasia to carcinoma. (Reprinted with permission from Beckmann CR, Ling FW, Barzansky BM, et al: *Obstetrics and Gynecology,* 2nd ed. Williams & Wilkins, Baltimore, 1995, p 448.)

gression to the periaortic nodes. The incidence depends on tumor grade and depth of myometrial invasion.

    d. Hematogenous spread to the lungs and liver is uncommon.

  6. Staging of endometrial carcinoma is described in Table 12-7.

B. Differential diagnosis. Postmenopausal perineal bleeding can originate from the gastrointestinal (GI) tract as well as reproductive tract processes (Box 12-1).

  1. GI tract causes include hemorrhoids, anal fissures, or colorectal carcinoma.

  2. Lower reproductive tract causes include atrophic vaginitis, vaginal fissures/tumors, vulvar lesions/tumors, and cervical lesions/tumors.

  3. Upper reproductive tract causes include atrophic endometritis, endometrial polyps, endometrial hyperplasia, and endometrial carcinoma.

C. Diagnosis

  1. GI tract etiology can be identified with a general physical examination,

Table 12-6. Risk Factors for Endometrial Carcinoma

Reproductive History	Systemic Diseases	Other Cancers
• Nulliparity	• Diabetes mellitus	• Breast carcinoma
• Late menopause	• Chronic hypertension	• Colon carcinoma
• Chronic unopposed estrogen	• Obesity	• Ovarian carcinoma

Table 12-7. FIGO* Surgical Staging of Endometrial Carcinoma (1988)

Stage	Grade
I	LIMITED TO THE UTERUS Ia G 1,2,3 Limited to endometrium Ib G 1,2,3 Invasion < 1/2 myometrium Ic G 1,2,3 Invasion > 1/2 myometrium
II	LIMITED EXTENSION BEYOND UTERUS IIa G 1,2,3 Endocervical gland involvement only IIb G 1,2,3 Cervical stromal invasion
III	EXTENSION WITHIN PELVIS III G 1,2,3 Invasion serosa/adnexa or positive peritoneal cytology IIIb G 1,2,3 Vaginal metastases IIIc G 1,2,3 Metastases to pelvic/para-aortic nodes
IV	DISTANT METASTASES IVa G 1,2,3 Invastion of bladder/bowel mucosa IVb Distant metastases/extra-abdominal or inguinal nodes

FIGO = International Federation of Gynecology and Obstetrics; *G 1,2,3* = histology shows grade 1, 2 or 3.

including rectal examination, stool guaiac, and proctosigmoidoscopy. Management depends on the specific pathology.

2. **Lower reproductive tract causes** can be identified with physical examination including pelvic examination, Papanicolaou (Pap) smear, and appropriate biopsies. **Management depends on the specific pathology.**

3. **Upper reproductive tract causes** can be identified only by a tissue diagnosis obtained by endometrial evaluation.

   a. **Endometrial biopsy** is helpful only if it is positive. This biopsy is highly inaccurate for diagnosing polyps and misses a significant number of hyperplasias. In addition, it does not allow for staging of cervical involvement.

   b. **Hysterosonography** is performed by infusing saline in the uterine cavity to identify endometrial polyps. An endometrial "stripe thickness" greater than 10 mm indicates higher risk of hyperplasia. However, tissue must still be obtained for histological studies.

   c. **Fractional dilation and curettage (D&C)** is the gold standard for evaluating postmenopausal bleeding. It is performed in two stages.

      (1) Initially, the endocervical canal is curetted obtaining the first specimen to rule out invasion of the cervix by carcinoma.

Box 12-1. Causes of Postmenopausal Bleeding

Exogenous estrogens	30%
Atrophic endometritis/vaginitis	30%
Endometrial cancer	15%
Endometrial/endocervical polyps	10%
Endometrial hyperplasia	5%
Miscellaneous	10%

---

(2) Then, the uterine cavity is curetted obtaining the second specimen to assess endometrial neoplasia or malignancy.

d. **Hysteroscopy** ideally is performed at the time of the fractional D&C, after obtaining the endocervical specimen. The endometrial cavity is visualized for polyps with operative resection immediately. Then the second specimen is obtained.

e. **Pap smears** have a poor sensitivity for endometrial neoplasia; only 40% of cases are identified.

D. Management

1. **Endometrial hyperplasia.** Management of endometrial hyperplasia is influenced by age of the patient, the tumor histopathology, and the patient's fertility desires.

   a. **Progestin therapy** is appropriate for postmenopausal patients who are not surgical candidates or premenopausal patients who desire fertility preservation. Medroxyprogesterone acetate (Provera) and megestrol acetate (Megace) are commonly used progestins.

      (1) Simple or complex hyperplasia **without atypia** predictably regresses with monthly cycling for the last 10 days of the cycle. Follow-up biopsy should be performed in 3 to 6 months.

      (2) Simple or complex hyperplasia **with atypia** has lower rates of response to progestin therapy. Follow-up biopsy should be performed in 3 months.

   b. **Surgical therapy** is indicated primarily for premenopausal patients who have hyperplasia with atypia and do not desire preservation of fertility or for postmenopausal patients.

      (1) **Total hysterectomy** is the treatment of choice. Either the abdominal or vaginal route may be used. The choice of approach depends on gynecological factors such as previous pelvic infections and adhesions, the presence of vaginal wall prolapse, or the presence of stress urinary incontinence.

      (2) A **D&C** alone may on occasion be therapeutic and curative with no further bleeding and normal histology on follow-up biopsy.

2. **Endometrial carcinoma.** Management of endometrial carcinoma is **primarily surgical** with other modalities as adjuvants, depending on tumor grade and stage at diagnosis.

   a. **Stage I lesions,** which involve only the uterine fundus, are managed with total abdominal hysterectomy (TAH), bilateral salpingo-oophorectomy (BSO), and cytological examination of peritoneal washings.

If the tumor grade is 2 or 3 (i.e., G2 or G3) or myometrial invasion is noted, selective pelvic and para-aortic lymph nodes are sampled.

b. **Stage II lesions,** which show only additional cervical involvement, are managed as advanced stage I cases. Preoperative whole pelvis radiation therapy is performed if gross cervical involvement is noted. Postoperative whole pelvis radiation with vaginal cuff implants is performed if nodal invasion was diagnosed or myometrial invasion was seen. Radical hysterectomy is no more advantageous than a simple TAH and radiation.

c. **Stage III and IV lesions,** which have wider metastases, are managed with a combination of TAH, BSO, progestin hormone therapy, chemotherapy, and radiation therapy.

d. **Recurrent lesions** are palliated by radiation for pelvic sites and by progestin or chemotherapy for extrapelvic lesions.

Review Test

Directions: Each of the numbered items or incomplete statements in this section is followed by answers or by completions of the statement. Select the ONE lettered answer or completion that is BEST in each case.

1. A 52-year-old woman has not had a menstrual period for 13 months. She complains of feelings of heat followed by upper body sweating that occurs unpredictably at any time of the day or night. Which one of the following conditions would be the most common underlying etiology her symptoms?

(A) Hypothalamic failure
(B) Hyperprolactinemia
(C) Ovarian follicle depletion
(D) Adrenal insensitivity
(E) Pituitary insufficiency

2. Which one of the following is an expected endocrinologic profile of a normal menopausal woman?

		Follicle-stimulating hormone	Luteinizing hormone
Estrogen	Progesterone		
(A) ↓	↓	↓	↓
(B) ↑	↓	↑	↓
(C) ↑	↑	↓	↓
(D) ↓	↓	↑	↑
(E) ↑	↑	↑	↑

3. A 55-year-old woman is 5 years postmenopause. She has an intact uterus and is taking daily conjugated estrogen replacement therapy (ERT) [0.625 mg]. Repetitive prospective studies have established that she is at higher risk for which one of the following conditions?

(A) Hypertension
(B) Endometrial hyperplasia
(C) Ovarian cancer
(D) Breast cancer
(E) Deep venous thrombosis (DVT)

4. A 60-year-old woman is 11 years postmenopause without any hormone replacement therapy. Her actual weight is 90% of her ideal body weight. Pelvic examination confirms an atrophic vaginal epithelium. For which one of the following conditions is she at higher risk?

(A) Decreased cortical bone
(B) Decreased vaginal pH
(C) Increased bladder capacity
(D) Increased low-density lipoprotein (LDL) cholesterol
(E) Generalized chills

5. A 64-year-old woman who is 13 years postmenopause presents with complaints of vaginal bleeding. She is not receiving any hormone replacement therapy. Which one of the following conditions is the most common single cause of her complaint?

(A) Endometrial carcinoma
(B) Endometrial polyps
(C) Endometrial hyperplasia
(D) Cervical carcinoma
(E) Atrophic vaginitis

6. A 58-year-old woman who is 150% of her ideal body weight has a 20-year history of adult-onset diabetes mellitus (DM). She recently underwent endometrial sampling for postmenopausal bleeding. The histology revealed moderately differentiated endometrial adenocarcinoma. If the carcinoma has already spread, which one of the following conditions is the most common pattern of spread?

(A) Lymphatic spread
(B) Direct extension to adjacent structures
(C) Exfoliation of malignant cells through oviducts
(D) Hematogenous spread

7. A 60-year-old woman experienced menopause 10 years ago. She has been diagnosed with endometrial carcinoma and has undergone an exploratory laparotomy with total abdominal hysterectomy (TAH) with bilateral salpingo-oophorectomy (BSO). The pathology report of the uterus shows a grade 2 tumor that has invaded one-third of the way through the myometrium. There is no cervical or vaginal involvement, but peritoneal washings show positive cytology. What is the stage of this cancer?

(A) Stage I
(B) Stage II
(C) Stage III
(D) Stage IV

329

Directions: The question below is negatively phrased, as indicated by a capitalized word such as NOT, LEAST, or EXCEPT. Select the ONE lettered answer or completion that is BEST.

8. All of the following conditions are risk factors for endometrial carcinoma EXCEPT

(A) hyperthyroidism
(B) obesity
(C) hypertension
(D) nulliparity
(E) diabetes mellitus (DM)

Answers and Explanations

1. The answer is C [I A 2, C 1].

Menopause occurs when insufficient ovarian follicles are present to maintain adequate estrogen levels. Endometrial proliferation is insufficient to yield menstruation and cease menses. Although hypothalamic failure and pituitary insufficiency could result in similar symptoms, they are much less common. Hyperprolactinemia and adrenal insensitivity are spurious detractors.

2. The answer is D [I C 1 b].

In normal menopause the final common pathway is ovarian follicle depletion. The hypothalamic-pituitary mechanism is still functional. Because menopause is basically end-organ failure, the normal hormonal products of that end-organ failure (estrogen and progesterone) are decreased. With an intact hypothalamus and pituitary, the gonadotropic stimulation increases in response to the low estrogen levels, resulting in increased follicle-stimulating hormone (FSH) and luteinizing hormone (LH) levels.

3. The answer is B [I E 2–4].

The only confirmed negative effect of postmenopausal estrogen replacement therapy (ERT) is endometrial hyperplasia, which can progress to endometrial carcinoma. This occurs mostly in patients who have had prolonged unopposed estrogen exposure. Possible complications of ERT in menopause have been studied in depth. Hypertension, ovarian cancer, breast cancer, and deep venous thrombosis (DVT) have not been confirmed as adverse outcomes of postmenopausal ERT.

4. The answer is D [I D 2 b].

This slender postmenopausal woman who is not receiving hormone replacement therapy has a low body-mass index, which suggests minimal peripheral body fat conversion of adrenal steroid to estrogens. The increase in low-density lipoprotein (LDL) cholesterol and decrease in high-density lipoprotein (HDL) cholesterol are potent mechanisms for the surge in heart disease in estrogen-deficient postmenopausal women. The impact on the reproductive tract is most apparent in terms of morbidity, but the effect regarding osteoporosis and cardiovascular disease is much greater in terms of mortality. Decreased cortical bone is incorrect because trabecular, not cortical, bone is decreased. Vaginal pH increases, not decreases; bladder capacity decreases, not increases; and hot flashes, not chills, are common.

5. The answer is E [II B; Box 12-1].

Vaginitis, endometritis, and exogenous estrogens are the most common causes of postmenopausal bleeding, which is an abnormal condition and must be investigated thoroughly. Endometrial or cervical carcinoma should be the assumed diagnosis until they are ruled out. Endometrial carcinoma, polyps, hyperplasia, and cervical carcinoma clearly must be ruled out.

6. The answer is B [II A 5 a].

The surgical staging of endometrial carcinoma reflects the most common route of spread. Direct extension to adjacent structures is the correct answer because stage I carcinoma describes the extent to which the tumor has directly invaded the myometrium. Lymphatic spread, oviduct exfoliation, and hematogenous spread are less likely methods of metastasis.

7. The answer is C [II A 6; Table 12-7].

Stage III is correct because there is a tumor-positive peritoneal cytology. Stage I is incorrect because, although the tumor has invaded the myometrium, there is evidence of further involvement in the positive peritoneal washings. Stage II is incorrect because there is no cervical involvement, and stage IV is incorrect because there is no distant metastases or involvement of the bladder or bowel.

8. The answer is A [II A 4; Table 12-6].

Hyperthyroidism has no relationship to the development of endometrial carcinoma. Obesity, hypertension, nulliparity, and diabetes mellitus (DM) are all well-recognized risk factors.

13

Pelvic Masses and Pelvic Pain

I. PREMENOPAUSAL PELVIC MASS

A. Causes of pelvic masses can include congenital, physiologic, and pathologic processes involving the following three organ systems located in the pelvis.

   1. Gastrointestinal (GI) causes include a colorectal tumor or diverticulosis, which can result in a left-sided inflammatory pelvic mass.

   2. Urinary tract causes include anomalies such as a pelvic kidney, ureterocele, or kidney tumor.

   3. Reproductive tract causes include the following:

   a. Processes involving the oviduct

   (1) Hydrosalpinx is caused by postinfection occlusion of both the proximal and distal oviducts, which results in serous fluid accumulation within a dilated oviduct.

   (2) Tubo-ovarian abscess (TOA) is an acute infectious pelvic mass that may involve any or all of the following: oviduct, ovary, broad ligament, bowel, and omentum.

   (3) Chronic pelvic inflammatory disease (PID) develops after the acute infectious process has resolved. The residual leaves an adherent pelvic mass that may involve any of the same organs involved in a TOA.

   (4) Paratubal cysts may be found within the mesosalpinx. **Hydatid cysts of Morgagni** are thin-walled pedunculated benign cysts attached to the distal oviduct. They are of paramesonephric origin and are usually small, but they can grow to 10 cm in size and can be very mobile.

   b. Processes involving the uterus

   (1) Pregnancy. Pregnancy is the **most common** cause of a pelvic mass in women who are in their reproductive years.

   (2) Leiomyomas (see III B)

   (3) Adenomyosis (see III C)

   c. Functional ovarian masses. These masses arise from excessive response to otherwise normal reproductive events.

   (1) Follicular cysts result from the persistence of an enlarged pre-

333

ovulatory follicle, which usually disappears spontaneously within 60 days. They are generally unilateral.

(2) Corpus luteum cysts result from resorption of blood from the central cavity of an enlarged cystic corpus hemorrhagicum, which usually spontaneously disappears if pregnancy does not occur. They are generally unilateral.

(3) Theca lutein cysts are the response of normal ovaries to excessively high β-human chorionic gonadotropin (β-hCG) levels (molar pregnancy, multiple gestation) and ovulation induction agents (clomiphene citrate, gonadotropins). They are generally bilateral and fluid filled, and they can be massive in size. Theca lutein cysts spontaneously disappear when the source of increased β-hCG levels (e.g., molar pregnancy, twins, clomiphene stimulation) is gone. Resolution may take many months.

(4) Luteomas of pregnancy are tumor-like nodules of lutein cells that may form in the ovaries during pregnancy. They are often multifocal and bilateral, and they can be massive in size. Luteomas of pregnancy totally regress after the pregnancy is over.

d. **Nonneoplastic, nonfunctional ovarian masses**

(1) Endometriomas are cysts on the ovary that result from accumulation of menstrual-like detritus from endometriosis. These "chocolate cysts" can enlarge to several centimeters in size.

(2) Polycystic ovaries are bilaterally mildly enlarged and may be found in patients with infertility, anovulation, obesity, and hirsutism. The ovaries feel smooth and have multiple small, fluid-filled cysts beneath a thickened capsule.

(3) Hyperthecosis of premenopausal ovaries may occasionally produce ovarian enlargement. Hyperthecosis results from proliferation of nests of stromal cells that produce excess androgen, which can result in hirsutism.

e. **Neoplastic ovarian lesions.** These lesions are most commonly epithelial tumors (80% of cases) followed next by the development of germ cell tumors (15% of cases). Table 13-1 summarizes the types of ovarian tumors.

(1) Serous cystadenomas are benign tumors that occur most commonly in 20- to 30-year-old women. Histologically, these tumors appear to be derived from ciliated tubal epithelium. They are commonly unilocular and may attain a large size. The malignant type accounts for 20% of all serous tumors.

(2) Mucinous cystadenomas are benign tumors with a histological appearance similar to endocervical columnar epithelium. They are generally multiloculated and are the largest tumors found in the human body (up to 150 pounds). **Pseudomyxoma peritonei** describes the intraperitoneal accumulation of thick mucin from this tumor. The malignant type accounts for 15% of all mucinous tumors.

(3) Transitional cell (Brenner) tumors are almost always benign, with only 2% being malignant. Histologically, they appear to be derived from transitional cell urothelium. They are usually small in size.

Table 13-1. Ovarian Tumors

Origin	Name	Histogenesis	Unique Finding	% Malignant
Coelomic Epithelial • 80%–85% of all ovarian tumors • Age at diagnosis older than 40 years	**Serous**	Cilated tubal epithelium	Psammoma bodies; Tumor marker: CA-125	20%
	Mucinous	Columnar endocervical epithelium	Pseudomyxoma peritonei; Tumor markers CA-125, CEA	15%
	Endometroid	Endometrial glands	Tumor marker: CA-125	95%
	Clear cell	Mesonephric tissue	Tumor marker: CA-125	98%
	Brenner	Transitional urothelium	Walthard cell rests	2%
Germ Cell • 10%–15% of all ovarian tumors • Age at diagnosis younger than 30 years	**Teratoma mature**	Many mature cell types	Rokitansky prominence	0%
	Teratoma immature	Fetal embryonic tissue	Tumor markers: α-FP, CA-125	100%
	Dysgerminoma	Primitive germ cells	Tumor marker: LDH	100%
	Gonadoblastoma	Dysgenetic gonads with Y chromosomes	Malignant only if there are associated dysgerminoma elements	0%
	Endodermal sinus	Extraembryonic tissue	Schiller-Duval bodies; Tumor-marker: α-FP	100%
	Embryonal carcinoma	Embryonic tissue	Tumor markers: α-FP, β-hCG	100%
	Nongestational choriocarcinoma	Extraembryonic tissue	Tumor marker: β-hCG	100%
Gonadal-Stromal • 3%–5% of all tumors • Age at diagnosis 50 years, with a range of 20–80 years	**Granulosa cell**	Ovarian gonadal cells	Cal-Exner bodies; estrogen production	< 5%
	Fibroma	Thecoma elements	Seen with Meigs' syndrome	< 5%
	Thecoma	Thecoma elements	Estrogen production	< 5%
	Sertoli-Leydig cell	Testicular gonadal cells	Crystals of Reinke Testosterone production	< 5%
	Lipid cell	Gonadal–stromal cells	Testosterone production	30%
	Gynandroblastoma	Both ovarian and testicular cell tissues	Testosterone production	100%

α-*FP* = alpha fetoprotein: β-*hCG* = beta-human chorionic gonadotropin; *CA-125* = cancer antigen 125; *CEA* = carcinoembryonic antigen; *LDH* = lactate dehydrogenase.

(4) Benign cystic teratomas (dermoid cysts) are relatively common, comprising 25% of all ovarian neoplasms. They derive from primordial germ cells and may contain any combination of well-differentiated ectodermal, mesodermal, and endodermal elements. Teeth, hair, and cartilage are often found in these cysts. Long pedicles allow these cysts to be palpated anterior to the uterus, even abdominally. **Struma ovarii** is a unique subtype in which thyroid tissue constitutes the entire neoplasm, resulting in hyperthyroidism in some cases.

B. Indicators of malignant potential

    1. Patient age is related to the chance of ovarian tumor malignancy (Box 13-1). Note that ovarian masses in even young patients can be malignant, and those in older women can be benign.

Box 13-1. Patient Age as Indicator of Ovarian Malignant Potential

Patient age	Chance of malignancy
Prepubertal years	10%
Reproductive years	15%
Postmenopausal years	50%

Box 13-2. Ultrasound in the Diagnosis of Ovarian Tumors

Findings suggesting benign tumor	Findings suggesting malignancy
Cystic	Solid
Simple cyst	Loculated cyst
Mobile	Fixed
Unilateral	Bilateral
Small	Large

---

2. **Ultrasound findings** can indicate suspicion of ovarian tumor malignancy (Box 13-2). Confirmation of malignancy is by histologic examination.

C. Diagnosis and management

1. **Pregnancy,** which is the most common cause of a premenopausal pelvic mass, can be easily ruled out by determining the patient's serum β-hCG level.

2. **Nonreproductive tract etiology** can be identified with imaging modalities such as sonography, intravenous pyelography (IVP), or barium enema. Management depends on the specific pathology.

3. **Functional ovarian etiology** may be suspected on the basis of history, patient age, and pelvic examination. This diagnosis is never appropriate in prepubertal or postmenopausal females. Ultrasound appearance of a simple, fluid-filled cyst without septa, solid components, or calcifications can strengthen the diagnosis. (However, if the patient is on combination oral contraceptive pills, the diagnosis of functional cyst is very unlikely.) **Conservative management** is recommended for the following diagnoses:

   a. **Follicular or corpus luteum cysts** can be managed by observation alone or by suppressing future cysts with combination oral contraceptive pills. A pelvic examination is repeated after the next menstrual cycle.

      (1) **If the mass regresses,** no further follow-up is needed.
      (2) **If the mass persists,** surgical management (generally laparoscopy) is indicated.

   b. Theca lutein cysts or pregnancy luteomas are managed conservatively with follow-up examination after the pregnancy is completed.

4. **All other pelvic masses** require surgical evaluation to establish a definitive tissue diagnosis.

   a. Ultrasound-guided cyst aspiration is controversial because of the possibility of rupturing a malignant mass and spilling tumor cells into the peritoneal cavity.

   b. Laparoscopy is the procedure of choice for patients who most likely have benign neoplasia. It requires specialized surgical skills, but it may be therapeutic as well as diagnostic. Endoscopic removal of the neoplasm can be accomplished without a large abdominal incision.

   c. Laparotomy is the procedure of choice if malignancy is suspected. Appropriate tumor staging steps should be followed to obtain peritoneal fluid for cytology, peritoneal biopsy specimens for staging, and tumor removal.

5. The **incision selected** should provide adequate exposure to perform whatever tasks are required. The cosmetic appearance assumes a lower priority if cancer is probable.

   a. Vertical midline incision is performed between the umbilicus and the symphysis pubis by cutting vertically through all layers from the skin into the peritoneal cavity. Exposure is maximal, and the incision can be extended into the upper abdomen, if necessary, for further exposure

   b. Pfannensteil's incision is performed suprapubically by cutting transversely through the skin and subcutaneous fat down through the rectus fascial sheath. The rectus muscles are separated from their raphe in the midline and then retracted laterally. Although this incision is cosmetically attractive and has a lower risk of dehiscence, it provides less surgical exposure.

   c. Maylard incision is performed suprapubically by cutting transversely through every abdominal wall layer from the skin to the peritoneal cavity. The rectus muscles are transected transversely. Exposure to the upper abdomen is greater than with Pfannensteil's incision, but it cannot be extended vertically.

6. **Suspected torsion of the ovary** is never managed conservatively, regardless of whether the mass is functional or neoplastic. This is a gynecological emergency in which delay could jeopardize ovarian viability.

   a. The **mechanism** is as described: The mass twists on its pedicle, thereby obstructing the blood supply and leading to possible ischemic injury. The ischemic pain results in a "uterine attack."

   b. Risk factors for torsion include size of the mass (i.e., > 6–8 cm in diameter) and mobility, which increases with the length of the mass pedicle.

   c. Symptoms and signs include sudden onset of acute, unilateral pelvic pain associated with abdominal tenderness and rebound.

   d. Management is emergency laparotomy. If the ovarian tissue is infarcted, surgical resection is indicated. If the tissue is still viable, the size of the mass should be reduced by resecting the ovarian neoplasm.

II. POSTMENOPAUSAL PELVIC MASS. A pelvic mass in a postmenopausal woman must be assumed to be an ovarian cancer until proven otherwise, although most postmenopausal ovarian neoplasms are benign.

A. Epidemiology. Ovarian cancer is the **second** most common gynecological malignancy. Median age at diagnosis is **69 years.**

1. **1% of all women** develop ovarian cancer.

2. **Ovarian cancer accounts for more deaths than all other primary pelvic cancers,** even though only 15%–20% of all gynecologic cancers arise from the ovary, because most ovarian cancers are stage III at diagnosis.

3. The **most common tumor type is epithelial** (85%), followed by germ cell tumors (5%), and then gonadal-stromal tumors.

B. Pathophysiology

1. **Epithelial carcinoma** may originate from serial disruptions of the ovarian germinal epithelium capsule as a result of repeated ovulations.

2. **Dysgerminoma and gonadoblastoma** are found more frequently in women with gonadal dysgenesis (45,X), as well as those with a Y chromosome (e.g., Turner's syndrome mosaicism: 45,XO/46,XY).

C. Risk factors

1. Age > 45 years

2. BRCA1 gene

3. Family history of ovarian cancer

4. Number of lifetime ovulations

5. Caucasian or Asian origin

6. Nulliparity, infertility, or late menopause

7. Industrialized society

8. Perineal talc use (possible)

D. Prevention. Protective factors for ovarian cancer appear to be conditions associated with fewer lifetime ovulations.

1. Use of oral contraceptive pills

2. Shorter duration of reproductive years

3. Conditions of chronic anovulation

4. History of breastfeeding

5. Multiparity

6. Tubal sterilization

E. Screening

1. The **pelvic examination** traditionally has been the method of screening asymptomatic patients for ovarian neoplasms. Although it has limited specificity and sensitivity, it remains the current method of choice.

2. **Ultrasound screening** has theoretical advantages in identifying pelvic masses and distinguishing the benign from the malignant. Color-flow

Doppler studies can assess patterns in vascular flow. However, randomized, prospective studies have not shown the cost effectiveness of sonography in screening asymptomatic patients for ovarian cancer (97% false positive rate).

F. **Classification** (see Table 13-1). The following summary points should be noted.

1. **Epithelial tumors** account for most ovarian neoplasms (50% of benign ovarian neoplasms and 85% of malignant ovarian neoplasms). They are thought to arise from the surface (coelomic) epithelium of the ovary. When malignant, they tend to occur in the sixth decade of life, and they have the worst prognosis of all ovarian neoplasms. Tumor markers include cancer antigen 125 (CA-125) and carcinoembryonic antigen (CEA).

   a. **Serous tumors are the most common epithelial tumor type.** These tumors are more often bilateral than other epithelial tumors, and histologically, they resemble ciliated tubal epithelium. **Psammoma bodies** are a unique finding. Serous adenocarcinomas are associated with the worst prognosis of all epithelial cancers.

   b. **Mucinous tumors** can grow to a weight of 150 pounds. Histologically, they resemble columnar endocervical epithelium. They are associated with **pseudomyoma peritonei** (accumulation of large amounts of intraperitoneal mucin-producing cells), which can result in recurrent bouts of bowel obstruction.

   c. **Endometrioid tumors** are uncommon and may be seen in conjunction with but not arising from endometriosis and endometriomas. Histologically, they resemble endometrial glands.

2. **Germ cell tumors** are the second most common type of ovarian cancers, constituting 5% of malignant ovarian tumors. They tend to occur in the second and third decades of life. Because of their lower grade and stage at diagnosis, they have a better prognosis than epithelial tumors. Tumor markers include lactate dehydrogenase (LDH), (α-fetoprotein (α-FP), and β-hCG.

   a. **Dysgerminomas are the most common malignant germ cell type.** These tumors, which can arise in dysgenetic gonads of ovarian dysgenesis, are analogous to the seminoma arising in male testis. When diagnosed, most commonly at age less than 30 years, 70% are stage Ia. With unilateral salpingo-oophorectomy alone, 5-year survival is 90%. Because these tumors are highly radiosensitive, recurrences can be treated with radiation therapy. Occasionally, LDH is secreted as a tumor marker.

   b. **Endodermal sinus tumors** are the **most rapidly growing** tumor known. They can occur in children as young as 13 months of age. **Schiller-Duval bodies** are a unique finding. α-FP is a recognized tumor marker.

   c. **Immature teratomas** arise from fetal embryonic tissues. They occur only in prepubertal or premenopausal females. When diagnosed, 70% are stage I. With unilateral salpingo-oophorectomy alone, 10-year survival is 70%. Tumor markers include α-FP and β-hCG.

3. **Gonadal-stromal tumors** are the least common ovarian neoplasms, and they often are **hormonally active.** They often act as low-grade malignancies.

    a. Granulosa tumors that produce estrogen are associated with precocious puberty in young girls (see Chapter 11), menstrual irregularities in women of reproductive years (see Chapter 11), and vaginal bleeding in postmenopausal women (see Chapter 12). When diagnosed, 90% are stage I. **Cal-Exner bodies** are a unique finding.

    b. Sertoli-Leydig cell tumors produce androgens and are often virilizing (see Chapter 11). **Crystals of Reinke** are a unique finding.

4. Metastatic tumors to the ovaries account for as many as 25% of ovarian malignancies and are usually **bilateral.** The most common primary sites are the breast, GI tract, or the endometrium. **Krukenberg's tumors** represent carcinomas of the stomach metastatic to the ovary.

G. Clinical findings

1. Symptoms are most often absent with early-stage ovarian cancer. When present, symptoms tend to be nonspecific.

    a. GI tract complaints such as nausea, abdominal cramping, or change in bowel habits are often the early symptoms of advanced stage disease. By this time, the disease may be widely disseminated throughout the peritoneal cavity.

    b. Abdominal distention and early satiety may be found when the mass is large enough to rise into the abdominal cavity.

    c. Postmenopausal bleeding may occur from endometrial hyperplasia stimulated by estrogen from a granulosa tumor.

    d. Virilization is found in 50% of patients who have an androgen-secreting Sertoli-Leydig cell tumor.

    e. Colicky pain is associated with torsion of a mobile ovarian tumor.

    f. Constant pain may be experienced with the distention of hemorrhage into a tumor.

2. Physical examination varies with the nature of the ovarian tumor.

    a. Fixed, bilateral masses are more common with malignancy, whereas mobile and unilateral masses are likely to be benign.

    b. Mobile tumors on long pedicles may move so freely that they are found in different locations at different times.

    c. A **nodular tumor exterior** is more suggestive of malignancy, whereas a smooth, regular surface is found with benign processes.

    d. Abdominal percussion may differentiate a large cyst from ascites. Percussion is dull over the entire abdomen with a large cyst, whereas with ascites the percussion note shifts when the patient changes position.

    e. Meigs' syndrome consists of ascites and hydrothorax in association with an ovarian fibroma or thecoma.

3. Preoperative workup should include the following tests:

    a. Papanicolaou (Pap) smear can screen for evidence of cervical dysplasia or malignancy.

    b. Titers of tumor markers should be obtained. These may include CA-125 and CEA in epithelial tumors; LDH, α-FP, and β-hCG in germ cell tumors; and estrogen and testosterone in hormonally active gonadal-stromal tumors. An elevated tumor marker alone does not diagnose ovarian cancer. **False-positive CA-125 levels** can be found in endometriomas, PID, leiomyomas, pregnancy, hemorrhagic ovarian cysts, and liver disease.

    c. **Useful imaging studies** include chest film to look for lung metastasis, plain film of the abdomen to identify calcifications, IVP to assess the urinary system, and barium enema to evaluate the lower GI tract.

    d. **Less helpful imaging studies,** the results of which may not significantly change management, include ultrasound and computed tomography (CT) scans.

H. Surgical staging (Table 13-2)

I. Mechanism. The mechanism of dissemination of ovarian cancer is varied.

    1. Implantation of exfoliated cells via peritoneal fluid is the **most common method of spread** involving the omentum, cul-de-sac, paracolic gutters, and liver capsule.

    2. Lymphatic spread to the pelvic and para-aortic nodes is found in 10% of patients who are thought to be stage I or II.

    3. Hematogenous spread is the **least common** method of metastasis. Sites involved may include the liver, skin, and lungs.

J. Management. Treatment of ovarian cancer is surgical regardless of cell type or stage of disease. Chemotherapy and radiation therapy are secondary treatments.

    1. Staging procedures must be part of any surgical approach and should include obtaining the following: peritoneal washings, biopsies of the peritoneum and diaphragm, and lymph node sampling, if necessary.

    2. Unilateral salpingo-oophorectomy may be indicated for selected

Table 13-2. FIGO Surgical Staging System for Ovarian Carcinoma (1987)

Stage	Grade	
I	LIMITED TO OVARIES	
	Ia	Limited to one ovary; no malignant ascites; capsule intact
	Ib	Limited to both ovaries; no malignant ascites; capsule intact
	Ic	Limited to ovaries; malignant ascites present; capsule not intact
II	LIMITED EXTENSION BEYOND OVARIES	
	IIa	Extension to uterus/tubes
	IIb	Extension to other pelvic tissues
	IIc	IIa or IIb with malignant ascites or positive peritoneal washings
III	EXTENSION WITHIN PELVIS	
	IIIa	Limited to true pelvis; negative nodes; positive peritoneal seeding
	IIIb	Same as IIIa, but implants < 2 cm diameter
	IIIc	Same as IIIa, but implants > 2 cm and/or positive nodes
IV	DISTANT METASTASES	
	Distant metastases	
	Pleural effusion	
	Parenchymal liver metastases	

FIGO = International Federation of Gynecology and Obstetrics

low-grade, stage Ia lesions in a young woman who wants to retain her fertility.

3. **Total abdominal hysterectomy** with bilateral salpingo-oophorectomy (TAH BSO), as well as infracolic omentectomy, is the mainstay of surgical therapy.

4. **Cytoreductive debulking surgery** is performed in patients with advanced cancer. The aim is to leave no residual tumor nodules larger than 1.5 cm.

5. **Chemotherapy** is generally recommended for all patients with ovarian cancers, with the exception of well-differentiated stage Ia tumors. The specific agents used depend on the tumor type.

6. **Radioisotope therapy** with intraperitoneal ^{32}P may benefit patients with stage Ic disease. Theoretically, the entire peritoneal cavity is treated, but distribution may not always be uniform.

7. **External-beam radiotherapy** has limited usefulness because the doses required are often associated with unacceptable bowel, liver, and kidney injury. However, dysgerminomas are uniquely sensitive to this therapy.

8. **Decreasing titers of tumor markers** can be used to follow tumor response to therapy.

III. ENLARGED UTERUS

A. The **differential diagnosis** (Table 13-3) is described as follows:

1. **Processes involving the uterine cavity. Pregnancy**—normal or abnormal (e.g., hydatidiform mole)—is the **most common cause** of an enlarged uterus in women of reproductive age.

2. **Processes involving the endometrium.** Advanced-stage endometrial carcinoma can cause an enlarged uterus, but it is usually found in older women with complaints of postmenopausal bleeding (see Chapter 12). Premalignant phases and even early overt carcinoma generally leave the uterus a normal size.

3. **Processes involving the myometrium.** The uterus may become en-

Table 13-3. The Enlarged Uterus

	Pregnancy	Adenomyosis	Leiomyoma	Malignancy
Age	15–45 years	Middle age	Middle age	Older age
Consistency	Soft	Boggy	Firm	Variable
Symmetrical	Yes	Variable	No	Variable
Tenderness	None	Variable	Variable	None
β-hCG	Positive	Negative	Negative	Negative

larged from benign and malignant lesions developing within the uterine smooth muscle wall.

B. Leiomyomas are the **most common uterine tumors** found in females with a prevalence of 25% in uteri of women older than 35 years of age. Most leiomyomas are smaller than 15 cm in size, but they may grow to 45 kg in weight.

1. **Histology.** Myomas are circumscribed but unencapsulated benign tumors of the uterine muscle wall (Figure 13-1). They contain fibrous connective tissue elements and are also known as **fibroids.**

2. **Risk factors.** Myomas are five times more common in **black women** than in white women. They contain more estrogen receptors than surrounding normal myometrium and are thus sensitive to changing estrogen levels. **Pregnancy** often causes myomas to grow in size, whereas after menopause they usually regress.

3. **Symptoms.** Most leiomyomas are asymptomatic, even large ones. When present, symptoms largely depend on tumor location and size (Table 13-4).

   a. **Abnormal menstrual bleeding** is the **most common clinical manifestation** and is found with a submucous myoma. Chronic blood loss anemia is a frequently associated finding.

   b. **Pain** is uncommon unless **carneous/red degeneration** or bleeding into the tumor occurs. The severity of the pain can mimic an acute abdomen. This occurs **most commonly with pregnancy.**

   c. **Pressure effects** are caused by large tumors distorting or obstructing either the urinary or GI tract. Symptoms can include constipation and urinary frequency.

   d. **Infertility** may result from constriction of the cervical canal, im-

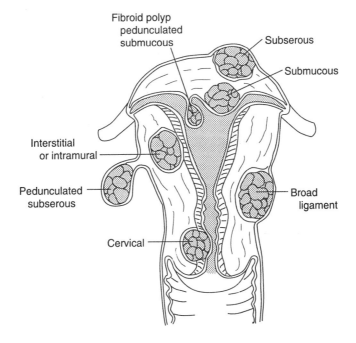

Figure 13-1. Common types of uterine leiomyomas. (Reprinted with permission from Beckmann CR, Ling FW, Barzansky BM, et al: *Obstetrics and Gynecology,* 2nd ed. Williams & Wilkins, Baltimore, 1995, p 440.)

Table 13-4. Uterine Leiomyomata

	Location	Symptoms	Diagnosis	Management
Submucosal	• Under endometrial basalis layer • Deforms uterine cavity contour • Possibly protrudes into uterine cavity	• Abnormal menstrual bleeding • Second trimester loss • Infertility	• Hysterosalpingogram (HSG) • Hysteroscopy • Fluid sonogram	*Surgical:* hysteroscopic resection
Subserosal	• Immediately beneath uterine serosa • Deforms external uterine contour • Protrudes into peroneal cavity	None unless large • then effects of pressure	• Pelvic examination • Laparoscopy • Sonogram	*Medical:* preop involution by GnRH agonist suppression *Surgical:* laparoscopic or laparotomy myomectomy
Intramural	• Within myometrial wall • Does not distort either the endometrium or serosa	None unless large • then effects of pressure	• Sonogram	*Medical:* preoperative involution by GnRH agonist suppression *Surgical:* laparoscopic or laparotomy myomectomy
Intraligamentous	• Protrudes into the broad ligament • Deforms external uterine contour	None unless large • then effects of pressure	• Pelvic examination • Sonogram	*Surgical:* resection a laparotomy
Pedunculated	• On pedicles of varying length and thickness • Usually attached to external uterine serosal surface • Seldom within the uterine cavity • Rarely prolapsing through external cervical os	Depends on location • Abnormal menstrual bleeding • Mobile mass	Hysteroscopy, HSG, or laparoscopy depending on location	*Surgical:* ligation of pedicle

GnRH = gonadotropin-releasing hormone

pingement on tubal ostia, endometrial distortion, or interference with uterine vascular supply.

    e. Second-trimester abortion can result from alteration of vascular supply to endometrial implantation sites from submucous myomas.

4. Examination. A bimanual pelvic examination reveals a firm mass. The uterus is typically nontender and asymmetrical. If the myoma is sufficiently enlarged, it can be palpated abdominally.

5. Imaging. Imaging studies that provide useful information on uterine contour and texture include standard abdominal or vaginal sonography. Uterine intracavitary myomas can be visualized by hysteroscopy, hysterosalpingography (i.e., x-ray studies using intrauterine injection of contrast media), and sonohysterography (sonographic imaging using intrauterine instillation of saline).

6. **Polycythemia.** Polycythemia has been described with leiomyomas secondary to an increase in erythropoietin.

C. **Adenomyosis** is the second most common benign cause of an enlarged, nonpregnant uterus. Its prevalence is 20% in hysterectomy specimens. Half of the patients with adenomyosis have coexistent leiomyomas. Endometriosis is found in 15% of these patients. Adenomyosis is correctly diagnosed preoperatively in only 10% of cases.

1. **Histology** is described as follows: <u>Islands of ectopic endometrial glands</u> and stroma are found within the myometrium without a direct connection with the endometrial cavity. They can be diffusely located throughout the myometrium, or they can be discrete and localized, forming an **adenomyoma.** Myometrial hypertrophy and hyperplasia around the islands cause globular enlargement of the uterine fundus. The endometrial glands are similar to the decidua basalis layer, and they show minimal cyclic bleeding.

2. **Risk factors** are described as follows: Adenomyosis is a disease of the later reproductive years and is <u>more common in multiparous</u> women. Regression of symptoms and findings is noted after the onset of menopause.

3. **Symptoms** are found in 70% of proven cases.
   a. **Abnormal menstrual bleeding** from an enlarged uterine cavity and interference with normal uterine contractions may lead to anemia.
   b. **Secondary dysmenorrhea** is related to the depth of myometrial penetration and arises from myometrial contractions induced by premenstrual swelling.
   c. **Infertility** can result from extension of adenomyosis into the isthmus of the oviduct, known as **salpingitis isthmica nodosa.** When this condition is bilateral, both oviducts can be obstructed.

4. **Examination** is often unremarkable except for fundal tenderness. The enlarged uterus may be globular in shape with uniform consistency.

5. **Imaging studies** have limited usefulness because of the diffuse intramural nature of the lesion. Magnetic resonance imaging (MRI) may identify large or diffuse lesions preoperatively.

D. **Stromal adenomyosis** is a benign condition of the uterus grossly similar to adenomyosis, but histologically the ectopic areas consist of only endometrial stroma without glandular elements. The malignant form of this lesion is the **endometrial stromal sarcoma.**

E. **Leiomyosarcoma** is the malignant form of a uterine leiomyoma occurring mostly in the early postmenopausal period.

1. **Histology** is similar to leiomyomas except leiomyosarcomas have more than five mitotic figures per 10 high-power fields. The **mitosis count** is the best indicator of tumor aggressiveness.

2. **Risk factors** are described as follows: Leiomyosarcomas are twice as

prevalent in black women as in white women. Malignant transformation of benign leiomyomas is extremely rare, occurring in only 0.1% of cases.

3. **Symptoms** are similar to those of leiomyomas with the exception of infertility.

4. **Examination** may reveal a rapidly enlarging asymmetrical uterus.

5. **Imaging studies** should include a chest radiograph to identify characteristic coin lesions of the lung. Metastasis is largely by the hematogenous route, with the lung the most frequent site. IVP identifies any impingement on the urinary tract.

F. **Management** of an enlarged uterus is based on the patient's age, suspected diagnosis, fertility desires, and degree of symptomatology, as well as the size and location of the mass.

1. **Pregnancy** can be easily ruled out by measuring the serum β-hCG level.

2. **Endometrial carcinoma** or its premalignant hyperplastic precursors should be ruled out with hysteroscopy and dilation and curettage (D&C) when clinically indicated.

3. **Conservative management** and observation is only appropriate if the clinical diagnosis of benign etiology is unequivocal. Most leiomyomas do not require treatment, especially if they are small and symptoms are minimal. Patients should have follow-up examinations every 6 months.

4. **Medical therapy** has not been shown to be effective in the long-term treatment of either myomas or adenomyosis.

    a. **Steroid hormones** have no beneficial effect. Estrogens may stimulate growth of myomas. Oral contraceptives usually worsen bleeding and pain with adenomyosis.

    b. **Gonadotropin-releasing hormone (GnRH) agonists** (e.g., leuprolide) can shrink myomas to variable degrees; however, enlargement occurs promptly after medication discontinuance.

       (1) Long-term use is inappropriate because of the serious side effects of **medical castration** (i.e., hot flashes, vaginal dryness, trabecular bone loss).

       (2) The main benefit of leuprolide is **premyomectomy shrinkage** to decrease intraoperative blood loss.

5. **Myomectomy** is indicated for myomas that are symptomatic in patients wishing to preserve fertility. Table 13-4 describes the surgical procedures appropriate for each myoma type. Cesarean delivery may be indicated for subsequent pregnancies if significant myometrial resection or endometrial penetration occurs. Recurrence of myomas is common.

6. **Hysterectomy** is curative for any leiomyomas. It is the only definitive therapy for adenomyosis.

7. **Surgical exploration** is imperative if malignancy is seriously suspected, because a tissue diagnosis is the only definitive way to exclude cancer. For uterine sarcomas, total abdominal hysterectomy, bilateral hysterectomy, and excision of resectable tumor are the cornerstones of treatment.

8. **Chemotherapy** for uterine sarcomas is used only as adjuvant therapy

after surgical extirpation of the primary lesions. When used as primary treatment, results have been dismal.

   9. **Radiation therapy** is largely used for localized sarcoma recurrence.

IV. PELVIC INFLAMMATORY DISEASE (PID)

   A. **Epidemiology**

   1. A **spectrum of inflammatory disorders** of the upper genital tract constitute PID including salpingitis, pelvic peritonitis, chronic pelvic adhesions, and TOA. Each year in the United States, 1 million women are treated for PID, leading to 150,000 surgical procedures.

   2. The **mechanism of dissemination** of microorganisms in pelvic infections is presented in Table 13-5. PID usually refers to infections ascending from the lower to the upper genital tract. Mechanisms of dissemination include the following:

   a. Organisms can ascend from the **cervix to the endometrium and endosalpinx,** attaching to columnar epithelium without deep invasion (e.g., chlamydia, gonococcus). This is characteristic of classic PID.

   b. Organisms can **invade lymphatics from the endometrium,** penetrating deep into the myometrium and parametrium (e.g., postabortion or postpartum infections).

   c. Organisms can be carried **from the lungs through the blood stream** to the pelvic organs [e.g., tuberculosis (TB)].

   3. **Infertility sequelae** of PID are related to the development of pelvic adhesions. The incidence of infertility after one or more episodes of un-

Table 13-5. Pelvic Infections: Mechanisms of Microorganism Dissemination

	Mechanism	Findings	Organisms	Examples
Ascending	Organisms ascend from cervix to endometrium and endosalpinx, attaching to columnar epithelium without deep invasion	Purulent salpingitis pouring pus into peritoneal cavity	· *Neisseria gonorrhoeae* · *Chlamydia trachomatis* · *Mycoplasma hominis* · *Ureaplasma urealyticum*	Classic pelvic inflammatory disease (PID) infections
Lymphatic	Organisms invade lymphatics from endometrium, penetrating deep into myometrium and parametrium	Cellulitis of the endometrium– myometrium– parametrium (endomyoparametritis)	70% anaerobes · Anaerobic cocci · Peptostreptocci · *Bacteroides* species 30% aerobes · Gram-negative enteric bacilli · Enterococci · Streptococci	Postpartum and postabortal infections
Hematogenous	Organisms are carried from the lungs through the blood stream to the pelvic organs	Salpingitis 100% Endometritis 80% Oophoritis 30%	*Mycobacterium tuberculosis*	Pelvic tuberculosis

treated or inadequately treated episodes of PID is as follows: 15% after one episode, 25% after two episodes, and 60% after three episodes.

B. Risk factors for PID (Table 13-6). Note that the highest risk subjects are young women who are sexually active with multiple partners.

C. Salpingitis-oophoritis. This is the classical presentation of PID.

1. **Etiology** is described as follows: Pathogenic organisms (see Table 13-5) are usually sexually transmitted. *Chlamydia trachomatis* infections often can be asymptomatic. Acute PID is frequently exacerbated by menses because of the breakdown of the protective barrier of cervical mucus.

2. **Symptoms** may be insidious, or acute onset of bilateral lower abdominal or pelvic pain may occur. Patients may have a sensation of pelvic pressure with back pain radiating down the legs and may have recently started their menses. Nausea with or without vomiting may be present.

3. **Examination** may reveal fever and tachycardia. Abdominal findings may vary from mild tenderness to distention, peritoneal signs, and ileus. Pelvic findings are mucopurulent cervical discharge with cervical motion tenderness. Adnexal tenderness usually is present with no masses palpated.

4. **Investigative findings** include increased white blood cell count (WBC) and sedimentation rate.
   a. Obtaining purulent fluid from the cul-de-sac by **culdocentesis** is diagnostic.
   b. **Cervical cultures** should be obtained but are not immediately available because the culture needs 24 hours to grow before it can be identified.
   c. **Sonography** is usually not remarkable unless an adnexal mass is present.
   d. **Laparoscopy,** with direct visualization of the oviducts, is the only definitive method of establishing the diagnosis.

5. **Differential diagnosis** includes disorders of any organ system within the pelvis. Possible diagnoses include the following:
   a. **Reproductive tract disorders** such as adnexal torsion, ectopic pregnancy, bleeding corpus luteum, and endometriosis

Table 13-6. Risk Factors for Pelvic Inflammatory Disease (PID)

Increased Risk	Decreased Risk
• Younger age	• Older age
• Multiple sexual partners	• Single sexual partner
• Increased intercourse frequency	• Decreased intercourse frequency
• Mucopurulent cervicitis	• Barrier contraceptives
• Prior episode of PID	• Steroid contraception
• Use of intrauterine device	

b. **GI tract disorders** such as appendicitis, diverticulitis, regional ileitis, and ulcerative colitis

c. **Urinary tract disorders** such as cystourethritis and pyelonephritis

6. **Management** of acute PID is **antibiotic therapy.** Surgery is rarely indicated.

    a. **Complicated PID** is managed on an inpatient basis (Box 13-3). Patients are kept at minimal activity, bowel rest is encouraged, and intravenous (IV) hydration is provided. Parenteral antibiotics (Box 13-4) are administered until clinical resolution has lasted for 48 hours.

    b. **Uncomplicated PID** is managed on an outpatient basis. Oral antibiotics recommended are shown in Box 13-5.

D. **Tubo-ovarian abscess (TOA)** is an uncommon complication of inappropriately or untreated PID. Not a true abscess, it is rather an inflammatory mass involving the oviduct, ovary, omentum, and bowel.

1. **Etiology** is described as follows: TOA is usually a sequela to acute pelvic inflammatory processes. The pathogenic organisms usually are not gonococcus but rather are secondary invaders such as anaerobic species, especially bacteroides.

2. **Symptoms** include severe pelvic and lower abdominal pain accompanied by nausea and vomiting. The patient may complain of painful defecation, severe back pain, or rectal pain.

3. **Examination** is usually striking. The patient usually has a high fever with tachycardia and may appear to be in septic shock.

    a. **Abdominal examination** may reveal guarding and rigidity.

    b. **Pelvic examination** is frequently difficult because of extreme tenderness.

    c. **Rectal examination** is the best method for palpation of a mass.

4. **Differential diagnosis** includes septic incomplete abortion, periappendiceal abscess, diverticular abscess, adnexal torsion, and degenerating leiomyoma.

5. **Management** depends on the severity of the disease and the response to therapy.

    a. **Conservative medical treatment** with multiagent parenteral antibiotics is the mainstay of therapy. Even large abscesses may resolve without the need for acute surgical intervention. Cefoxitin-doxycycline or clindamycin-gentamicin has high response rates.

Box 13-3. Indications for Inpatient Treatment

- Uncertain diagnosis
- First episode in a nulligravida
- Failure of outpatient therapy
- Intrauterine device in the uterus
- Evidence of pelvic abscess
- Temperature $\geq$ 39°C or 102.2°F
- Poor tolerance of oral medication

Box 13-4. Inpatient antibiotic options include any one of the following:

- **Cefoxitin** 2 g IV q6 h   plus **Doxycycline** 100 mg q12h IV or PO
- **Cefotetan** 2 g IV q12h   plus **Doxycycline** 100 mg q12h IV or PO
- **Clindamycin** 900 mg IV q8h   plus **Gentamycin** 2 mg/kg IV, then 1.5 mg/kg q8h IV

Box 13-5. Outpatient antibiotic options are:

- **Cefoxitin** 2 g IM plus probenecid 1 g PO, or
- **Ceftriaxone** 250 mg IM, or equivalent **cephalosporin**

plus

- **Doxycycline** 100 mg PO bid × 14 days, or
- **Tetracycline** 500 mg PO qid × 14 days

---

    b. Percutaneous or cul-de-sac drainage is appropriate if fever persists despite adequate antibiotic coverage and patients are not septic.

    c. Emergency laparotomy is required with deterioration of the patients' condition or abscess rupture. TAH BSO is generally indicated, but unilateral adnexectomy may be appropriate for unilateral disease.

E. Chronic pelvic inflammatory disease (PID). Chronic PID implies tissue changes in the parametria, tubes, and ovaries. Adhesions of the peritoneal surfaces to the adnexa and fibrotic changes in the tubal lumen are usually present.

    1. Etiology is described as follows: Chronic PID is usually a sequela of inadequately treated or untreated acute PID.

    2. Symptoms may include chronic pelvic pain, infertility, dyspareunia, history of ectopic pregnancy, and abnormal uterine bleeding.

    3. Examination reveals tenderness on movement of the cervix, uterus, or adnexae. Adnexal masses may be enlarged sterile hydrosalpinges or tubo-ovarian adhesion complexes. Lower abdominal tenderness is frequently found.

    4. Differential diagnosis includes endometriosis, inflammatory bowel disease, and adenomyosis. The definitive diagnosis is made by laparoscopy or laparotomy.

    5. Management is often disappointing.

      a. Long-term **antibiotic treatment** is seldom of value.

      b. Symptomatic relief with **mild analgesics** may help patients cope with the chronic pain.

      c. Conservative limited **surgical procedures** may be helpful for infertility treatment, but they seldom provide pain relief.

      d. TAH BSO may be the only option for significant pain relief. **Estrogen replacement therapy (ERT)** [see Chapter 12] is indicated for these patients whose ovaries are removed. Progestins are not needed because the uterus is removed.

    F. Fitz-Hugh-Curtis syndrome. This is a sequela of PID in which acute, profuse pelvic purulence extends into the upper abdomen. It leads to a perihepatitis with liver capsule inflammation but without parenchymal involvement. Fibrinous exudate results in "violin-string adhesions" extending from the liver to pelvic-organ visceral peritoneum. Right upper quadrant pain may mimic cholecystitis, pyelonephritis, or viral pneumonia.

V. ECTOPIC PREGNANCY is diagnosed when pregnancy implantation occurs outside of the uterine cavity.

    A. Epidemiology

        1. Ectopic pregnancy is the third leading cause of pregnancy-related **maternal death** in the United States. It is responsible for 10% of all maternal mortality.

        2. **Incidence is increasing,** with reported cases quadrupling in the past 20 years from 1 in 200 to 1 in 40 live births.

        3. The **hazards for subsequent pregnancies** are significant. A repeat ectopic pregnancy is experienced by 50% of patients. Only 50% of patients will deliver a live infant.

        4. The **most likely site** for ectopic pregnancy is the oviduct (95%), with eight times as many implantations occurring in the distal ampulla than in the proximal isthmus. Cornual (2%) and abdominal pregnancies (1%) are uncommon. Cervical and ovarian pregnancies are rare (Figure 13-2).

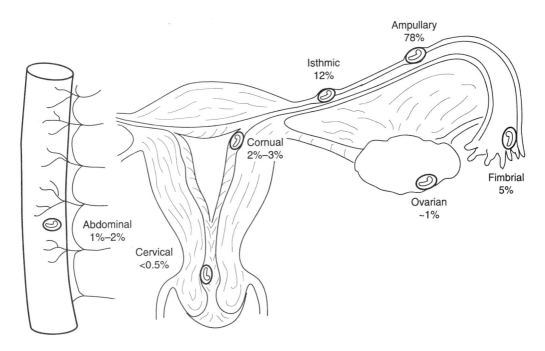

Figure 13-2. Incidence of types of ectopic pregnancy by location. (Reprinted with permission from Beckmann CR, Ling FW, Barzansky BM, et al: *Obstetrics and Gynecology,* 2nd ed. Williams & Wilkins, Baltimore, 1995, p 322.)

B. Risk factors (Box 13-6). <u>Previous PID is the</u> most common risk factor. Note the common theme of etiologies resulting in tubal scarring or adhesions. Risk factors are found in only 20% of women who experience ectopic pregnancy.

C. Mechanism. The mechanism of implantation is presented in Table 13-7. Whereas the normal endometrium provides trophoblastic access to abundant blood supply, Nitabuch's layer prevents deeper villus penetration. The oviduct lacks not only abundant blood supply but also the ability to prevent villus penetration.

D. Clinical findings. Clinical findings are variable depending on how early the diagnosis is made, the location of the implantation, and whether rupture has occurred.

    1. With an **unruptured ectopic pregnancy,** the **classic symptom triad** is <u>amenorrhea</u>, <u>abnormal vaginal bleeding</u>, and <u>abdominal pain</u>. The <u>classic signs</u> are <u>adnexal or cervical motion tenderness</u>. <u>Uterine enlargement is not usually appreciated</u>. <u>Fever is rare</u>.

    2. With a **ruptured ectopic pregnancy,** findings parallel the degree of <u>internal bleeding and hypovolemia</u>. <u>Abdominal guarding and rigidity</u> are usually indicative of significant intraperitoneal bleeding. <u>Orthostatic blood pressure (BP) and pulse changes indicate substantial blood loss</u>.

E. Differential diagnosis. This includes both gynecological and nongynecological entities.

    1. **Reproductive tract** causes could be <u>spontaneous abortion</u>, <u>molar pregnancy</u>, <u>ruptured corpus luteum</u>, <u>acute PID</u>, adnexal torsion, or degenerating leiomyoma.

    2. **Nonreproductive tract** causes include acute appendicitis, <u>pyelonephritis</u>, <u>pancreatitis</u>, <u>diverticulitis</u>, <u>regional ileitis</u>, or <u>ulcerative colitis</u>.

F. Diagnostic testing. <u>Endocrine tests</u>, <u>sonography</u>, and <u>laparoscopy</u> are used in the diagnosis of ectopic pregnancy.

Box 13-6. Risk Factors for Ectopic Pregnancy

- Previous PID (eight times increased risk)

- Previous ectopic pregnancy (50% increased risk)

- Tubal ligation in the past 2 years

- Previous tubal surgery

- Intrauterine device in place

- Prolonged infertility

- Diethylstilbestrol (DES) exposure in utero

PID = pelvic inflammatory disease

Table 13-7. Mechanism of Implantation: Intrauterine and Tubal Pregnancy

Site of Implantation	Degree of Decidual Reaction	Initial Villi Penetration	Resistance to Deeper Villi Penetration?	Access to Vascular Supply
Uterine endometrium	Extensive	Through a normal endometrial mucosa	Further villus invasion is halted by the zone of fibrinoid degeneration (Nitabuch's layer) in deeper layers of decidua basalis.	Good
Tubal ampulla	Minimal	Through profuse endosalpingeal mucosa plicae	A *poorly developed tubal muscularis* offers little resistance to further villus entry of the subserosal adventitial space. The tubal mucosa and lumen are preserved. Lower chance of tubal rupture.	Poor
Tubal isthmus	Minimal	Through minimal endosalpingeal mucosa plicae	A *well-developed tubal muscularis* resists further villus penetration. The tubal mucosa and lumen are destroyed. Significant chance of tubal rupture.	Poor

1. **A rapid β-hCG test** with a sensitivity of at least 5 mIU/ml should be performed. A value less than 5 mIU/ml can virtually exclude ectopic pregnancy. The normal β-hCG doubling time is 58 hours. Most ectopic pregnancies have either a prolonged doubling time or a noticeable plateau.

2. **Pelvic sonography** should be performed to look for an intrauterine gestational sac. The **discriminatory threshold** is the critical international reference preparation (IRP; see Chapter 3 I C 2 b) β-hCG value above which a normal gestational sac can be found (Table 13-8). Failure to find a gestational sac when either of these thresholds is reached is presumptive evidence of an ectopic pregnancy.

3. **Laparoscopy** is usually both diagnostic and also therapeutic. It allows complete visualization of the pelvic structures, although an early unruptured ectopic may not always be found.

4. **Culdocentesis** (i.e., placing a needle through the posterior fornix into the cul-de-sac) is seldom performed. Culdocentesis is helpful if the aspiration is grossly bloody. However, results of the culdocentesis may be negative with a true hemoperitoneum if the cul-de-sac is obliterated in patients who have had PID.

5. **Serum progesterone** levels of greater than 25 ng/ml virtually assure an intrauterine pregnancy, whereas levels lower than 15 ng/ml are suspicious of an abnormal pregnancy, either intrauterine or ectopic. A limitation of this test is its prolonged turnaround time.

Table 13-8. Discriminatory Threshold for Ectopic Pregnancy

Sonography Mode	Gestational Age	Discriminatory Threshold
Transvaginal	35 days	1500 mIU/ml
Transabdominal	42 days	6500 mIU/ml

G. **Management.** Treatment is based on whether the oviduct is ruptured, patient desires regarding future fertility, and the condition of the contralateral oviduct.

1. The choice of **surgical approach** is based on the stability of the patient's vital signs.

   a. **Laparotomy** is indicated if the patient is hemodynamically unstable with a significant hemoperitoneum. The bleeding must be rapidly stopped.

   b. **Operative laparoscopy** is the procedure of choice in the stable patient. The procedure is performed on an outpatient basis, and postoperative morbidity is markedly less than that with laparotomy.

2. The choice of **tubal procedures** is directed by the site of implantation, size of the mass, and degree of tubal damage.

   a. **Linear salpingostomy** is indicated for an ampullary ectopic pregnancy less than 5 cm in size. The antimesenteric border is incised, the trophoblastic tissue is hydrodissected free, and the incision is allowed to close secondarily. Follow-up with serial β-hCG titers is needed to rule out the 5% incidence of a persistent ectopic pregnancy.

   b. **Segmental resection** is indicated for an isthmic ectopic pregnancy in which the tubal lumen is usually severely distorted. The tubal segment containing the ectopic mass is resected. Reanastomosis of the tubal stumps can be performed at a later time.

   c. **Salpingectomy** is the procedure of choice when the normal tubal anatomy is clearly destroyed or there is no desire for future fertility.

3. **Methotrexate** is being used successfully for the medical management of ectopic pregnancies. Criteria include a β-hCG titer less than 6000 mIU/ml and the unruptured ectopic mass of less than 3 cm diameter. Methotrexate, a folic acid antagonist, destroys any rapidly growing tissues. A single intramuscular (IM) dose is given after liver enzyme studies have been used to screen for liver disease.

H. **Follow-up studies.** Long-term observation is important to avert preventable complications.

1. **Serial β-hCG titers** are required at weekly intervals after conservative surgery or medical therapy and repeated until the values return to nonpregnant values. Additional courses of methotrexate may be required until a satisfactory β-hCG response is detected.

2. **Blood type and Rh** determination should be made to identify if the patient is Rh$_o$(D) negative. Rh$_o$(D) immune globulin is indicated to prevent isoimmunization if the atypical antibody test is negative.

Review Test

Directions: Each of the numbered items or incomplete statements in this section is followed by answers or by completions of the statement. Select the **ONE** lettered answer or completion that is **BEST** in each case.

1. A routine pelvic examination indicates that a 25-year-old woman has an asymptomatic 5-cm pelvic mass. Laboratory tests reveal a negative β-human chorionic gonadotropin (β-hCG). Which of the following conditions is the most likely diagnosis?

(A) Dermoid cyst
(B) Corpus luteum cyst
(C) Hydrosalpinx
(D) Pelvic kidney
(E) Serous cystadenoma

2. Which one of the following characteristics of ovarian masses is more suggestive of a benign than malignant etiology?

(A) Loculations
(B) Bilaterality
(C) Solid consistency
(D) Mobility
(E) Large size

3. A 40-year-old woman is being interviewed as a new patient. She states that when she was 15 years old, her mother was diagnosed with ovarian cancer and died of the malignancy within the next year. The woman has no information as to the specific tumor type. Which one of the following tumor types would be the most likely?

(A) Metastatic
(B) Epithelial
(C) Germ cell
(D) Gonadal-stromal

4. A 32-year-old woman is undergoing an annual physical examination. You identify an enlarged uterus on bimanual examination. No adnexal masses are noted. Rectovaginal examination is unremarkable. Which one of the following conditions is the most likely cause of this enlarged uterus?

(A) Leiomyoma
(B) Pregnancy
(C) Adenomyosis
(D) Endometriosis
(E) Carcinoma

5. A 43-year-old woman with a known history of uterine leiomyomas presents to the outpatient office complaining of lower abdominal and pelvic pain. On pelvic examination you find her uterus is 12-week size with irregular contour and tenderness to palpation. Which one of the following kinds of degeneration is the most likely etiology of these findings?

(A) Myxomatous
(B) Calcareous
(C) Cystic
(D) Carneous
(E) Hyaline

6. An 18-year old female college student comes to the student health service complaining of bilateral lower abdominal and pelvic pain. On pelvic examination you note mucopurulent cervical discharge and cervical motion tenderness. She states she has had the same symptoms twice before but never was treated. She inquires whether her symptoms will adversely affect future fertility. What is the likelihood that she will experience infertility when she attempts to conceive?

(A) 5%
(B) 10%
(C) 25%
(D) 35%
(E) 50%

7. A 21-year-old woman presents to the emergency department with vaginal bleeding and lower abdominal-pelvic pain. Her last normal menstrual period was 7 weeks ago. On bimanual pelvic examination you note cervical motion tenderness and left adnexal tenderness. You cannot palpate any definite masses. A qualitative urinary pregnancy test is positive. You order a transvaginal pelvic sonogram and quantitative β-human human chorionic gonadotropin (β-hCG) titer. An intrauterine gestational sac using transvaginal sonography should be seen above which of the following β-hCG titer threshold values?

(A) 500 mIU/ml
(B) 1000 mIU/ml
(C) 1500 mIU/ml
(D) 3500 mIU/ml
(E) 6500 mIU/ml

Directions: Each of the numbered items or incomplete statements in this section is negatively phrased, as indicated by a capitalized word such as NOT, LEAST, or EXCEPT. Select the ONE lettered answer or completion that is BEST in each case.

8. All of the following steps are basic principles in the surgical management of a pelvic mass EXCEPT

(A) obtaining adequate exposure
(B) using a cosmetic incision
(C) obtaining a tissue diagnosis
(D) performing all procedures in one operation
(E) avoiding iatrogenic spread of malignant cells

9. All of the following conditions are risk factors for ectopic pregnancy EXCEPT

(A) previous salpingitis
(B) endometriosis
(C) previous ectopic pregnancy
(D) previous tubal pregnancy
(E) intrauterine device (IUD) present in uterus

Directions: The set of matching questions in this section consists of a list of four to twenty-six lettered options (some of which may be in figures) followed by several numbered items. For each numbered item, select the ONE lettered option that is most closely associated with it. To avoid spending too much time on matching sets with large numbers of options, it is generally advisable to begin each set by reading the list of options. Then, for each item in the set, try to generate the correct answer and locate it in the option list, rather than evaluating each option individually. Each lettered option may be selected once, more than once, or not at all.

Questions 10–15

For each of the following ovarian tumors, select the classic pathological finding that is appropriate.
(A) Psammoma bodies
(B) Crystals of Reinke
(C) Schiller-Duval bodies
(D) Pseudomyxoma peritonei
(E) Cal-Exner bodies
(F) Rokitansky's prominence

10. Mature teratoma

11. Mucinous tumor

12. Granulosa tumor

13. Sertoli-Leydig tumor

14. Serous tumor

15. Endodermal sinus tumor

Answers and Explanations

1. The answer is B [I A 3 c (2), C 3 a].

After ruling out pregnancy with a measurement of the β-human chorionic gonadotropin (β-hCG) level, the most likely cause of a pelvic mass in a premenopausal woman during her reproductive years is a functional ovarian cyst such as a corpus luteum cyst. These cysts arise from the normal cycle of folliculogenesis and ovulation. If the patient was on ovulation suppression through steroid contraception, then a dermoid cyst would be highly likely as a nonfunctional, neoplastic enlargement of the ovary. Hydrosalpinx, pelvic kidney, and serous cystadenoma are appropriate in the differential diagnosis, but are less likely.

2. The answer is D [Box 13-2; I C].

A mobile mass is more likely to be nonmalignant than one that is fixed. Assessment of the nature of an ovarian mass comes essentially from clinical findings on pelvic examination and from imaging studies. Definitive diagnosis is only from tissue examination because the false-positive and false-negative rates of these findings are high. Loculations, bilaterality, solid consistency, and large size are all associated with malignancy.

3. The answer is B [II A, F].

Classifications of ovarian tumors can be long and tedious, with many types being rare and unusual. Approximately 80%–85% of all ovarian tumors are of coelomic epithelial type. Metastatic tumors are found only 25% of the time, germ cell tumors are found in 10%–15% of cases, and gonadal-stromal tumor types are found just 3%–5% of the time.

4. The answer is B [III A 1].

Whatever the chief complaint or physical finding in a woman in her reproductive years, the possibility of pregnancy should be considered with an enlarged uterus. Pregnancy is the most common cause of an enlarged uterus in women between the ages of 15 and 45 years. If pregnancy is not confirmed, leiomyomas, adenomyosis, endometriosis, or carcinoma could be considered.

5. The answer is D [III B 3; Table 13-4].

Degenerative changes of leiomyomas result from alterations in the blood supply of the tumor. The bleeding into the tumor of carneous degeneration causes pain and tenderness. This is almost always pregnancy-associated when the myoma growth may be rapid. Myxomatous, calcareous, cystic, and hyaline forms of degeneration do not cause tenderness.

6. The answer is C [IV A 3].

The scenario is classic for acute salpingo-oophoritis with chlamydia and/or gonorrhea ascending from the lower to the upper genital tract. Pelvic adhesions from pelvic inflammatory disease (PID) are a significant cause of tubal occlusion or fimbrial agglutination resulting in infertility. Approximately 25% of women are infertile after two inappropriately treated PID episodes.

7. The answer is C [V F; Table 13-9].

The discriminatory threshold is the β-human chorionic gonadotropin (β-hCG) value below which a gestational sac could not be expected to be found by sonography. Because transvaginal sonography has a higher resolution than transabdominal sonography, it would be expected to identify a gestational sac at an earlier gestational age by the transvaginal route. The critical level is 1500 mIU/ml for transvaginal sonography. The critical level is 6500 mIU/ml for transabdominal sonography.

8. The answer is B [I A 3 d, C 4–5].

A surgical approach is the definitive management of nonfunctional ovarian pelvic masses. Using a cosmetic incision is the correct answer (but incorrect statement) because, although anatomic placement of the incision is a consideration, it should not outweigh the other goals, including the patient's life and health. Using an adequate incision, obtaining a tissue diagnosis, avoiding multiple procedures, and avoiding iatrogenic tumor spread are all important basic surgical principles.

9. The answer is B [V B; Table 13-7].

An ectopic pregnancy results when implantation occurs outside of the uterine cavity. The oviduct is the site for 95% of ectopic pregnancies. Anything that would prevent normal transit of the zygote through the fallopian tube would be a risk for ectopic pregnancy. Endometriosis is the correct answer (but incorrect statement) because, although it is associated with infertility and pelvic pain, endometriosis is not associated with ectopic pregnancy. Previous salpingitis, previous ectopic pregnancy, previous tubal surgery, and current use of an intrauterine device (IUD) are all risk factors for ectopic pregnancy.

10–15. The answers are 10-F, 11-D, 12-E, 13-B, 14-A, 15-C [I A 3 e; Table 13-1].

Mature teratomas are germ cell tumors of the ovary. They are always benign, and they tend to occur in the early reproductive years. Rokitansky's prominence is the location within the tumor in which numerous kinds of tissue from various organ systems may be found. This can include bone, cartilage, retina, hair, and sebaceous tissue.

Mucinous tumors are epithelial tumors of the ovary that can grow extremely large. Pseudomyxoma peritonei is a rare condition characterized by the progressive accumulation of mucin within the peritoneal cavity, the consequence of slow leakage of mucin and tumor cells. Treatment is difficult, with reaccumulation of the mucin noted frequently, requiring multiple surgical procedures.

Granulosa tumors are rare ovarian tumors of gonadal-stromal origin. They are capable of synthesizing a variety of steroid hormones, with 75% of patients having evidence of estrogen excess. Histologically, these tumors have the characteristic Cal-Exner bodies.

Sertoli-Leydig tumors are gonadal-stromal ovarian tumors that are almost always benign. They can be found in women of all ages and often are hormonally active, producing androgens. Histologically, these tumors have the characteristic crystals of Reinke.

Serous tumors are epithelial tumors that can be either benign or malignant. Serous carcinomas are the most common type of ovarian cancer. Histologically, these tumors have the characteristic psammoma bodies.

Endodermal sinus tumors are of germ cell origin and are always malignant. They are the most rapidly growing tumors known. Histologically, these tumors have the characteristic Schiller-Duval bodies.

14

Sexuality

I. INTRODUCTION

A. Sexuality is the most emotionally weighted human physiologic function. It is subject to many societal taboos and regulations, which often apply more to women's than men's sexual behavior. Adequate sexual functioning is a complex interaction of hormonal events and psychosocial relationships.

B. Sexual health is defined by the World Health Organization (1975) as:

1. Capacity to enjoy and control sexual and reproductive behavior in accord with social and personal ethics.

2. Freedom from fear, shame, guilt, and misconceptions that inhibit sexual response and can impair sexual relationships.

3. Freedom from organic disorders, disease, and deficiencies that may interfere with sexual or reproductive functions.

II. NORMAL FEMALE SEXUAL RESPONSE (Table 14-1). Although many sexual responses in females are basically similar to those in males, some profound differences are evident.

A. Desire phase (libido)

1. Desire is **increased or decreased** by higher brain centers via a balance of the **dopamine-sensitive** excitatory center and the **serotonin-sensitive inhibitory center.**

2. **Testosterone dependence,** which maintains the threshold of response, is initially determined by prenatal programming.

B. The **excitement or arousal phase** (Figure 14-1) is mediated by the **parasympathetic nervous system,** with sensory connections through the pudendal nerve and motor connections close to reflex centers for bladder and bowel control.

1. **Gender-specific differences** must be understood to prevent false expectations between partners.

Table 14-1. Human Female Sexual Response

	Mediated by	Physiologic Mechanism	Gender Differences	
			Female	**Male**
Desire	Testosterone (Central nervous system)	**Excitation** is dopamine dependent; **Inhibition** is serotonin dependent	No significant differences in desire	
Excitement	Parasympathetic (Autonomic nervous system)	Vasocongestion is the primary response	• *Individual variability* in rapidity of response • Tactile and psychic stimuli important • Slower • Not easily inhibited	• Predictably *rapid* response • Visual stimuli important • More rapid • Easily inhibited
Plateau	Parasympathetic (Autonomic nervous system)	Vasocongestion is the primary response	No significant differences in mechanism	
Orgasm	Sympathetic (Autonomic nervous system)	Reflex clonic muscular contractions are the primary response	• *Individual variability* • Multiple orgasm potential • Easily inhibited	• Predictably *similar* • Limited to single orgasm • Not easily inhibited
Resolution	Return to basal physiologic state	Reversal of vasocongestion	Slow	Rapid
Refractory		Time needed to refill seminal vesicles	Nonexistent in females	Occurs only in males

   a. **Females** respond more to tactile and psychic stimuli. For many females, sexual interest and response are affected by the emotional tone of the relationship. Females tend to have more individual variability than males in how they experience sexuality.

   b. **Males** respond more than females to visual stimulation. Males can more easily separate sexuality from a relationship, and lack of nurturing may not have a negative impact.

2. **Pelvic vascular engorgement in females** is evidenced by the following changes:

   a. **Clitoral enlargement or tumescence** occurs as the clitoris doubles in size.

   b. **Lubrication** caused by paravaginal arteriole dilation results from:

      (1) Seeping of vascular transudate across vaginal epithelium

      (2) Estrogen dependence via maintenance of vaginal mucosa

   c. **Ballooning and tenting** of the proximal vagina occurs as the vaginal barrel lengthens up to 50%.

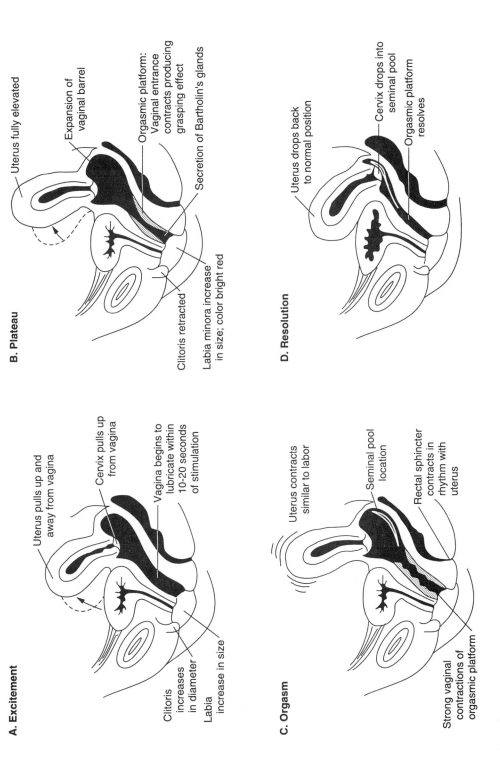

A. Excitement

Uterus pulls up and away from vagina

Cervix pulls up from vagina

Vagina begins to lubricate within 10-20 seconds of stimulation

Clitoris increases in diameter

Labia increase in size

B. Plateau

Uterus fully elevated

Expansion of vaginal barrel

Orgasmic platform: Vaginal entrance contracts producing grasping effect

Secretion of Bartholin's glands

Clitoris retracted

Labia minora increase in size; color bright red

C. Orgasm

Uterus contracts similar to labor

Seminal pool location

Rectal sphincter contracts in rhythm with uterus

Strong vaginal contractions of orgasmic platform

D. Resolution

Uterus drops back to normal position

Cervix drops into seminal pool

Orgasmic platform resolves

Figure 14-1. Stages of the female sexual response cycle: (A) Excitement; (B) Plateau; (C) Orgasm; (D) Resolution. (Reprinted with permission from Beckmann CR, Ling FW, Barzansky BM, et al: *Obstetrics and Gynecology*, 2nd ed. Williams & Wilkins, Baltimore, 1995, pp 286–288.)

    d. Engorgement of the labia minora and majora occurs.

  3. Pelvic vascular engorgement in males is evidenced by erection of the penis (engorgement and increase in size).

  4. Extragenital changes

    a. Increased pulse and blood pressure (BP)

    b. Increased generalized muscle tension

    c. Extrapelvic vascular dilation (e.g., breast swelling, nipple erection, areolar engorgement, skin flush)

C. The **plateau phase** is characterized by the progression and intensification of excitement (see Figure 14-1) and is also mediated through the **parasympathetic** nervous system. It includes:

  1. Retraction of the erect clitoris into the clitoral hood

  2. Formation of an **orgasmic platform,** engorging and swelling of the outer one-third of the vagina, decreasing the inner diameter by 40%, and gripping the penis

  3. Elevation and ballooning of proximal two-thirds of the vagina

  4. Increase in uterine size

  5. Further labial engorgement

D. The **orgasmic phase** (see Figure 14-1) is mediated by the **sympathetic nervous system** at the peak of generalized muscle tone. It requires that the sensory threshold be exceeded through adequate duration and intensity of stimulation.

  1. Regulation of the orgasmic phase is via the following:

    a. Stimulation of the periclitoral sensory nerve endings. (Penile stimulation of the clitoris is usually less intense than manual stimulation; many women require additional manual stimulation for orgasm to occur.)

    b. Lowering the threshold by voluntarily contracting the pelvic muscles (e.g., as in Kegel exercises)

  2. Reflex clonic contractions occur initially in the orgasmic platform and levator sling.

    a. Frequency of contractions is five to ten per minute, with considerable variation in degree among women.

    b. Intensity subsides quickly and is followed by contractions of the uterus and anal sphincter.

    c. Gender-specific differences

      (1) Females have more significant individual orgasmic variability than males.

      (2) Females may have **multiple orgasms.**

E. The **resolution phase** is described in Figure 14-1. During this phase, the following occurs:

  1. Clitoral detumescence

  2. Abatement of orgasmic platform

  3. Release of muscle tension

4. Diminished vaginal ballooning
5. Gender-specific differences
   a. **Resolution is rapid for males,** usually taking only a few minutes.
   b. Resolution is **slower for females,** taking up to 30 minutes.

F. The **refractory phase (period of inability to be aroused) occurs only in males** (females have potential for multiple orgasms) and is of variable duration, lasting from minutes to days (usually longer with advancing age).

III. CLASSIFICATION OF SEXUAL PROBLEMS. Sexual **concerns** (largely intrapsychic), if not resolved, can result in sexual **difficulties** (largely interpersonal and relational), which can then progress to true sexual **dysfunctions** (impaired sexual response).

A. **Sexual concerns** relate to issues bothering **only the patient.** They are common and can usually be managed by the primary care physician.

1. **Normalcy-related issues** (e.g., "am I normal if ... ?"). These issues involve sexual thoughts, fantasies, or behaviors about which the patient has concerns about being abnormal. There is a wide range of normality in sexual functioning. Treatment is education and reassurance.

2. **Body image—related issues.** These concern negative perceptions regarding sexual attractiveness as a result of either genetic endowments (too little or too much), illness (chronic or acute), or surgery (ablative or ostomy procedures). The degree of patient anxiety and concern may have little correlation with the objective reality of physical appearance or the extent of surgical trauma.

3. **Life cycle—related issues.** The most common of these concerns are related to marital sexuality (e.g., sexual performance, reproductive limitation), sex education of children, and adolescent sexuality. Other concerns involve loss of companionship from divorce or death and changes that occur with aging.

B. **Sexual difficulties** arise from issues that result in **couple conflict.** These may relate to unresolved sexual concerns. Such difficulties frequently arise between partners who differ about what is "normal" sexual behavior, and they may concern gender-related differences in approach to sexuality. These common problems are often suitable for management by a primary care physician. Conjoint couple counseling is frequently helpful. Aspects of sexual conflict may include:

1. **Timing** of sexual encounters, which relates to conflicts concerning frequency (i.e., number of times per week), timing during the day (i.e., morning or evening), or spontaneity (i.e., planned or spontaneous)

2. **Nature** of the sexual act itself, which relates to conflicts concerning lighting (lights on or off), repertoire (usual mode or variations), duration (time for foreplay or afterplay), or kind(s) of coital positions

C. **Sexual dysfunctions** are characterized by impairment of inborn physiological sexual reflexes: desire, arousal, and orgasm. They are common, with a prevalence of 50% in married couples, and may be present even when women report positive marital satisfaction. Sexual dysfunctions are classified according to the earliest phase in which disruption is experienced: desire, arousal, or orgasm. Problems may begin with orgasmic difficulties, which subsequently may affect arousal, finally leading to loss of desire.

1. **Desire disorder.** Hypoactive sexual desire is apathy for and lack of enjoyment of sexual opportunities. This is the second most frequent female sexual complaint (Box 14-1). It should not be interpreted as a lack of ability to respond physiologically.

   a. **Possible causes** of desire disorders include:

      (1) **Organic factors** (e.g., postcastration low levels of sex steroids)

      (2) **Medication effects** (e.g., from antihistamine, antidepressant, antipsychotic, or antihypertensive agents)

      (3) **Psychological factors** (e.g., poor quality of relationship with sexual partner, depression, sequelae of sexual trauma, fear of pregnancy)

   b. **Management.** This dysfunction is the most resistant to treatment because of the interweaving of complex psychological and relationship issues. Fewer than 50% of patients show definite improvement. Referral to a qualified sex therapist or counselor is essential.

2. **Arousal disorder.** This dysfunction is characterized physiologically by a failure of the vaginal lubrication response and lack of pelvic engorgement. Normal desire may be present, however.

   a. **Estrogen deficiency,** either postoophorectomy or postmenopausal, **is the most common cause.**

   b. **Management** of hormone deficiencies and medication side effects is simple to correct. The rate of successful treatment is 80%.

3. **Lack of orgasm.** Stimulation must be sufficiently long and intense to allow adequate opportunity for orgasm. One-half of women do not experience orgasm through penile thrusting alone but require direct clitoral stimulation. Orgasm is under voluntary control, and thus learned inhibition can occur. Anorgasmia can be divided into two categories, and treatment for each type is usually successful.

   a. **Primary anorgasmia** is diagnosed when a woman has never experienced an orgasm through any means. Approximately 10% of adult women in the United States have never been orgasmic. Self-stimulation is often recommended to achieve the first orgasm.

Box 14-1. Prevalence of Female Sexual Complaints

Dyspareunia	50%
Decreased desire	20%
Partner problem	10%
Decreased lubrication	10%
Vaginismus	5%
Anorgasmia	5%

b. **Secondary anorgasmia** is diagnosed when a woman has had periods of normal orgasmic functioning. All causes of desire–arousal disorders may result in secondary anorgasmia, and these should be explored during treatment.

c. **Management** is directed at enhancing sensory stimulation and decreasing a woman's involuntary inhibition. Treatment is successful in up to 90% of women.

4. **Coital pain** is the **most common sexual complaint** verbalized during office visits. Etiology may be organic or psychogenic. Most cases are secondary to difficulty with vaginal lubrication. This condition warrants a thorough workup, with treatment focusing on the identified cause.

a. **Vaginismus** is a painful reflex spasm of the paravaginal thigh adductor muscles. It is the **only sexual dysfunction that can be diagnosed on physical examination.** The cause is almost always **psychogenic.** A history of sexual trauma or sexual rigidity is often noted. Treatment is stepwise "desensitization" with gradual accommodation of vaginal dilators of increasing size and is often highly successful.

b. **Dyspareunia** is defined as pain related to intercourse. It is important to distinguish whether pain occurs during entry, with deep thrusting, or following intercourse.

(1) **Physical causes** of painful sex are given in Table 14-2. Treatment is directed at the specific physical cause identified.

(2) **Psychological contributions** can be significant, involving a vi-

Table 14-2. Causes of Dyspareunia

	Introitus	Clitoris	Vagina	Uterus/Adnexae
Congenital	Intact hymen	NA	Septum	NA
Infectious	Vulvitis Bartholinitis	Vulvovaginitis	Vulvovaginitis	Acute pelvic inflammatory disease (PID)
Chemical irritation	Soaps Powders Perfumes	Soaps Powders Perfumes	Douching	NA
Hypoestrogenic state	Genital epithelial atrophy	Genital epithelial atrophy	Genital epithelial atrophy	NA
Adhesions or scarring	Episiotomy	Lichen sclerosis	NA	Chronic PID Endometriosis
Trauma	Acute injury	Acute injury	Acute injury	NA
Vascular	NA	NA	Inadequate lubrication	Pelvic congestion syndrome
Psychogenic	NA	NA	Vaginismus	NA

NA = not applicable.

cious pain–tension cycle. Anticipated pain causes tenseness, which results in pain that worsens the anxiety, which intensifies the pain.

IV. CLINICAL APPROACH TO SEXUAL PROBLEMS

A. **Physician objectives**

1. **Identifying patient concerns** through active listening. Do not interrupt the patient, judge, or solve. Show concern and serious attention. Affirm the legitimacy of the patient's concerns through reflective statements. Allow 5–10 minutes to ascertain the situation.

2. **Categorizing the nature of the problem** (e.g., sexual concern, sexual difficulty, or sexual dysfunction). Provide appropriate permission, reassurance, or limited information.

3. **Determining if you plan to manage or refer.** Diagnosis and management of problems with organic and pharmacological causes is appropriate for a physician.

4. **Implementing therapeutic interventions.** Select patients who are appropriate for referral to a sex therapist.

B. **Nomenclature** of sexual dysfunction

1. **Primary dysfunction.** The satisfactory experience of the entire sexual response cycle has never been met.

2. **Secondary dysfunction.** All phases of the cycle were experienced in the past, but are no longer experienced.

3. **Situational dysfunction.** The sexual response cycle functions in some but not all situations.

C. **Obtaining a sexual history** should be part of developing an initial data base for every new patient. Sexual concerns should be treated as legitimate problems. Making assumptions about a patient's sexual lifestyle and sexual practices should be avoided.

1. **Reasons why physicians may avoid inquiring about sexual issues** include:

a. Conflicts about their own sexual problems

b. Personal discomfort with their own sexuality

c. Time restraints in managed care settings

2. **Reasons why patients may avoid bringing up sexual issues** include:

a. Personal discomfort with sexual topics

b. Feelings that the physician is not interested

c. Not wanting to waste the physician's time

3. **Guidelines for sexual history taking** include:

a. Support the validity of patients' concerns, both verbally and nonverbally.

b. Do not assume that all patients are married or heterosexual.

c. Maintain your own values, but do not let them make unwarranted intrusion into the interview.

d. Use lay terminology, and avoid medical lingo.

4. **Screening questions** to ask every new patient include:

   a. "Are you sexually active?"

   b. "Is the sexual relationship satisfying for you?"

   c. "Do you think the sexual relationship is satisfying for your partner?"

   d. "Do you have any concerns about your sexual life or functioning?"

5. **Follow-up areas of questioning** if the screen is positive include:

   a. What does the patient perceive as the problem?

   b. What were the patient's previous sexual experiences like?

   c. How do the patient's sexual expectations differ from reality?

   d. What is the nature of the patient's relationship with her sexual partner?

   e. How is the patient feeling about the rest of her life (i.e., is depression a factor)?

D. **Factors affecting prognosis**

1. Long-duration problems are harder to resolve than those of acute onset.

2. Primary dysfunctions are more difficult to solve than secondary ones.

3. Relationship issues are harder to solve than medication-related effects.

4. Psychiatric illness and self-esteem issues may confound therapy.

E. **Life events** may affect sexual functioning.

1. **Pregnancy.** Most studies have shown a decrease in sexual interest, frequency of intercourse, and orgasmic ability with progression through the trimesters of pregnancy. However, the need of a pregnant woman to be held and stroked increases with pregnancy.

2. **Postpartum recovery** may be associated with episiotomy or incisional pain, along with discomfort from lactational vaginal atrophy.

3. **Recent onset of sexual activity** after death or divorce may create the need for adjustments to new expectations and behaviors with new sexual partners.

4. **Postoperative recovery** may be associated with incisional pain as well as a negative impact on body image.

5. **Postmenopausal low estrogen levels** may lead to genital epithelial atrophy and cause mood changes.

V. SEXUAL ASSAULT

A. **Rape** is sexual activity between a victim and an assailant that occurs under coercion and includes the element of force or the threat of physical harm.

1. **Incidence.** Rape is the most underreported violent crime in the United States, with 80% of cases not reported. By the age of 21, one in five women experiences sexual assault. Rape is more prominent in urban areas, and the rate is increasing at 10% per year.

2. **Familiarity of location or assailant.** Nearly 20% of rape victims can identify their assailant by name. Approximately 50% of all rapes occur in the victim's home, and 80% occur within the victim's own neighborhood.

B. Basic types of rape

1. **Power rape** is the most common (50%) type, and is usually **premeditated** and preceded by fantasies.

   a. The motivation is to demonstrate **control** of a victim rather than to inflict injury.

   b. It may involve **multiple assailants.**

   c. The assailant is frequently a **repeat offender** who may ask the victim if she enjoyed it.

2. **Anger rape** is the next common (40%) type, and it is usually **impulsive and episodic.**

   a. The motivation is to **humiliate and degrade** the victim.

   b. It may be triggered by a **stressful situation,** with the victim being merely a convenient object on which to vent rage.

   c. There is a greater chance of **physical injury.**

3. **Sadistic rape** is the least common (5%) of all types, and is often **premeditated** with **ritualized genital torture** or **mutilation.**

   a. It may result in the victim's **death.**

   b. Assailants often have a history of domestic violence and are more likely to be psychotic.

C. Clinical approach

1. **"Rape–trauma" syndrome** describes psychological sequelae to the victim that may persist long after the healing of physical trauma has taken place. Loss of control over her life during the period of the assault is central.

   a. **Immediate (acute phase) reactions** of the victim can vary from loss of emotional control to an apparently well-controlled behavior pattern. The victim simultaneously experiences shock, disbelief, fear, guilt, and shame. Physical complaints may include headache and chronic pelvic pain as well as eating and sleep disturbances. Emotional problems may involve depression, anxiety, and mood swings.

   b. **Delayed (organization phase)** reactions from rape may last for months or even years. They include nightmares, phobic reactions, fear, flashbacks, and survivor guilt (post-traumatic stress syndrome), in addition to gynecologic and menstrual complaints.

   c. **Immediate assistance in regaining control is needed.** Examples of how the physician can relate to the victim to help her regain control include:

      (1) Obtain permission and consent before starting the interview, examination, and specimen collection.

      (2) Emphasize that she is not to blame for the attack.

      (3) Allow her to discuss her feelings and current perceptions of her situation.

      (4) Explain the symptoms she may experience and advise her about where to seek help.

   d. **Long-term follow-up** includes:

      (1) Follow-up visits for counseling, depending on the phase of delayed reaction

(2) Referral to legal aid and rape victim support groups

(3) Providing rape "hot-line" numbers for counseling and support

2. Medical evaluation. Injuries are sustained by 40% of rape victims.

   a. Stabilization of vital signs must be dealt with first.

   (1) Informed consent must be obtained. In addition to fulfilling legal requirements, this process assists the victim in regaining control of her body and her life.

   (2) Major injuries requiring operative repair or hospitalization must be assessed. Injuries are sustained by 40% of rape victims, with 1% of a severe nature.

   b. History taking. The words *rape* and *sexual assault* are legal terms that should not be used in medical records.

   (1) A chaperone should be present during history taking and examination to reassure the victim and provide support.

   (2) The patient should be asked to state in her own words what happened, including details of the act(s) performed. Identification of the attackers should be requested.

   (3) A past and current obstetric and gynecologic history concerning infections, date of last menstrual period (LMP), use of contraception, and pregnancy should be obtained.

   c. Physical examination (see V C 3)

   (1) Search carefully for bruises, abrasions, or lacerations about the neck, back, buttocks, and extremities.

   (2) Document injuries with drawings or photographs appropriately labeled with the patient's name.

   (3) Perform a gentle pelvic examination to assess the status of reproductive organs and collect samples from the cervix and vagina for *Neisseria gonorrhoeae* and *Chlamydia trachomatis*.

   (4) Use a Wood light to find semen on the patient's body, because dried semen fluoresces under such a lamp.

   (5) Obtain baseline laboratory specimens for serology, human immunodeficiency virus (HIV) and pregnancy tests, urine drug screen, and blood alcohol.

   (6) Administer tetanus toxoid if the skin is broken from trauma.

   d. Infectious disease prophylaxis

   (1) Hepatitis B immune globulin followed by the standard three-dose immunization series

   (2) Empiric therapy for chlamydial, gonococcal, and trichomonal infections and bacterial vaginosis

   (a) Ceftriaxone 125 mg IM in a single dose plus

   (b) Metronidazole 2 g PO in a single dose plus

   (c) Doxycycline 100 mg PO bid for 7 days

   e. Pregnancy prevention ("morning after pill"). The risk of pregnancy after sexual assault is 2%–4%.

   (1) Combination oral contraceptive pills (OCPs) should be administered **immediately,** followed by two tablets in **12 hours.** The dosage is two tablets of high-progestin OCPs or four tablets of low-progestin OCPs.

   (2) When administered within 72 hours, the failure rate is 1%.

(3) Prophylactic antiemetics may be indicated, because nausea occurs in 50% of patients.

3. **Legal concerns.** Sexual assault assessment kits are available that list the necessary steps and the items to be obtained so as much information can be prepared for forensic purposes as possible.

  a. **Collection of physical evidence** should be performed at the time of physical examination (see V C 2 c).

   (1) Obtain informed consent.

   (2) Document the physical and emotional condition of the patient.

   (3) Document evidence of force and tissue injury.

   (4) Document evidence of sexual contact.

   (a) Examine clothes and skin for loose hair, stains, and debris that may be used as evidence.

   (b) Obtain vaginal secretions looking for motile sperm and presence of acid phosphatase, and DNA evaluation.

   (c) Obtain head and pubic hair specimens by combing and clipping.

   (d) Obtain a saliva specimen for ABO blood group secretory status.

  b. **Label all materials and specimens,** turn them over to the proper authorities, and retain a receipt for the patient's chart.

Review Test

Directions: Each of the numbered items or incomplete statements in this section is followed by answers or by completion of the statements. Select the ONE lettered answer or completion that is BEST in each case.

1. Which one of the following conditions is the most common complaint of a sexual nature verbalized by women in outpatient visits?

(A) Decreased lubrication
(B) Dyspareunia
(C) Decreased desire
(D) Vaginismus
(E) Anorgasmia

2. Which one of the following characteristics of sexual dysfunction is associated with a high chance of successful therapy?

(A) Long duration of dysfunction
(B) Situational dysfunction
(C) Association with medication
(D) Primary dysfunction

3. Which one of the following causes of sexual dysfunction is most likely to have a psychogenic etiology?

(A) Diabetes mellitus (DM)
(B) Arthritis
(C) Hypertension
(D) Vaginismus
(E) Endometriosis

4. Which one of the following actions is the most important step in management of a rape victim after ensuring that her vital signs are stable?

(A) Obtaining a saliva specimen for blood typing
(B) Assisting the victim to regain feelings of control in her life
(C) Performing a gentle pelvic examination with a chaperone present
(D) Drawing blood for serology
(E) Performing a pregnancy test

5. Which one of the following treatments is the recommended pregnancy prevention protocol for a rape victim?

(A) Medroxyprogesterone acetate (Depo-Provera) intramuscularly (IM)
(B) Subcutaneous implants of l-norgestrel (Norplant)
(C) Combination of oral contraceptive tablets, two tablets orally stat and again in 12 hours
(D) Placement of an intrauterine device (IUD)
(E) Menstrual extraction

Directions: Each of the numbered items or incomplete statements in this section is negatively phrased, as indicated by a capitalized word such as NOT, LEAST, or EXCEPT. Select the ONE lettered answer or completion that is BEST in each case.

6. All of the following characteristics of a normal sexual response cycle are shared by both females and males EXCEPT

(A) refractory phase
(B) orgasmic phase
(C) excitement phase
(D) desire phase
(E) plateau phase

7. All of the following are true statements about rape EXCEPT

(A) most occur outside the victim's neighborhood
(B) it is the most underreported violent crime in the United States
(C) it is more prominent in urban areas
(D) most victims are female
(E) it involves force or threat of harm

Directions: The set of matching questions in this section consists of a list of four to twenty-six lettered options (some of which may be in figures) followed by several numbered items. For each numbered item, select the ONE lettered option that is most closely associated with it. To avoid spending too much time on matching sets with large numbers of options, it is generally advisable to begin each set by reading the list of options. Then, for each item in the set, try to generate the correct answer and locate it in the option list, rather than evaluating each option individually. Each lettered option may be selected once, more than once, or not at all.

Questions 8–12

For each of the following physiological characteristics, select the appropriate phase of the normal female sexual response cycle.
(A) Refractory phase
(B) Orgasmic phase
(C) Excitement phase
(D) Desire phase
(E) Plateau phase

8. It is mediated by dopamine

9. Lubrication occurs

10. It is not shared by both genders

11. The clitoris retracts under its hood

12. The threshold is lowered by Kegel exercises

Answers and Explanations

1. The answer is B [III C 4 b].

Painful intercourse (dyspareunia) is the most common female sexual complaint. Studies show that up to 25% of women in outpatient visits have sexual problems or concerns. Decreased lubrication, decreased desire, vaginismus, and anorgasmia are all valid complaints of women, but they are noted with much less frequency than dyspareunia.

2. The answer is C [IV D].

Discontinuing a pharmacological agent in favor of a different medication is often very successful because sexual dysfunction can arise from psychogenic or organic causes. Treatment of organic causes with a reversible nature has high success rates. Dysfunctions of long duration, situational dysfunction, and dysfunction of a primary nature are less likely to be successful in treatment.

3. The answer is D [III C 4 a].

Vaginismus is characterized by painful reflex spasms of the paravaginal thigh adductor muscles, which prevents insertion of the penis into the vagina. It is largely of psychogenic origin and is very successfully treated by the patient gradually placing dilators of increasing size into her vagina. Diabetes mellitus (DM), arthritis, and hypertension are known organic causes of sexual dysfunction. Endometriosis may cause painful intercourse.

4. The answer is B [V C 1 c].

The most significant long-term impact of rape on a woman is the loss of control that she feels over her body. Addressing this need should underlie all interaction with the victim. Obtaining a saliva specimen, a pelvic examination, and a blood serology are important steps to take, but they should not override the issue of restoring control. Performing a pregnancy test is premature, unless the victim was already pregnant.

5. The answer is C [V C 2 e].

The high-dose oral contraceptives create an endometrium that is unfavorable to implantation, with a failure rate of 1% and nausea occurring in 50% of women. Pregnancy prevention or contragestation should be offered to the rape victim. Medroxyprogesterone acetate and subcutaneous implants are effective contraceptives; contragestagens [e.g., mefipristone (RU-486)] are not. Placing an intrauterine device (IUD) and menstrual extraction have been used as contragestational agents, but are not as reliable as high-dose oral contraceptives.

6. The answer is A [II F].

The refractory phase is found only in males; it is the period during which they are unable to be aroused. The female and male sexual response cycles are similar in sequence but may be different in the way they are experienced. The orgasmic phase, the excitement phase, the desire phase, and the plateau phase are all phases of the sexual response cycle experienced by both genders.

7. The answer is A [V A 2].

Nearly 80% of rapes occur within the victim's own neighborhood. Rape is primarily a crime of violence; sexuality is secondary. It involves involuntary sexual activity between the victim and the assailant as a result of force or threat of physical harm. Rape is the most underreported violent crime in the United States. It is more prominent in urban areas, and most victims are female.

8–12. The answers are 8-D [II A], 9-C [II B], 10-A [II F], 11-E [II C], 12-B [II D].

The desire phase of the sexual response cycle is enhanced by the mediation of dopamine but is inhibited by serotonin. Lubrication occurs in the excitement phase and is a consequence of transudation of fluid in the vagina from the paravaginal arterioles. The refractory phase is not shared by both genders; it exists only in males. The clitoris retracts under its hood in the plateau phase, with progression and intensification of the changes of the excitement phase. The threshold of the orgasmic phase is lowered by voluntary pelvic muscle contractions such as Kegel exercises.

15

The Female Breast

I. NORMAL BREAST DEVELOPMENT

A. Anatomy. The anatomy of the breast involves four major tissues (Figure 15-1).

1. **Glandular tissue** produces the milk secretions. Acinar secretory cells, which have the potential to produce milk, are arranged to form an **alveolus** (Figure 15-2). When the myoepithelial cells that surround each alveolus contract, milk is ejected into **ducts**. Large numbers of alveoli, with their ducts, form **lobules**. Groups of lobules join to form one of the 12 to 20 **conical lobes** of each breast.

2. **Ductal tissue** transports the milk secretions to the nipples. Groups of alveoli empty their secretions into distal **lactiferous ducts**. Many lactiferous ducts from each lobule unite to form a **major duct** for each lobe. Each major duct widens to form an **ampulla** as it reaches the areola. Each ampulla narrows to form a separate opening on the **nipple.**

3. **Fibrous tissue** supports the breast. Chest wall superficial fascia condenses to form multiple **fascial bands** or ligaments. The fascial bands (i.e., **Cooper's ligaments**) extend from the chest wall to the skin and support the subcutaneous tissue. Tumor-induced distortion of the fascial bands leads to skin dimpling.

4. **Fatty tissue,** which comprises 85% of the substance of the breasts, provides the bulk and characteristic shape. Fat lies within and between glandular/ductal tissue of the breast lobes.

B. Developmental changes in the breast are noted throughout the life cycle (see Figure 15-1).

1. **Embryonic breast development** starts in utero as early as day 35, when ectodermal precursors arise from the pair of ventral ridges extending from each forelimb to each forearm. Normally, the multiple pairs of breast buds disappear, and one pectoral pair remains.

2. **At birth,** the breast units are complete with alveoli and lactiferous ducts. Neonatal breasts can secrete "witch's milk" as a result of stimulation of maternal hormones.

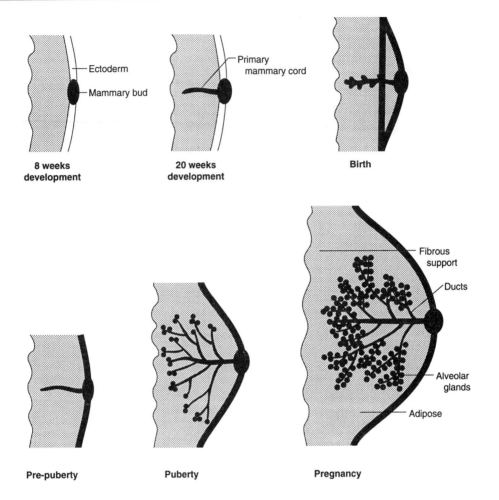

Figure 15-1. Developmental changes to the breast throughout the life cycle. (Reprinted with permission from Speroff L, Glass RH, Kase NG: *Clinical Endocrinology and Infertility,* 5th ed. Williams & Wilkins, Baltimore, 1994, p 549.)

3. **At puberty,** breast development is known as **thelarche.**

   a. **Proliferation** of all breast components occurs, including the number of acinar/alveolar units, ductal size and branching, and the size of the nipples and areola. However, the amount of stromal fat has the greatest impact on breast size and contour. In addition, the nipple smooth muscle becomes sensitive to tactile stimulation during puberty.

   b. **Many hormones** contribute to adolescent breast development. **Estrogen** stimulates duct growth, nipple size, and fatty stromal growth. **Progesterone** stimulates lobuloalveolar development. **Prolactin controls lactation.** Other necessary hormones include adrenal steroids, insulin, growth hormone, and thyroxin.

4. **During the reproductive years,** periodic menstrual breast changes occur that reflect the hormonal milieu. However, the changes are variable depending on the individual woman.

   a. **In the premenstrual phase,** the acinar cells undergo hypertrophy

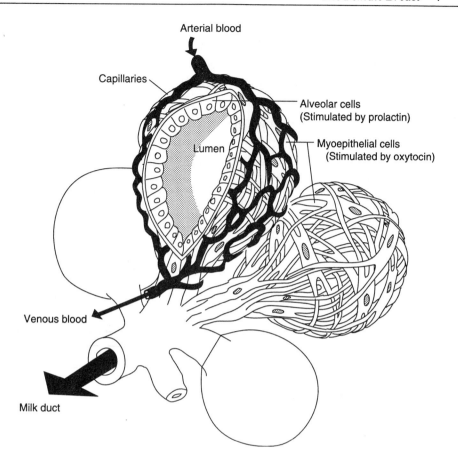

Figure 15-2. Diagram of a cluster of alveoli, the basic units of the mammary gland. (Reprinted with permission from Gabbe SG, Niebyl JR, Simpson JL (eds): *Obstetrics—Normal and Problem Pregnancies,* 2nd ed. Churchill Livingstone, New York, 1991, p 177.)

and hyperplasia. The ductal lumen increases in diameter. Overall breast size and turgor increase.

   b. In the postmenstrual phase, the acinar cells decrease in size and number. The ductal lumen diminishes in diameter. The breast size and turgor decrease.

5. **After menopause,** decreasing sex steroid levels cause the breasts to undergo gradual involution. The acinar elements decrease in number and size. The ductal tissue recedes, and the adipose tissue loses its turgor.

II. NORMAL LACTATION

A. **Normal lactational breast changes**

1. **Breast hypertrophy** occurs with pregnancy. Each breast increases in size by approximately 400 g. Blood flow to the breast doubles over the nonpregnant state. The breast components that increase include blood vessels, myoepithelial cells, and connective tissue. Fat deposition, as well as retention of water and electrolytes, also increases.

2. **Stages of lactation** include **mammogenesis, lactogenesis,** and **galactopoiesis.** Table 15-1 summarizes the significant aspects of these stages.

B. **Human breast milk.** Normal constituents of human milk are summarized in Table 15-2. The composition of breast milk is similar regardless of race, age, parity, breast size, or laterality of breast.

C. **Characteristics.** Immunological characteristics of human breast milk strengthen the immature neonatal immune system.

1. **Passive immunity** is supplied in the form of **immunoglobulin A (IgA) antibodies,** which provide specific protection against enteric bacteria. Maximal transfer occurs in the first week of life.

2. **Active immunity** is supplied by the transfer of high levels of leukocytes (up to 100,000 cells/ml of human milk). Most leukocytes are mononuclear cells and macrophages, including T cells and B cells.

D. **Clinical problems with lactation**

1. **Congestive mastitis** is synonymous with **breast engorgement.**
   a. **Symptoms and signs.** Onset is usually on day 2 or 3 postdelivery, with both breasts swollen, tender, tense, and warm. Axillary adenopathy can be found, with mild temperature increase common.
   b. **Management** depends on breastfeeding plans. Bromocriptine, al-

Table 15-1. Stages of Lactation

	Definition	Onset	Initiating Events	Essential Hormones
Mammogenesis	Preparing breasts for milk secretion by breast growth and development	Puberty	*Increasing levels* of estrogen and progesterone	Estrogen: ductal tissue growth and budding Progesterone: maturation of alveolar ducts Prolactin, growth hormone, insulin, cortisol: differentiation of glandular cells into secretory and myoepithelial cells
Lactogenesis	Initiation of milk secretion in alveoli	Postpartum after placenta is removed	*Declining levels* of estrogen, progesterone, and human placental lactogen	Prolactin: stimulates synthesis of casein lactose and milk fatty acids
Galactopoiesis	Maintenance of established milk secretion	After each emptying of ducts and alveoli	Periodic suckling	Oxytocin: contracts the myoepithelial cells to empty the alveolar lumen Prolactin: stimulates continued secretory replacement of ejected milk

Table 15-2. Normal Constituents of Human Milk

Constituent	Main Moiety
Water	Main component comprising 85% of milk by weight
Carbohydrate	Lactose (glucose and galactose)
Protein	Casein and α-lactalbumin
Lipids	Palmitic and oleic acid
Enzymes	Amylase, catalase, peroxidase, and lipase to help in digestion of breast milk
Immunology	IgA antibodies to protect against enteric bacteria T- and B-cell lymphocytes to provide active immunity

though effective as a lactational suppressant, is no longer used in this capacity because of an alleged risk of strokes.

(1) If lactation is desired, the breasts should be manually emptied after infant feeding. Emptying the breasts stimulates more milk production.

(2) If lactation is not desired, the breasts should be firmly bound with a breast binder. Ice packs and analgesics may be helpful. Breast stimulation should be avoided. Without emptying of the alveoli, milk secretion soon ceases, and the breasts dry up.

[handwritten: Staph aureus from infant's nostrils] **2. Infectious mastitis** arises from nipple trauma followed by the introduction of *Staphylococcus aureus* from the infant's nostrils into the nipple ducts.

   a. Symptoms and signs. Onset is usually after the first postdelivery week. Involvement is usually unilateral, often with only one quadrant or lobe of the breast affected. The area is tender, reddened, swollen, and hot, with purulent nipple drainage if an abscess forms. High fevers can occur, and patients usually appear ill.

[handwritten: Cloxa dicloxa Cephalosporins] **b. Management is multifaceted.** Antibiotics recommended include cloxacillin, dicloxacillin, or a cephalosporin. Breastfeeding should be continued. Local heat, breast support, and analgesics are helpful. If an abscess is present, it should be incised and drained.

III. BREAST MASSES

A. Breast self-examination (BSE) should be performed monthly by all women older than 20 years. The best time during the month for BSE is just after a woman's menstrual period.

   1. The **upright position** is used for inspecting the breasts in the mirror. The procedure should be started with the arms held at the side, then with the arms raised up. Finally, the supraclavicular and axillary areas should be palpated for nodes.

   2. The **lying down position** is used to palpate each quadrant against the chest wall with the flat of the fingers. The upper, outer quadrant is the site of 45% of breast cancers. The nipples and areolas should be felt for lumps and secretions.

B. Breast examination

1. **Visual inspection**

   a. A **good light should be used** when looking for **lumps, dimpling, or wrinkling** of the skin on the breast and axillae.

   b. The **patient should be placed in a sitting position,** first with arms at her sides, then with arms pressed on her hips while tensing her pectoralis muscles, and finally with arms held above the head.

2. **Bimanual palpation of breasts.** The patient should be examined in the following positions:

   a. **Sitting position,** leaning forward with hands on knees

   b. **Supine position,** with arms relaxed at side

3. **Palpation of the axillae and breasts** is performed using fingers.

4. **Palpation of the nipples** is performed using the thumb and forefinger.

5. **Palpation of the supraclavicular areas** is performed using fingers.

C. Breast imaging methods of confirmed value

1. **Mammography** is the gold standard for screening and can be sensitive to calcifications and tumor sizes of 1 mm in diameter.

   a. **Biopsy is the only definitive diagnosis for breast cancer** (see IV). Mammography can only raise the index of suspicion of a tumor (Figure 15-3).

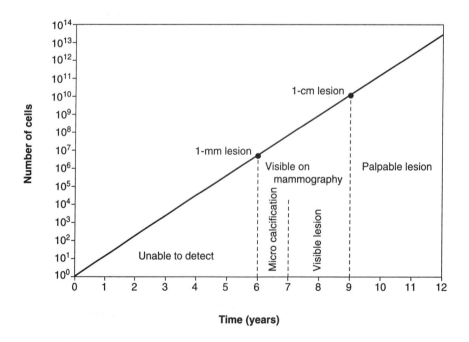

Figure 15-3. Mammographic and clinical detection of breast mass, assuming a cancer doubling time of 100 days. (Adapted with permission from Beckmann CR, Ling FW, Barzansky BM, et al: *Obstetrics and Gynecology,* 2nd ed. Williams & Wilkins, Baltimore, 1995, p 240.)

    b. Guidelines for mammography screening are given in Table 15-3. The age for starting routine mammography screening is controversial; opinions conflict regarding the role of x-ray exposure in inducing cancerous changes in younger women versus the likelihood of detecting a cancer.

    c. The technique used for mammography requires compression of the breasts for optimal visualization of masses using the standard craniocaudal and lateral views.

  2. Sonography is best for differentiating solid from cystic lesions. It is not recommended for breast cancer screening.

D. Breast imaging methods of unconfirmed value

  1. Diaphanography assesses the **light transillumination** differential between normal and abnormal areas of the breast.

  2. Thermography assesses the **heat production** differential between normal and abnormal breast areas.

E. Surgical diagnostic methods for assessing breast masses

  1. Fine-needle aspiration (FNA) can provide a diagnosis in 90% of breast masses. In this office procedure, a 22-gauge needle is used to aspirate fluid, and anesthesia is not required. If the cytology results show that the fluid is clear and the mass disappears, no further follow-up is required, except a single mammography screening.

  2. Core biopsy makes use of a 14-gauge needle to obtain a tissue core of a solid breast mass. If breast cancer or a specific benign condition is not detected by core biopsy, open biopsy is necessary.

  3. Open biopsy, the time-honored method, is usually performed in an operating room under local anesthesia. Use of open biopsies is decreasing as FNA and core biopsy becomes more widespread. **Absolute indications** for open biopsy include the following:

    a. Cystic mass not collapsed on FNA

    b. Bloody fluid obtained on FNA

    c. Spontaneous serous or serosanguinous nipple discharge

    d. Suspicious mammogram

F. Common benign breast disorders

  1. Fibrocystic changes are clinically apparent in 50% of women, most often between the ages of 20 and 50 years. The lesions are usually multiple,

Table 15-3. Guidelines for Mammography Screening

Guideline	Age
If significant risk factors	Before age 35 years
Baseline study	Ages 35–40 years
Repeat every 1–2 years	Ages 40–49 years
Annual mammography	Age 50 years and older

Bilateral

MBI

Multiple   irregular

bilateral, and irregular associated with pain and tenderness. They are the **most common of all benign breast conditions.**

    a. Histology shows epithelial proliferation within the ducts plus stromal fibrosis sometimes leading to cyst formation. If the lesions are associated with atypia, the risk of malignant transformation is increased.

    b. Symptoms are cyclic bilateral breast pain, which is usually located in the upper, outer quadrant. Often poorly localized, the pain may radiate to the shoulders and upper arms. It occurs as a result of breast stromal edema, ductal dilation, and some inflammatory response.

    c. Signs include excessive nodularity with ill-defined thickness or "lumpiness" with rubbery consistency.

    d. The **mechanism** of fibrocystic changes is an exaggerated physiological response to cyclic levels of ovarian hormones (i.e., increased estrogen and decreased progesterone). Therefore, fibrocystic changes improve with pregnancy, lactation, and menopause, but worsen during perimenopause.

    e. Management requires first ruling out malignancy by mammography and aspiration of the dominant cyst. Reduction of dietary methylxanthines (caffeine) along with supplemental vitamin A may be helpful. Oral contraceptives and nonsteroidal anti-inflammatory drugs (NSAIDs) can suppress symptoms in many patients. Diuretics are of temporary benefit for premenstrual mastalgia. Medications used with varying degrees of success include progestins, tamoxifen, and bromocriptine.

2. Fibroadenomas are the **most common benign female breast tumors.** These sharply circumscribed, smoothly rounded, slippery, mobile nodules, which are up to 15 cm in diameter, are usually solitary and slow growing. They frequently occur in women under 25 years of age.

    a. Histology shows proliferation of both fibrous and glandular tissue.

    b. Management may be conservative for nonpalpable, small masses identified as fibroadenomas by mammography or sonography. Other lesions require **surgical excision** for definitive diagnosis and cure.

3. Intraductal papillomas appear as small, palpable masses adjacent to the areola that are accompanied by serosanguinous nipple discharge. They are most common in older premenopausal women and are often associated with fibrocystic changes.

    a. Histology shows proliferation of ductal epithelium, which is primarily benign, but may rarely be malignant.

    b. Management requires identification of the involved duct and **surgical biopsy.**

4. Duct ectasia may be manifest as tender, hard, erythematous masses adjacent to the areola in association with burning or itching. A thick, greenish-black discharge may be present in dilated ducts with inspissated secretions in perimenopausal or postmenopausal women.

    a. Histology shows dilated, distended terminal collecting ducts obstructed with inspissated, lipid-containing epithelial cells. Lesions are mostly benign but may rarely be malignant.

    b. Management requires identification of the involved duct and surgical biopsy.

  5. Galactoceles are cystic, centrally located swellings that develop shortly after lactation ceases. Cystic duct dilations fill with thick, milky fluid. They can occur in multiple sites in the breast around times of lactation.

    a. Histology shows a dilated duct distended with inspissated milk material.

    b. Management involves simple needle aspiration. If the mass recurs, **excisional biopsy** may be necessary.

  6. Fat necrosis may form a rare lesion that appears as a tender, firm mass that does not increase in size. It is associated with breast trauma, and ecchymosis may be seen. If untreated, the mass usually gradually disappears. The lesion is often accompanied by skin or nipple contraction, mimicking carcinoma.

    a. Mammography may show multiple, small stippled calification.

    b. Management involves simple needle aspiration. If the mass recurs, **excisional biopsy** may be necessary.

  7. Cystosarcoma phyllodes appears as a firm, smooth, generally slow-growing mass measuring 5 cm or more in size. It is most common in the fifth decade of life. The majority of masses are benign, but 10% can be malignant. The malignant forms are the **most common breast sarcoma.**

    a. Histology shows fibroepithelial elements characterized by a predominance of connective tissue hypercellularity with increased pleomorphism and mitotic activity.

    b. Management is **total excision** with a wide margin of healthy tissue.

IV. BREAST CANCER

  A. Epidemiology. Breast cancer is the **most common invasive cancer** in women (Figure 15-4). A woman has a 1 in 12 chance of developing breast cancer during her lifetime (Figure 15-5). The incidence increases with age; two-thirds of malignancies occur in women older than 50 years. Breast cancer is a systemic disase that may recur many years after initial diagnosis. The relative risk (RR) of breast cancer in women is 100 times higher than in men. The risk of breast cancer in the average American woman equals the risk of lung cancer in a heavy smoker, whether male or female.

  B. Risk factors (Table 15-4) identify only 25% of women who eventually develop breast cancer. Factors associated with the greatest increase in RR are:

    1. BRAC1 or BRAC2 gene (RR of 14)

    2. Two first-degree relatives with breast cancer (RR of 5)

    3. Benign breast disease with atypical hyperplasia (RR of 4)

  C. Types of breast cancer (Table 15-5 and Figure 15-6). The majority of malignant breast tumors are adenocarcinomas, but microscopically they represent a heterogenous group of tumors.

    1. Ductal carcinoma. Most carcinomas originate in the epithelium of the collecting ducts.

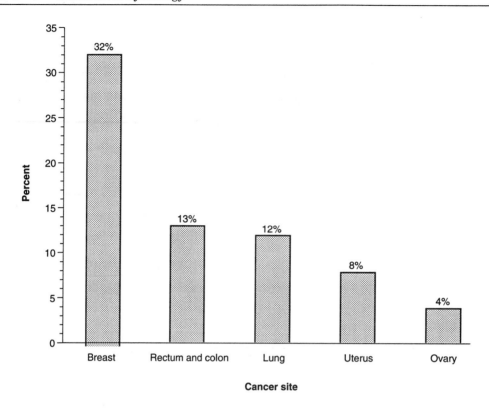

Figure 15-4. Comparative incidence of leading cancers in women in the United States as of 1993. (Reprinted with permission from Speroff L, Glass RH, Kase NG: *Clinical Endocrinology and Infertility,* 5th ed. Williams & Wilkins, Baltimore, 1994, p 562.)

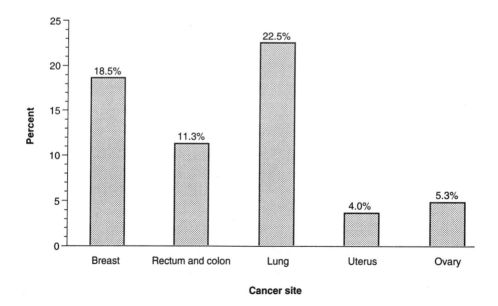

Figure 15-5. Distribution of cancer deaths by site in women in the United States as of 1993. (Adapted from Speroff L, Glass RH, Kase NG: *Clinical Endocrinology and Infertility,* 5th ed. Williams & Wilkins, Baltimore, 1994, p 562.)

Table 15-4. Risk Factors for Breast Cancer

Genetic	Environmental	Reproductive	Morphologic
• Age older than 40 years	• High dietary fat	• Nulliparity	• Ovarian cancer
• Positive family history	• Moderate alcohol use	• Delayed childbearing	• Uterine cancer
• North American white	• Breast irradiation (>90 rads)	• Early menarche	• Breast cancer (contralateral)
• BRCA gene	• Breast trauma	• Late menopause	• Atypical hyperplasia

Table 15-5. Types of Breast Cancer

Breast Cancer Type	Percent	Unique Characteristic
Infiltrating ductal type	80%	Arises in the epithelial lining of large or intermediate ducts
Lobular infiltrating type	10%	Arises from the epithelium of the terminal ducts of the lobules
Inflammatory type	3%	Most malignant type with findings of tenderness erythema and edema
Paget's type	1%	Can be misdiagnosed as dermatitis

    a. In situ ductal carcinoma (5% of tumors). The lesion has not penetrated the basement membrane, and a definite mass is not palpable.

        (1) This type of breast cancer is usually diagnosed by microcalcification identified on mammography.

        (2) Multifocal areas of carcinoma are found in the same breast in up to 10% of women.

        (3) Primary treatment is simple mastectomy.

    b. Infiltrating ductal carcinoma is the most common breast malignancy (80%). These lesions, having broken through the basement membrane, are histologically invasive.

        (1) The more common, histologically **heterogeneous** cell types are grossly firmer and diffuse. Masses composed of these cells have a **worse** prognosis.

        (2) The less common, histologically **uniform** cell types are grossly softer, mobile, and well delineated. Masses composed of these cells have a **better** prognosis.

  2. Lobular carcinoma. These carcinomas originate in the terminal lobular ducts.

    a. In situ lobular carcinoma (3%). The lesion has not penetrated the basement membrane, and a definite mass is not palpable.

        (1) Mammographic findings are not characteristic.

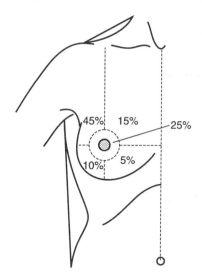

Figure 15-6. Frequency of breast cancer at various anatomic sites. (After DeCherney AH, Pernoll ML (eds): *Current Obstetrics and Gynecologic Diagnosis and Treatment,* 8th ed. Appleton & Lange, East Norwalk, Conn., 1994, p 1123.)

    (2) Malignant potential is less than with in situ ductal carcinoma, and the latent period to gross invasion is longer, up to 20 years. When the lesion does become invasive, the subsequent cancers are ductal, not lobular.

    (3) Bilateral disease is common, and frequently it is multifocal.

  b. Infiltrating lobular carcinoma (9%). Lesions are histologically invasive, having broken through the basement membrane.

    (1) The carcinoma tends to have multicentric origin in the same breast and to involve both breasts more often than infiltrating ductal carcinoma.

    (2) Histology shows uniform small, round neoplastic cells that infiltrate the stroma in a "single file" fashion.

3. Inflammatory carcinoma (2%). This is the **most malignant form of breast cancer.**

  a. Clinically, a rapidly growing, indistinct, painful mass that enlarges the breast is apparent.

  b. The inflammatory changes, caused by tumor blockage of dermal lymphatics, can be mistaken for an infectious process.

  c. Metastases tend to occur early and widely, leading to low cure rates.

4. Paget's carcinoma (1%). This form of breast cancer can be mistaken for a dermatitis. Clinical findings such as eczema of the nipple or bacterial infection lead to delay in diagnosis.

  a. The presenting symptoms are itching and burning of the nipple.

  b. The basic lesion is usually an infiltrating intraductal carcinoma that invades the epidermis.

  c. The prognosis is often good.

D. Methods of metastasis. Breast cancer is considered a systemic disease at diagnosis as a result of its relatively long preclinical growth phase and high tendency to metastasize. The disease may recur many years after initial diagnosis.

1. Initial invasion is into surrounding tissues, then into lymphatic and vascular space.

2. **Axillary nodes** are the **most common site of regional metastasis,** with internal mammary nodes, the next more frequent type of spread.

3. **Lung and liver** are the **most common sites of distant metastasis.**

E. **Staging of breast cancer** (Table 15-6) is based on the TNM classification. The tumor size and characteristics are described (T), regional lymph node involvement is documented (N), and distant metastases are noted (M). The higher the stage at diagnosis, the lower the risk for cure, and the poorer the prognosis.

F. **Prognostic factors**

1. **Axillary node status.** The number of positive nodes is the most important prognostic factor for survival. The initial size of the lesion is the single best predictor of likelihood of positive axillary nodes. Yet even patients with negative nodes have a 25% chance of recurrrent disease.

2. **Receptor status.** Receptor-positive tumors are usually more well differentiated and exhibit less aggressive clinical behavior than receptor-negative tumors, which seldom respond to hormone manipulation. Hormone therapy has a 60% response if estrogen receptors are positive and an 80% response if both estrogen and progesterone receptors are present.

3. **DNA content.** Disease-free survival rates are significantly better in diploid tumors (i.e., those with normal DNA content) than in aneuploid cancers.

G. **Treatment.** Treatment is based on the presence or absence of estrogen or progesterone receptors, the extent of disease, and biological aggressiveness. Curative treatment is anticipated only for stage I or II disease. Palliation is the only option for stage IV patients.

Table 15-6. Clinical and Surgical Staging of Breast Carcinoma*

Stage	Criteria
I	Tumor <2 cm in diameter Nodes, if present, felt to be benign No distant metastases
II	Tumor 2–5 cm in diameter Nodes, if palpable, not fixed No distant metastases
III	Tumor >5 cm or any size with skin or chest wall invasion Positive supraclavicular No distant metastases
IV	Distant metastases present

*From American Joint Committee on Cancer based on TNM (Tumor, Nodes, Metastasis) criteria

1. **Surgery.** With the recognition that breast cancer is often systemic, the therapeutic emphasis has changed to less radical surgery and increased radiation and chemotherapy. Partial mastectomy plus axillary dissection (recovering at least 15 nodes) followed by radiation therapy appears to be equivalent to modified radical mastectomy for stage I and II patients.

2. **Chemotherapy.** Adjuvant therapy is appropriate for all axillary node–positive patients as well as selected young, node-negative patients. Premenopausal women have improved survival with cyclophosphamide, methotrexate, 5-fluorouracil (5-FU), and doxorubicin. The major effect of multiagent chemotherapy is prolonging the disease-free interval rather than improving overall survival. Postmenopausal women respond better to tamoxifen but need to be watched closely for endometrial hyperplasia. Patients with estrogen and progesterone receptor-positive tumors respond well to antiestrogen therapy and premenopausal oophorectomy.

3. **Radiation therapy.** Radiation therapy is used for treatment of potentially curable stage I and stage II disease, as well as for palliation of locally advanced cancers with distant metastases.

4. **Breast cancer and pregnancy.** Approximately 2% of breast carcinomas are diagnosed during pregnancy, often after a significant delay in diagnosis. Pregnancy has little impact on prognosis, and abortion does not improve survival. FNA and open biopsy are risk-free and should be utilized for appropriate lesions. During the first and second trimesters, prompt treatment, including mastectomy and axillary dissection, should be performed as soon as possible after diagnosis. Third trimester temporizing to enhance fetal maturity may be appropriate in selected cases prior to instituting definite cancer therapy.

Review Test

Directions: Each of the numbered items or incomplete statements in this section is followed by answers or by completions of the statement. Select the ONE lettered answer or completion that is BEST in each case.

1. Which one of the following tissues is the most significant component of the female breast, giving it size and characteristic shape?

(A) Glandular tissue
(B) Ductal tissue
(C) Fibrous tissue
(D) Fatty tissue

2. Which one of the following statements regarding breast development is correct?

(A) Completion of breast unit development occurs at puberty
(B) Breast precursors arise from mesodermal origin
(C) Proliferation of breast components at puberty is called pubarche
(D) Multiple pairs of breast buds are present in embryonic life

3. Which one of the following is the most significant constituent of human breast milk by weight?

(A) Carbohydrate
(B) Water
(C) Protein
(D) Lipid
(E) Enzymes

4. Which one of the following is the predominant immunoglobin (Ig) in human breast milk?

(A) Immunoglobulin M (IgM)
(B) IgE
(C) IgA
(D) IgG
(E) IgF

5. Which one of the following breast quadrants has the highest incidence of breast cancers being diagnosed?

(A) Upper outer
(B) Lower outer
(C) Upper inner
(D) Lower inner

6. Which one of the following is the standard imaging method for assessing breast disease?

(A) Sonography
(B) Diaphanography
(C) Thermography
(D) Nuclear magnetic resonance
(E) Mammography

7. Which one of the following conditions is a risk factor for breast cancer?

(A) Multiparity
(B) Late menarche
(C) Delayed childbearing
(D) High carbohydrate diet
(E) Fibroadenoma

8. Which one of the following conditions is an indication for fine-needle aspiration (FNA) of the breast?

(A) Multiple cystic masses
(B) Solid breast mass
(C) Serosanguinous nipple discharge
(D) Suspicious mammogram

Directions: The sets of matching questions in this section consist of a list of four to twenty-six lettered options (some of which may be in figures) followed by several numbered items. For each numbered item, select the ONE lettered option that is most closely associated with it. To avoid spending too much time on matching sets with large numbers of options, it is generally advisable to begin each set by reading the list of options. Then, for each item in the set, try to generate the correct answer and locate it on the option list, rather than evaluating each option individually. Each lettered option may be selected once, more than once, or not at all.

Questions 9–11

For each of the following characteristics, select the appropriate physiologic breast function.

(A) Mammogenesis
(B) Lactogenesis
(C) Galactopoiesis

9. Maintained by emptying the alveoli

10. Requires rapidly declining levels of multiple hormones

11. Requires high level of multiple hormones

Questions 12–16

For each of the following characteristics, select the type of benign breast disorder that is appropriate.

(A) Fibrocystic disease
(B) Fibroadenoma
(C) Intraductal papilloma
(D) Mammary duct ectasia
(E) Galactocele

12. Inspissated secretions

13. Cystic dilation of ducts

14. Abnormal nipple discharge

15. Hormonally related symptoms

16. Lesion may be up to 15 cm in size

Answers and Explanations

1. The answer is D [I A 4].

Fatty tissue comprises 85% of the substance of the average woman's breast. The female breast is also composed of glandular tissue, ductal tissue, and fibrous tissue.

2. The answer is D [I B 1].

Breast development occurs in human females starting in early embryonic life and continues into puberty and through each menstrual cycle. Many embryonic breast buds form along the milk line; normally, all but one pectoral pair disappear. Completion of breast unit development occurs before birth, not at puberty. Breast precursors arise from ectodermal, not mesodermal, origin. Proliferation of breast components at puberty is called thelarche. Pubarche is the development of pubic hair.

3. The answer is B [II B; Table 15-2].

Human breast milk is composed of each of the options listed for this question. However, 85% of the milk by weight is water.

4. The answer is C [II C 1].

The most common immunoglobin (Ig) found in the body secretions is IgA. This is also true of breast milk. IgA is maximal in the secretions of the first week of life, and it protects the neonate specifically against enteric bacteria.

5. The answer is A [III A 2].

Breast cancer occurs more often in the upper, outer quadrant of the breast than any other, probably because it includes the tail of the breast that continues up into the axillae. Approximately 45% of breast cancers are identified in this location.

6. The answer is E [III C 1].

Many imaging techniques have been proposed and studied to improve the early identification of breast cancers. None has proven as successful as mammography, which is sensitive to tumor sizes as small as 1 mm. Sonography is helpful in differentiating solid from cystic lesions. Diaphanography assesses differences in light transillumination; thermography, differences in heat production; and nuclear magnetic resonance, differences in tissue magnetic fields. All are of unproven value in breast cancer detection.

7. The answer is C [IV B; Table 15-4].

One of the most significant risk factors for breast cancer is delayed childbearing. A woman who has a child before the age of 18 years has one-third the risk of breast cancer as a woman who has a child after the age of 35 years. Nulliparity, not multiparity, is a risk factor. Early menarche, not late menarche, is also a risk factor. A high-fat diet rather than a high-carbohydrate diet is associated with breast cancer. Fibroadenoma is unrelated to breast cancer risk.

8. The answer is A [III E 3].

Multiple cystic masses is the correct answer. Fine-needle aspiration (FNA) has become the method of choice for investigating cystic breast masses. If the masses collapse, the cytology of the aspirated fluid is negative, and mammography is negative, no surgery is indicated. Open breast biopsy in the operating room is the time-honored method for diagnosing breast masses. Solid breast masses, serosanguinous nipple discharge, and suspicious mammogram are all indications for core biopsy or open breast biopsy.

9–11. The answers are: 9-C, 10-B, 11-A [II A 2; Table 15-1].

Emptying the alveoli is the stimulus for galactopoiesis, which is the maintenance of established milk secretion initiated by periodic suckling of the infant at the breast.

Rapidly declining levels of multiple hormones [e.g., estrogen, progesterone, human placental lactogen (hPL)] are the stimulus for lactogenesis, which is the stimulation of milk secretion into the alveoli initiated by the expulsion of the placenta after delivery.

High levels of multiple hormones (e.g., estrogen, progesterone, prolactin growth hormone) are required for mammogenesis, which is the preparation (i.e., growth, development) of the breasts for milk secretion that occurs at puberty.

12–16. The answers are: 12-D [III F 4], **13-E** [III F 5], **14-C** [III F 3], **15-A** [III F 1], **16-B** [III F 2].

Inspissated secretions are frequently the main finding in premenopausal women with mammary duct ectasia. Surgical biopsy reveals benign plasma cell infiltration.

Cystic dilation of ducts filled with thick, milky fluid is seen in lactating women with galactoceles. These can be multiple in location but are benign.

Abnormal nipple discharge is the presenting complaint in premenopausal women with intraductal papillomas. They can be either benign or malignant.

Hormonally related symptoms are common with fibrocystic disease. Tenderness is bilateral, and multiple sites are frequently involved.

Lesions up to 15 cm in size are found with fibroadenomas, which are the most common benign female breast tumor.

16

Infertility

I. TERMINOLOGY

A. Fertility is the ability to conceive after 12 months of penis-in-vagina intercourse without contraception. In normal fertile couples, 50% conceive within 3 months, 75% within 6 months, and 90% within 12 months.

B. Infertility is a term used to indicate that a couple has a reduced capacity to conceive compared with the general population. It is applied when conception has not occurred after 12 months of penis-in-vagina intercourse without contraception. In the United States, infertility is prevalent in 10% of couples. The emotional impact of infertility can be significant.

   1. Classification
      a. Primary infertility is identified in couples in whom a pregnancy has never been established.
      b. Secondary infertility is identified in couples who have previously conceived but are currently unable to do so.

   2. The definition of infertility applies to two kinds of couples:
      a. Hypofertile couples, who ultimately conceive but require more time or assistance
      b. Sterile couples, who never conceive

C. Fecundability is the likelihood of conception occurring in a population of couples within a given period of time, usually 1 month. Fecundability is inversely related to advancing age of the female partner (Figure 16-1).

II. REQUIREMENTS FOR NORMAL FERTILITY. For conception to occur, six fertility components must be present (Table 16-1). Abnormalities in each component can result in infertility and should be considered by the clinician evaluating a couple.

III. CAUSES OF INFERTILITY (relative proportions in parentheses)

A. Ovulation does not occur (10%–15%).

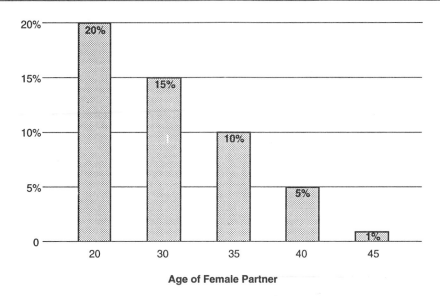

Age of Female Partner

Figure 16-1. Fecundability by age of female partner.

Table 16-1. Requirements for Normal Fertility

Fertility Prerequisite	Physiologic Requirement
1. Ovulation occurs	Hypothalamic-pituitary-ovarian axis must be intact
2. Fallopian tube is patent and functional	Fimbria must be able to sweep egg into patent, functional oviduct
3. Spermatozoa are present and functional	Testes must produce mature, functional gametes
4. Coitus is timely and suitable	Intercourse must take place at midcycle placing sperm in the vagina
5. Cervical mucus is favorable	Mucous quality must facilitate sperm entry and storage
6. Endometrium is receptive	Uterine lining must be hormonally ready for implantation

1. **Possible causes** include polycystic ovarian (PCO) disease, hyperprolactinemia, hypogonadotropic hypogonadism, and hypothyroidism.
2. **Diagnosis** can be established by a variety of means.
    a. A history of **unpredictable, irregular cycles,** which is presumptive evidence of anovulation
    b. A **basal body temperature (BBT)** chart (Figure 16-2) showing absence of mid-cycle elevation. (In ovulatory cycles the BBT rises and remains elevated 0.5°F–0.8°F for at least 11 days during the luteal phase. This elevation results from the thermogenic effect of progesterone.) The BBT should be obtained after 6 or more hours of sleep, prior to ambulating.

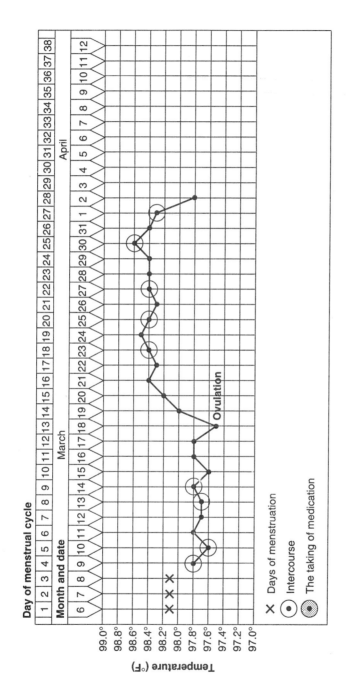

Figure 16-2. A basal body temperature record. The mid-cycle rise in temperature is caused by the progesterone effect. (After Beckmann CR, Ling FW, Barzansky BM, et al: *Obstetrics and Gynecology*, 2nd ed. Williams & Wilkins, Baltimore, 1995, p 392.)

c. A serum **progesterone** level < 3 ng/ml in what should be the mid-luteal phase

d. An **endometrial biopsy** in what should be the luteal phase showing proliferative changes without evidence of progesterone effect

B. **Fallopian tube is neither functional nor patent (30%–40%).**

1. **Possible causes** include adhesions from previous pelvic inflammatory disease (PID), ruptured appendix, peritonitis from any cause, endometriosis, or ectopic pregnancy.

2. **Diagnosis** can be radiologic or operative.

   a. **Hysterosalpingogram (HSG)** shows proximal or distal occlusion of an oviduct by outlining internal anatomy through infusion of a radio-opaque medium. Lack of patency is suggested by failure of media spilling into the cul-de-sac.

   b. **Laparoscopy** can assess external contours and peritoneal surfaces of the uterus and oviducts to identify agglutinated fimbria and adhesions. This is usually the last diagnostic test performed because of its expense. General anesthesia and full operating room facilities are required.

C. **Spermatozoa either are not present or are not functional (30%–40%).**

1. **Possible causes** include constantly increased scrotal temperature, smoking, high alcohol intake, epididymitis, exposure to toxins, varicocele, or endocrine disorders.

2. **Diagnosis** is by semen analysis (see IV A 2).

D. **Coitus either is not timely or is not performed properly.** This is an uncommon cause of infertility.

1. **Possible causes** include engaging in intercourse too infrequently, failing to time intercourse with mid-cycle ovulation, ejaculating outside the vagina, using spermicidal agents inadvertently, and not allowing the seminal pool to remain in the vagina.

2. **Diagnosis** is obtained by a careful history.

E. **Unfavorable cervical mucus (10%)**

1. **Possible causes** include a lack of estrogen stimulation around the time of ovulation. This low-estrogen effect results in thick mucus through which the sperm cannot pass.

2. **Diagnosis** was once made by a mid-cycle **postcoital test** (PCT). Cervical mucus was aspirated 2–4 hours postcoitus and evaluated grossly, to determine the ability of the mucus to stretch (spinbarkeit), and microscopically, to determine the number of sperm and assess motility. The PCT is now only of historical interest because intrauterine insemination is used to bypass unfavorable cervical mucus.

F. **Unreceptive endometrium** (also known as **luteal phase defect**)

1. **Possible causes** include decreased follicle-simulating hormone (FSH) levels, abnormal patterns of luteinizing hormone (LH) secretion, or decreased response of the endometrium to progesterone.

2. **Diagnosis** is by endometrial biopsy, which is performed 2–3 days before the expected menses. A luteal phase defect is diagnosed by a lag of 2 or more days in endometrial histology compared with the known cycle day. This finding must be consistent and be found in at least two cycles. Significant questions exist concerning two issues: (1) whether such histological lag is a normal variation and (2) if such a lag is present, whether it actually causes infertility.

IV. **DIAGNOSTIC EVALUATION** is a two-phase process and follows a comprehensive history, including sexual history, as well as a complete physical examination.

A. **Phase one. Inexpensive and noninvasive tests** should first be performed. **Initial treatment** should focus on anovulation or abnormal semen analysis before proceeding to invasive testing. If the initial tests are normal, more invasive tests may be necessary.

1. **Ovulation documentation**

a. If cycles are regular by history, obtain a midluteal progesterone level for indirect evidence of ovulation (> 10 ng/ml) as well as to document normal luteal function. A BBT chart may also provide indirect evidence of ovulation.

b. If cycles are irregular or absent, begin ovulation induction even though occasional ovulatory cycles may occur.

2. **Semen analysis**

a. The semen specimen should be obtained 2–7 days after coitus and examined within 30–60 minutes. Semen volume and sperm concentration, morphology, and motility should be evaluated. Normal values are shown in Table 16-2.

b. At least 75% of fertile men have at least one abnormal characteristic, and 25% have two abnormalities. It is more important to consider the number of abnormal parameters rather than the extent of abnormality in a single parameter.

c. If the semen analysis is abnormal, the semen analysis should be repeated on two or three occasions at least 1 month apart. Semen quality may vary over time, and the spermiogenesis cycle is 74 days.

3. **Selected laboratory tests**

Table 16-2. Normal Semen Analysis Values

Characteristic	Value
Semen volume	2–5 ml
Sperm concentration	>20 million/ml
Sperm motility	>50%
Normal forms	>30%
pH	7.2–7.8

    a. Baseline tests include complete blood count (CBC), urinalysis, cervical Papanicolaou (Pap) smear, and fasting blood glucose.

    b. Ovarian reserve is assessed if the female partner is over 35 years age by obtaining an **FSH** level on the third day of the cycle. An elevated level (> 12 mIU/ml) indicates impending ovarian failure.

    c. Tubal disease risk is assessed by obtaining a *Chlamydia* **immunoglobulin G (IgG) antibody** level. If this value is negative, the risk of tubal disease is less than 5%.

    d. Ovarian endometrioma is ruled out by a **pelvic sonogram.**

B. Phase two. If indicated, more expensive, invasive, and painful tests may be necessary.

    1. HSG

        a. Schedule the procedure during the first week following menses. Consider prophylactic doxycycline to prevent exacerbation of previous PID and nonsteroidal anti-inflammatory drugs (NSAIDs) to prevent stimulation of painful uterine cramping.

        b. Use water-soluble media to better visualize tubal mucosa to establish if tubal disease is proximal or distal.

        c. False-positive findings may occur with tubal spasm, suggesting proximal obstruction that is not present.

        d. Proceed to controlled ovarian hyperstimulation and intrauterine insemination if unexplained infertility exists (i.e., ovulation is documented and normal findings are found on HSG, FSH, *Chlamydia* IgG, sonogram).

    2. Diagnostic laparoscopy. This expensive, invasive procedure is indicated only if the HSG shows tubal disease or if the sonogram shows endometrioma.

        a. Schedule the procedure in the follicular phase of the cycle.

        b. Infuse indigo carmine dye transcervically into the peritoneal cavity at laparoscopy to confirm tubal patency.

        c. Perform tubal reconstruction or salpingectomy depending on the extent of tubal disease found at laparoscopy.

    3. Unexplained infertility. If all these preliminary tests are normal, the diagnosis is "unexplained infertility." Approximately 15% of infertile couples fall into this category.

        a. If no further workup or treatment is performed and the couple is managed expectantly, the monthly pregnancy rate is 2%. The spontaneous pregnancy rate within 3 years is 60%.

        b. If no pregnancy occurs within 3 years, the likelihood of subsequent pregnancy drops markedly.

V. MANAGEMENT

A. Anovulation. Ovulation induction using medical therapy can increase fecundability to approach that of normal fertile couples. Success is noted in more than 90% of patients.

1. **Bromocriptine** is effective in inducing ovulation if hyperprolactinemia is the cause.

2. **Clomiphene citrate** is usually used initially in all other instances. It is a synthetic, weak estrogen that competes with endogenous estrogen for estrogen-binding sites in the hypothalamus. As clomiphene blocks the endogenous estrogen negative feedback, it leads to enhanced gonadotropin-releasing hormone (GnRH) release. The agent is administered for 5 days in the early follicular phase. A low dose (50 mg) is used initially, increasing until there is evidence of ovulation. The dose is then continued for 3–6 months with intercourse during mid-cycle. Ovulation is successful in 70% of women, with a pregnancy rate of 50%.

3. **Human menopausal gonadotropin** (hMG) stimulation of ovarian follicles, combined with mid-cycle human chorionic gonadotropin (hCG) [to trigger ovulation], is used for patients who are resistant to clomiphene. Ovarian response must be monitored closely by serum estrogen levels and sonographic assessment of follicle number. Ovulation is successful in 90% of women, with a pregnancy rate of 50%.

4. **GnRH** is an alternative to hMG. It has the advantage of lower rates of hyperstimulation but the disadvantage of requiring either intravenous (IV) or subcutaneous (SQ) pulsatile infusion.

5. **Hyperstimulation,** from clomiphene and hMG, can result in multiple ovarian follicles being stimulated by higher doses of medication. Twin pregnancy rates are 8% with clomiphene and 20% with hMG. Excessive ovarian stimulation can produce large theca lutein cysts with transudation of ovarian fluid, resulting in ascites and hemoconcentration. Treatment is conservative, allowing spontaneous involution.

6. **Partial ovarian destructive** procedures such as laparoscopic electrocautery or laser drilling are effective in inducing ovulation in women with PCO syndrome who fail to respond to medical therapy. These procedures destroy androgen-producing ovarian stroma, but periovarian adhesions are a significant risk.

B. **Tubal disease.** Distal obstruction (85%) is more common than proximal obstruction (15%).

1. **If pelvic tuberculosis** with tubal disease is found on HSG, tubal reconstructive surgery should be avoided, because patients should be considered sterile. The diagnosis should be confirmed with an endometrial biopsy, and appropropriate antibiotic therapy should be instituted.

2. **If any distal tubal disease** is found on HSG, laparoscopy should be performed. If tubal disease is surgically correctable, lysis of adhesions, fimbrioplasty, or other reconstructive procedures is indicated. If tubal disease is beyond repair, both tubes should be surgically removed, because in vitro fertilization (IVF) success rates are diminished if damaged oviducts remain.

3. **If proximal tubal obstruction** is found on HSG, hysteroscopically directed or fluoroscopically guided transcervical catheterization should be performed to attempt recanulation of the cornual areas.

C. **Semen quality problems**

1. **Intrauterine insemination (IUI).** This is used with oligozoospermia, mild-to-moderate semen abnormalities, and unexplained infertility. IUI is associated with higher pregnancy rates if combined with clomiphene stimulation of ovulation than if used in natural ovulatory cycles. The procedure is performed on the day of ovulation. Sperm are washed (to remove seminal prostaglandins that can produce severe uterine cramping) and then centrifuged. Sperm separation procedures produce specimens with improved motility and morphology. The sperm pellet (in 0.5 ml of solution) is then placed high in the uterine cavity.

2. **Intracytoplasmic sperm injection (ICSI).** This is used with severe semen abnormalities. A single sperm is injected into the oocyte in vitro. Fertilization rates of 60% are achieved regardless of sperm motility, with 30% pregnancy rates. Delivery rates are comparable to those of conventional IVF.

3. **Donor insemination.** A last resort, this technique is used with azospermia or failed ICSI. Psychological comfort of both partners is important to ensure marital stability. Donors must be screened for general health and genetic diseases. Laboratory screening for sexually transmitted diseases (STDs) is crucial.

D. **In vitro fertilization (IVF)**

1. IVF is used with severe tubal disease, severe endometriosis, and male factor problems or unexplained infertility.

2. Follicle development can be either stimulated (by clomiphene or hMG) or unstimulated. Oocyte retrieval is by ultrasound-guided transvaginal follicle aspiration.

3. After 6–12 hours of preincubation, sperm are added to oocytes in a culture medium. Day 3–5–cleaving embryos are transferred on day 3–5 into the uterus. Unused embryos may be frozen and thawed for later use.

4. Pregnancy rates of 40% can be expected for each IVF cycle for up to three or four cycles, with delivery rates of 35%.

VI. ENDOMETRIOSIS

A. Endometriosis is found in up to 40% of infertile women. A proposed mechanism for infertility causation involves increased intraperitoneal macrophages that enter the oviduct and phagocytose sperm. A cause-and-effect relationship has not yet been established. Endometriosis may be a result of infertility, rather than a cause.

B. No medical therapy increases fertility rates with endometriosis. In absence of tubal disease, surgical resection or ablation of peritoneal endometrisis is controversial.

C. Pregnancy rates with surgical management of tubal disease are 60% if the damage is moderate and 35% if it is severe.

Review Test

Directions: Each of the numbered items or incomplete statements in this section is followed by answers or by completions of the statement. Select the ONE lettered answer or completion that is BEST in each case.

1. Which one of the following conditions is a complication of medical induction of ovulation?

(A) Increased congenital anomalies
(B) Ovarian hyperstimulation
(C) Increased embryonic demise
(D) Gestational diabetes
(E) Hirsutism

2. Which one of the following semen analysis values is abnormal?

(A) Semen volume = 5 ml
(B) Sperm concentration = 30 million/ml
(C) Sperm motility = 50%
(D) Normal forms = 60%
(E) pH = 6.5

3. Which one of the following procedures is the appropriate management when an abnormal semen analysis is identified?

(A) Artificial insemination by donor
(B) Repeat semen analysis
(C) Artificial insemination with split ejaculate
(D) Adoption
(E) Antibiotic therapy

Directions: Each of the numbered items or incomplete statements in this section is negatively phrased, as indicated by a capitalized word such as NOT, LEAST, or EXCEPT. Select the ONE lettered answer or completion that is BEST.

4. All of the following are methods of detecting ovulation EXCEPT

(A) basal body temperature (BBT)
(B) endometrial biopsy
(C) urine luteinizing hormone (LH) test
(D) serum estrogen
(E) molimina

Directions: The set of matching questions in this section consists of a list of four to twenty-six lettered options (some of which may be in figures) followed by several numbered items. For each numbered item, select the ONE lettered option that is most closely associated with it. To avoid spending too much time on matching sets with large numbers of options, it is generally advisable to begin each set by reading the list of options. Then, for each item in the set, try to generate the correct answer and locate it in the option list, rather than evaluating each option individually. Each lettered option may be selected once, more than once, or not at all.

Questions 5–7

For each of the following characteristics, select the appropriate method of assessing uterine/tubal disease.

(A) Hysterosalpingogram (HSG)
(B) Hysteroscopy
(C) Laparoscopy

5. Expensive and invasive procedure

6. Outpatient procedure without anesthesia

7. Procedure for resecting uterine cavity defects

Answers and Explanations

1. The answer is B [V A 5].

Medical induction of ovulation is accomplished by oral clomiphene citrate, which is an antiestrogen, or parenteral human menopausal gonadotropin (hMG). The only true complication of these agents from the options given is ovarian hyperstimulation, which is a potentially life-threatening condition. The other major complication of induction of ovulation is multiple pregnancy. Increased congenital anomalies, increased embryonic demise, gestational diabetes, and hirsutism are all false and do not represent complications of ovulation induction.

2. The answer is E [III C; Table 16-2].

Male factor etiology is present in approximately 50% of infertile couples. The normal semen pH range is 7.2 to 7.8. The more acidic the pH is, the more hostile it is to healthy sperm. Semen volume of 5 ml, sperm concentration of 30 million/ml, sperm motility of 50%, and normal forms of 60% are all within normal semen analysis parameters.

3. The answer is B [IV A 2, V C].

Normal semen quality may vary considerably over time, suggesting that a diagnosis of male factor infertility should be deferred until consistently abnormal results are confirmed through repeated semen analysis. Artificial insemination and adoption are premature until abnormal semen analysis values have been confirmed. Antibiotic therapy is appropriate only for confirmed infection.

4. The answer is D [III A 2 c].

Anovulation is one of the major etiologies of infertility. Identification of ovulation is an important part of the infertility workup. Serum estrogen is the correct answer (but incorrect statement) because the progesterone, not estrogen level, identifies whether ovulation has occurred. Basal body temperature (BBT), endometrial biopsy, urine luteinizing hormone (LH) test, and molimina are all methods of detecting ovulation.

5–7. The answers are: 5-C [IV B 2], **6-A** [IV B 1], **7-B** [V B 2].

The most expensive and invasive procedure for assessing the uterus and fallopian tubes is laparoscopy. The procedure, which inspects the external anatomy of the pelvic organs, is performed in an operating room with general anesthesia.

A procedure that can be performed on an outpatient basis without anesthesia is the hysterosalpingogram (HSG). Radio-opaque dye is infused transcervically into the uterus, and radiographs are taken to outline the internal anatomy of the uterus and fallopian tubes.

Resecting of the uterine cavity defects can be accomplished by using an operative hysteroscope. This procedure must be performed in an operating room under anesthesia.

COMPREHENSIVE EXAMINATION

Directions: Each of the numbered items or incomplete statements in this section is followed by answers or completions of the statement. Select the ONE lettered answer or completion that is BEST in each case.

1. Which question best differentiates whether a pregnancy belongs under the category of parity or abortus in reproductive history taking?

(A) Was a live fetus expelled?
(B) Was a gestational sac or embryo found on ultrasound?
(C) Did the pregnancy terminate intentionally or spontaneously?
(D) Were any birth defects present?
(E) What was the gestational age of the pregnancy?

2. Which is the most prevalent indication for primary cesarean deliveries in the United States?

(A) Malpresentation
(B) Cephalopelvic disproportion (CPD)
(C) Fetal distress
(D) Placenta previa
(E) Chorioamnionitis

3. A 20-year-old woman who comes to the emergency department at 10 weeks' gestation has a history of vaginal bleeding and cramping along with passage of some tissue. She continues to bleed, and a vaginal sonogram shows existing intrauterine debris. You perform a suction dilation and curettage (D&C). Which procedure is an essential part of the routine follow-up care of this patient?

(A) Rh blood typing status
(B) Hysterosalpingogram (HSG)
(C) Cervical cultures
(D) Antiphospholipid antibody screen
(E) Thyroid studies

Questions 4 and 5

A 25-year-old woman (gravida 3, para 2) is undelivered at term. She is Rh-negative. Her Rh-positive husband is the father of her three children, all of whom were Rh-positive. She did not receive 28-week antepartum $Rh_o(D)$ immunoglobulin (RhoGAM).

4. What is the chance that the woman has already developed $Rh_o(D)$ isoimmunization?

(A) 0.2%
(B) 2%
(C) 15%
(D) 30%
(E) 50%

After delivery, the woman is discharged from the hospital without receiving $Rh_o(D)$ immunoglobulin (RhoGAM) postpartum.

5. What is the risk that the woman will develop $Rh_o(D)$ isoimmunization?

(A) 0.2%
(B) 2%
(C) 15%
(D) 30%
(E) 50%

6. A 30-year-old woman comes to you for prenatal care. On taking her history, you learn that she had rheumatic fever as a child and has residual heart disease. From which of the following cardiac lesions does she most likely suffer?

(A) Mitral insufficiency
(B) Mitral stenosis
(C) Aortic stenosis
(D) Aortic insufficiency
(E) Pulmonary stenosis

7. A 23-year-old woman has heavy, dark hair on her forearms and lower legs but not on her chest or abdomen. She has normal secondary sexual characteristics with regular menses and normal general, breast, and pelvic examinations. These findings are most consistent with which of the following conditions?

(A) Hypertrichosis
(B) Hirsutism
(C) Defeminization
(D) Virilization

8. An 18-year-old primipara underwent an emergency primary cesarean delivery at 39 weeks' gestation. Although she progressed in labor until her cervix was 7 cm dilated, her cervix did not dilate further over 3 hours despite regular, strong uterine contractions (UCs). Now in her third postoperative day, she has spiked a fever [temperature to 103°F (39.4°C)]. Her lungs are clear, and her wound is clean and dry. However, her uterus is tender to palpation. Which statement regarding the diagnosis and treatment of her current situation is correct?

(A) Endometrial cultures should be obtained before giving antibiotics
(B) Parenteral antibiotics should be continued until the patient is afebrile for 48 hours
(C) Appropriate antibiotics should target a single organism
(D) Offending infectious agents are generally pathogenic organisms
(E) Infectious agents are seldom anaerobic

9. A 55-year-old woman complains of loss of appetite but increasing abdominal girth. On abdominal examination, there is evidence of shifting dullness to percussion. On pelvic examination, diffuse fixed masses extending to the pelvic sidewalls are palpated. Which of the following patterns of spread is most common to the form of cancer that is most likely present?

(A) Lymphatic spread
(B) Direct extension
(C) Exfoliation of malignant cells
(D) Hematogenous spread

10. A 23-year-old woman (gravida 2, para 1) undergoes routine prenatal laboratory screening. She has no symptoms referable to the urinary tract. However, the urine culture is positive, with more than 100,000 colony-forming units (CFUs) of *Escherichia coli*. Which of the following is the most significant obstetrical complication if the woman is not appropriately treated?

(A) Preterm delivery
(B) Hydrops fetalis
(C) Spontaneous premature membrane rupture
(D) Intrauterine growth restriction (IUGR)
(E) Postpartum hemorrhage

11. A 25-year-old woman is seen for her first prenatal visit at 12 weeks' gestation by dates. She complains of severe nausea and vomiting. Her fundal height is 16-week size, but no fetal heart tones are heard with a doppler stethoscope. A sonogram shows an enlarged uterus but no fetus or placenta. The uterus appears to be filled with cystic structures. With this condition, metastasis to which of the following sites would be associated with a good prognosis?

(A) Bone
(B) Lung
(C) Brain
(D) Liver

12. A 21-year-old sexually active woman has a cervical Papanicolaou (Pap) smear that is consistent with a low-grade squamous intraepithelial lesion. Colposcopic visualization of the cervix reveals mosaicism, punctation, and white epithelium. Which of the following is a risk factor for the identified condition?

(A) Tobacco smoking
(B) Positive family history
(C) Early menarche
(D) Use of spermicidal or barrier contraception
(E) Caucasian race

13. A 26-year-old woman (gravida 1, para 0) with a 2-year history of infertility has ovulation induction with clomiphene citrate. Now pregnant with twins, she is at 15 weeks' gestation. Ultrasound examination shows a single anterior placenta but a membrane separates the uterus into two sacs. This woman at greatest risk for which of the following obstetrical complications?

(A) Postpartum uterine atony
(B) Spontaneous premature rupture of membranes (PROM)
(C) Iron-deficiency anemia
(D) Preterm labor and birth
(E) Pregnancy-induced hypertension

14. Twenty-four hours ago, a 19-year-old woman gave birth to a 3200-gram male neonate by a spontaneous vaginal delivery. She would like to breastfeed her son. Her prenatal panel indicates an absence of rubella antibodies. Before administering a postpartum rubella immunization, you will inform her of which of the following facts?

(A) She should avoid pregnancy for 3 months after immunization
(B) She should avoid breastfeeding after the immunization
(C) The vaccine uses a killed virus
(D) Passive immunity occurs immediately after immunization
(E) The immunization is free of side effects

15. A 22-year-old woman (gravida 1, para 0) presents to the emergency department with a history of vaginal bleeding and 15 weeks' gestation by dates. On examination, her fundus is to the umbilicus. Her blood pressure (BP) is 150/95 mm Hg, and she has 2+ proteinuria. She has no history of hypertension. Which of the following is the most likely diagnosis?

(A) Recent onset of chronic hypertension
(B) Mild preeclampsia
(C) Multiple gestation
(D) Molar pregnancy

16. A 33-year-old woman (gravida 4, para 2, abortus 1) with a 5-year history of chronic hypertension comes to the maternity unit at 29 weeks' gestation. She reports that she has not felt the baby move in 12 hours and expresses concern that her baby might be dead. A 3-hour 100-gram oral glucose tolerance test (OGTT) shows three elevated values. Her blood glucose values have been within the target range. Which of the following methods most accurately confirms fetal demise?

(A) Absence of fetal movement by maternal report
(B) Absence of fetal cardiac motion on sonography
(C) Absence of fetal cardiac activity by external sonocardiography
(D) Absence of fetal heart tones by Doppler auscultation
(E) Absence of fetal movement by sonography

17. A 67-year-old woman complains of vulvar itching. On examination, you find a 6 × 8-mm left vulvar lesion. The pathological report obtained on biopsy describes full-thickness involvement of the epithelium with basal cells. The basement membrane is intact without any invasion. Which mode of treatment is recommended?

(A) Skinning vulvectomy
(B) Simple vulvectomy
(C) Radical vulvectomy
(D) Radiation therapy

18. A concerned mother brings her 15-year-old daughter for evaluation, stating that the girl has never had a menstrual period. The girl is 54 inches tall and has a webbed neck. As an infant, she was diagnosed with coarctation of the aorta. Which of the following descriptions applies to this patient?

(A) Breasts present, uterus present
(B) Breasts present, uterus absent
(C) Breasts absent, uterus absent
(D) Breasts absent, uterus present

19. A 31-year-old woman (gravida 2, para 2) presents to the emergency department with acute onset of intense, left-lower abdominal and pelvic pain. On pelvic examination, you find an exquisitely tender 8-cm left adnexal mass. Which etiological factor is the most significant risk factor for the condition described?

(A) Cause of the mass
(B) Sonographic appearance
(C) Duration of the mass
(D) Patient age
(E) Size of the mass

20. An 18-year-old primigravida initiates prenatal care at 15 weeks' gestation. A prenatal panel is performed. The cell profile reveals the following: hemoglobin of 8.5 g/dl, hematocrit of 25%, and a mean corpuscular volume (MCV) of 75 fl. Which of the following statements regarding this condition is correct?

(A) It is the most prevalent anemia in pregnant women
(B) An increased total iron-binding capacity is diagnostic
(C) It is associated with an increased mean corpuscular hemoglobin
(D) A decrease in hemoglobin precedes the loss of bone marrow iron stores
(E) With iron therapy, the first response parameter is an increasing level of hemoglobin

21. A 29-year-old woman comes to your office stating that her last menstrual period (LMP) was 4 months ago. Her previous menstrual cycles have been normal and predictable. A qualitative urine pregnancy test is negative. You administer 150 mg of progesterone-in-oil intramuscularly (IM), and she experiences normal withdrawal bleeding within 7 days. Which of the following statements regarding this patient is correct?

(A) The ovarian follicles are exhausted
(B) The follicle-stimulating hormone (FSH) level is markedly increased
(C) The response to gonadotropin-releasing hormone (GnRH) stimulation is negative
(D) The hypothalamus has failed
(E) The endometrium has been estrogen-primed

22. A 31-year-old woman (gravida 2, para 1) has a positive atypical antibody titer screen on her first-trimester prenatal laboratory testing. It was identified as being directed against a red blood cell (RBC) antigen associated with hemolytic disease of the newborn. Which question is the most significant in developing a management plan?

(A) What is the level of the antibody titer?
(B) What is the mother's ABO blood type?
(C) What is the gender of the fetus?
(D) When did the isoimmunization occur?
(E) Are the father's RBCs antigen-positive for the atypical antibody?

23. A 22-year-old primipara who is 48 hours postpartum is not feeling well and complains of chills. On examination, you find that her temperataure is 102°F (38.9°C). Which of the following is the most common risk factor for the condition she probably has?

(A) Cesarean delivery
(B) Manual removal of placenta
(C) Prolonged labor
(D) Anemia
(E) Premature rupture of membranes (PROM)

24. A 25-year-old woman came to the emergency department after passing vesicular tissue vaginally. She underwent a suction curettage under general endotracheal anesthesia. Histological evaluation of the tissue shows proliferative trophoblastic cells with edematous placental villi but no blood vessels. The most common clinical history found with this condition is

(A) bleeding before 16 weeks' gestation
(B) hyperthyroidism
(C) preeclampsia before 24 weeks' gestation
(D) severe hyperemesis
(E) passage of vesicles vaginally

25. A 36-year-old woman (gravida 3, para 2, abortus 1) complains of irregular, unpredictable menstrual bleeding at intervals varying from 5 to 35 days. The amount of bleeding varies from minimal spotting to heavy bleeding with clots. A qualitative urine pregnancy test is negative. Which of the following tests would be the most helpful in evaluating the cause of this condition?

(A) Papanicolaou (Pap) smear
(B) Pelvic ultrasound
(C) Hysterosalpingogram (HSG)
(D) Dilation and curettage (D&C)
(E) Laparoscopy

26. A 20-year-old woman (gravida 1, now para 1) at 39 weeks' gestation underwent a scheduled primary low-segment transverse cesarean section under general anesthesia for a footling breech presentation in labor at 3-cm dilation with membranes intact. Five hours postcesarean, her temperature is 102°F (38.9°C). Which of the following is the most appropriate management?

(A) Pelvic examination
(B) Intravenous (IV) heparin
(C) Pulmonary exercises
(D) IV antibiotics
(E) Blood cultures

27. A 19-year-old woman, a student at the local university, complains of bilateral lower abdominal and pelvic pain. Her last menstrual period (LMP) was 5 days ago. On laparoscopy, she has inflamed, edematous oviducts bilaterally. Which of the following is a criterion for inpatient management of this woman?

(A) Costovertebral angle tenderness
(B) Cervical motion tenderness
(C) Positive cervical culture
(D) Evidence of pelvic abscess
(E) Increased sedimentation rate

28. A 32-year-old woman (gravida 0, para 0) has been unable to conceive for the past 12 months despite regular intercourse. She has irregular menses and complains of leakage of milky fluid from her nipples. A serum prolactin level is elevated. Which pharmacological agent is most likely to be helpful?

(A) Opiates
(B) Phenothiazines
(C) Bromocriptine
(D) Butyrophenones
(E) Methyldopa

29. A 30-year-old woman (gravida 1, para 1) just delivered twin female neonates at 32 weeks' gestation. The presentation of the twins was cephalic-cephalic, and she underwent a vaginal delivery. You examine the fetal membranes and find two separate placentas. Which statement is most likely to be true of this pregnancy?

(A) The dividing membrane between the sacs has four layers
(B) The twin girls are identical
(C) The risk of birth defects and anomalies is high
(D) Zygote cleavage occurred on day 14 post-conception
(E) The pregnancy was a consequence of ovulation induction

30. A 17-year-old woman is seen in the emergency department for unilateral left-sided abdominal-pelvic pain. A quantitative serum β-human chorionic gonadotropin (β-hCG) level is 4500 mIU/ml. No intrauterine gestational sac is apparent on transvaginal sonography. However, on sonogram a left-sided pelvic mass is noted consistent with an unruptured ampullary ectopic pregnancy measuring 4 cm in length. Which of the following is the surgical procedure of choice?

(A) Laparoscopic salpingectomy
(B) Laparotomy with linear salpingostomy
(C) Laparoscopic segmental resection of oviduct
(D) Laparoscopic linear salpingostomy

Directions: Each of the numbered items or incomplete statements in this section is negatively phrased, as indicated by a capitalized word such as NOT, LEAST, or EXCEPT. Select the ONE lettered answer or completion that is BEST in each case.

31. A 24-year-old woman (gravida 2, para 1) was admitted to the maternity unit 3 hours ago with regular uterine contractions (UCs). Pelvic examination revealed her cervix to be 5 cm dilated and 80% effaced with the fetal head at −1 station. A repeat examination a few minutes ago revealed no change in her cervical dilation and effacement. Her UCs are now occurring every 5–6 minutes and lasting for 15–20 seconds. With regard to management, the appropriate next step involves any of the following factors EXCEPT

(A) phosphorylation of myosin
(B) β-adrenergic agonists
(C) activation of myosin light-chain kinase
(D) prostaglandin $F_{2\alpha}$
(E) oxytocin

32. A 34-year-old woman (gravida 4, para 3) at 28 weeks' gestation undergoes a 1-hour 50-gram glucose challenge with a resulting value of 150 mg/dl. Values of a subsequent 3-hour 100-gram oral glucose tolerance test (OGTT) are: fasting, 85 mg/dl; 1-hour, 195 mg/dl; 2-hour, 170 mg/dl; and 3-hour, 120 mg/dl. All of the following statements concerning this pregnancy complication are correct EXCEPT

(A) it is usually diagnosed in the first half of pregnancy
(B) it is the most common type of diabetes in pregnancy
(C) it resolves after pregnancy is terminated
(D) it is usually managed by diet therapy alone
(E) it may include newly unmasked type I and II diabetes mellitus (DM)

33. An 18-year-old woman comes to the emergency department complaining of lower abdominal and pelvic pain. She states that her last menstrual period (LMP) was 10 weeks ago, but she experienced minimal vaginal bleeding 3 hours ago. A qualitative urine β-human chorionic gonadotropin (β-hCG) test is positive. A culdocentesis is negative. Which of the following is LEAST helpful in making a diagnosis?

(A) Negative culdocentesis
(B) Positive β-hCG test
(C) Amenorrhea
(D) Vaginal bleeding
(E) Abdominal pain

34. A 21-year-old woman complains of an irritating vaginal discharge. On pelvic examination you find mucopurulent cervical discharge. A Gram stain shows inflammatory cells but no gram-negative diplococcus bacteria. All of the following statements concerning the organism that is probably causing the cervical discharge are correct EXCEPT

(A) it is seldom asymptomatic
(B) it causes acute urethral syndrome
(C) it produces inflammatory oviduct changes
(D) it causes hypertrophic cervical inflammation
(E) it causes infertility

35. When obtaining a reproductive history, all of the following are satisfactory confirmations of a pregnancy that enable it to qualify under the gravida (G) category EXCEPT

(A) late onset of menses
(B) positive pregnancy test
(C) ultrasound showing an embryo or fetus
(D) embryo that was passed
(E) pathology report showing villi

36. A 29-year-old woman (gravida 3, para 2) is 62 inches tall and weighs 250 pounds. A 1-hour 50-gram oral glucose tolerance test (OGTT) obtained at her first prenatal visit at 12 weeks' gestation was 120 mg/dl. A repeat glucose screen performed at 27 weeks' gestation was 160 mg/dl. A subsequent 3-hour 100-gram OGTT was positive. All of the following are significant factors in the pathogenesis of this condition EXCEPT

(A) human placental lactogen (hPL)
(B) pancreatic islet cell insufficiency
(C) placental insulinase
(D) increased levels of free cortisol
(E) increased levels of progesterone

37. A 37-year-old primigravida who had a prolonged evaluation for primary infertility is at 31 weeks' gestation. This pregnancy was the result of in vitro fertilization. She presents to the maternity unit stating fluid gushed from her vagina as she was standing in the checkout line in the local grocery store. The fluid ran all over the floor. An appropriate workup includes all of the following EXCEPT

(A) a digital examination to assess cervical dilation
(B) a speculum examination to assess for pooling in the posterior fornix
(C) cervical/vaginal cultures for group B streptococcus
(D) an assessment of fetal well-being
(E) an assessment of maternal vital signs

38. A 17-year-old woman (gravida 2, para 2) who delivered a 3800-gram male neonate 40 minutes ago has continued to bleed moderately since the delivery. Even though the uterine fundus feels well contracted, the placenta has not separated. Which of the following is the LEAST likely cause of this condition?

(A) Succenturiate lobed
(B) Placenta increta
(C) Bilobed placenta
(D) Placenta percreta
(E) Placenta accreta

39. A 31-year-old woman (gravida 1, para 0) presents at 30 weeks with confirmed preterm premature rupture of membranes (PPROM) having irregular uterine contractions (UCs). Her temperature is 100°F (37.8°C), and her uterus is tender to palpation. The fetal monitor tracing is reassuring, and the fetal presentation is cephalic. Appropriate management would include all of the following EXCEPT

(A) administration of intramuscular (IM) betamethasone
(B) obtaining of cervical cultures
(C) administration of subcutaneous (SQ) terbutaline to stop labor
(D) administration of parenteral antibiotics
(E) use of continuous electronic fetal monitoring (EFM)

40. A 38-year-old woman (gravida 7, para 6) is 7 cm dilated in the active phase of labor. Pregnancy complications include chronic hypertension and gestational diabetes mellitus (GDM). Membrane rupture occurred spontaneously 20 minutes ago, and continuous electronic fetal monitoring (EFM) is underway utilizing a direct internal scalp electrode. Baseline fetal heart rate (FHR) is 110 beats/min, and variability is diminished. Uterine contractions (UCs), which are being monitored with an external tocodynamometer, are occurring every 2–3 minutes and lasting for 45–60 seconds. With each contraction, the FHR drops rapidly to 130 beats/min but returns to 110 beats/min immediately after the contraction is over. All of the following are appropriate interventions in this situation EXCEPT

(A) decreasing the intravenous (IV) infusion rate
(B) changing maternal position
(C) decreasing uterine activity
(D) administering high-flow oxygen
(E) performing a vaginal examination to rule out prolapsed cord

41. A 29-year-old woman (gravida 3, para 0, abortus 2) is in active labor. Abruptly, the continuous internal electronic fetal monitor patterns show a fetal bradycardia that remains at 80 beats/min despite appropriate conservative interventions. You conclude the fetus must be delivered rapidly and consider using obstetrical forceps for an operative vaginal delivery. To accomplish a safe forceps delivery, all of the following prerequisites must be present EXCEPT

(A) the cervix must be at least 8 cm dilated
(B) the head must be engaged
(C) orientation of the head must be known
(D) membranes must be ruptured
(E) the bladder should be empty

42. A 23-year-old nulligravida woman complains of a variety of symptoms that are present only during the second half of her menstrual cycle. She states that she experiences no symptoms during the first week of her cycle. However, when the symptoms are present, they are disabling. You might expect this woman to manifest all of the following EXCEPT

(A) headache
(B) heavy menses
(C) nausea
(D) breast tenderness
(E) mood changes

43. A 45-year-old woman (gravida 5, para 5) complains of pelvic pressure and loss of urine with coughing and sneezing. You perform a pelvic examination and note that the cervix can be seen at the introitus without the patient increasing intra-abominal presssure. In addition, you note a bulging of the anterior vaginal wall. All of the following are risk factors for this condition EXCEPT

(A) ascites
(B) genetic predisposition
(C) previous pregnancies
(D) chronic cough
(E) endometriosis

44. A 23-year-old woman (gravida 2, para 1) is at 33 weeks' gestation as confirmed by early first-trimester sonogram. She came to the office stating that she has not felt her baby move as much as usual. You perform a nonstress test (NST), which reveals a baseline fetal heart rate (FHR) of 140 beats/min and no accelerations or decelerations of the FHR. However, the baseline FHR variability is decreased. All of the following are associated with this FHR finding EXCEPT

(A) sedatives
(B) chronic hypoxemia
(C) fetal arrhythmia
(D) fetal prematurity
(E) fetal sleep

45. A 65-year-old woman complains of abdominal-pelvic cramping and a sensation of fullness after eating only small amounts of food. Pelvic examination reveals fixed, bilateral masses that feel nodular to palpation. A carcinoembryonic antigen (CEA) titer is elevated. All of the following are risk factors for her condition EXCEPT

(A) positive family history
(B) Caucasian race
(C) late menopause
(D) use of oral contraceptives
(E) perineal talc powder

46. A 36-year-old woman (gravida 4, para 2, abortus 1) is admitted to the maternity unit in labor with a cervical dilation of 5 cm. Continuous electronic fetal monitoring (EFM) is underway using an external sonocardiograph. The baseline fetal heart rate (FHR) is 175 beats/min. All of the following conditions are associated with this EFM pattern EXCEPT

(A) maternal fever
(B) maternal hyperglycemia
(C) fetal hypoxia
(D) fetal prematurity
(E) β-adrenergic agonists

Directions: The set of matching questions in this section consists of a list of four to twenty-six lettered options (some of which may be in figures) followed by several numbered items. For each numbered item, select the ONE lettered option that is most closely associated with it. To avoid spending too much time on matching sets with large numbers of options, it is generally advisable to begin each set by reading the list of options. Then, for each item in the set, try to generate the correct answer and locate it on the option list, rather than evaluating each option individually. Each lettered option may be selected once, more than once, or not at all.

Questions 47–53

For each one of the following characteristics, select the type of genetic disorder that is most often associated with it.
(A) Autosomal dominant
(B) Autosomal recessive
(C) Sex-linked
(D) Cytogenetic
(E) Polygenic

47. It is related to advanced maternal age

48. It needs genes from both parents to be expressed

49. It contributes mostly to biochemical or enzymatic disorders

50. Unaffected offspring will not transmit disease

51. There is no male-to-male transmission

52. It causes mostly gross anatomic lesions

53. Its recurrence rate is approximately 2%

Questions 54–58

For each of the following treatments, select the appropriate type of female urinary incontinence.
(A) Sensory irritation incontinence
(B) Motor urge incontinence
(C) Overflow incontinence
(D) Total incontinence
(E) Genuine stress incontinence

54. Intermittent catheterization

55. Estrogen replacement therapy (ERT)

56. Anticholinergics

57. Bladder retraining

58. Antibiotics

Questions 59–63

Select the electronic fetal monitoring (EFM) periodic change associated with each of the following characteristics.
(A) Accelerations
(B) Early decelerations
(C) Variable decelerations
(D) Late decelerations

59. Mediated by sympathetic nervous system

60. A response to umbilical cord compression

61. Never is reassuring

62. A response to fetal movement

63. A response to fetal head compression

Questions 64–66

Match each of the following pelvic infectious organisms with its appropriate route of dissemination.
(A) Lymphatic spread
(B) Hematogenous spread
(C) Endometrial/salpingeal
(D) Body fluids

64. Chlamydial pelvic inflammatory disease (PID)

65. Postabortion *Escherichia coli* infection

66. Pelvic tuberculosis (TB)

Questions 67–71

For each of the following causes of fetal demise, select the diagnostic modality that is most appropriate.
(A) Toxoplasmosis, rubella, cytomegalovirus, and herpes (TORCH) studies
(B) Fetal autopsy
(C) Anticardiolipin antibodies
(D) Kleihauer-Betke test
(E) Fetal karyotyping
(F) Total body radiograph
(G) Atypical antibody titer

67. Fetomaternal bleed

68. Fetal aneuploidy

69. Maternal isoimmunization

70. Osteochondrodysplasia

71. Gross anatomic anomalies

Questions 72–76

For each of the characteristics identified, select the diagnostic category of first trimester loss that best applies.
(A) Inevitable abortion
(B) Missed abortion
(C) Completed abortion
(D) Threatened abortion
(E) Incomplete abortion

72. Managed by scheduled dilation and curettage (D&C)

73. Diagnosed by heavy bleeding, cramping, and passage of tissue followed by minimal bleeding and cramping

74. Managed by observation and serial β-human chorionic gonadotropin (β-hCG) determinations.

75. Diagnosed by heavy bleeding, cramping, and a dilated internal cervical os with no passage of tissue

76. Diagnosed by heavy bleeding, cramping, and a dilated internal cervical os with passage of tissue

Questions 77–88

For each laboratory test identified, select the direction of normal change in pregnancy.
(A) Increased
(B) Decreased
(C) Unchanged

77. Serum blood urea nitrogen (BUN)

78. Urine protein

79. Glomerular filtration rate (GFR)

80. Creatinine clearance (CrCl)

81. Serum uric acid

82. Fibrinogen

83. Albumin

84. Alkaline phosphatase

85. Prothrombin time (PTT)

86. Cholesterol

87. Bilirubin

88. γ-glutamyl transferase (GGT)

Questions 89–94

For each of the following characteristics, select the type of intrauterine growth restriction (IUGR) with which it is most often associated.
(A) Symmetric IUGR
(B) Asymmetric IUGR
(C) Both of the above

89. Amniotic fluid that is usually normal

90. Occurrence primarily because of fetal causes

91. Occurrence because of late pregnancy insults

92. Decreased abdominal circumference (AC)

93. Normal femur length (FL)

94. Diagnosis by ultrasound

Questions 95–100

For each of the following molecular moieties identified, select the option that best describes its relationship to transport across the placenta.
(A) Crosses by active transport
(B) Crosses by simple diffusion
(C) Does not cross the placenta
(D) Crosses by facilitated diffusion

95. Insulin

96. Amino acids

97. Thyroxine

98. Glucose

99. Ketones

100. Glucagon

Answers and Explanations

1. The answer is E [Chapter 8 I A 5]. The most critical criterion in distinguishing parity from abortus is the gestational age at which the pregnancy terminated. Determining whether a live fetus was expelled, whether a gestational sac or embryo was found on ultrasound, whether the pregnancy was terminated intentionally or spontaneously, and whether any birth defects were present are important parts of the reproductive history and should be obtained for all patients.

2. The answer is B [Chapter 6 VI C 2 a (1)]. Cephalopelvic disproportion (CPD) is the most prevalent indication for primary cesarean delivery, which is defined as the procedure being performed for the first time. The total cesarean rate in the United States is 20%–25%. In reality, CPD is in a general category that arises from failure of dilation in the active phase of stage I of labor or failure of descent in stage II of labor. The causes may be true disproportion of the fetal head to the maternal pelvis, abnormal fetal presentation, or abnormal attitude of the fetal head. Although malpresentation, fetal distress, and placenta previa are indications for primary cesarean delivery, they are not as prevalent as CPD. Chorioamnionitis is not an indication for a cesarean delivery in and of itself.

3. The answer is A [Chapter 3 I E 1, 2, 4 b]. Prevention of Rh isoimmunization by administering $Rh_o(D)$ immunoglobin (RhoGAM) to women at risk is an important part of complete care. This requires maternal Rh blood typing status to determine if the mother is Rh negative. Few first-trimester pregnancy losses are caused by uterine anomalies [diagnosed by hysterosalpingogram (HSG)], cervical infections (diagnosed by cervical cultures), antiphospholipid syndrome (diagnosed by antiphospholipid antibody screen), or thyroid disorders (diagnosed by thyroid studies).

4–5. The answers are: 4-B, 5-C [Chapter 3 VI C, D 3, F 1; Table 3–10]. Spontaneous bleeding from the fetoplacental unit to the mother can occur at any time during pregnancy. The risk of such bleeding increases as the pregnancy progresses. The risk of spontaneous isoimmunization before term is 2% in a susceptible mother (i.e., Rh-negative with an Rh-positive fetus) who has not received $Rh_o(D)$ immunoglobin prophylaxis. The chance that this woman would have developed $Rh_o(D)$ isoimmunization if she had received prophylactic $Rh_o(D)$ immunoglobin at 28 weeks is 0.2%. The risk of mixing fetoplacental blood into the mother's circulation is obviously highest during delivery and during placental separation in the third stage of labor. The risk of spontaneous isoimmunization after delivery is 15% in a susceptible mother (i.e., Rh-negative with an Rh-positive fetus) who did not receive $Rh_o(D)$ immunoglobin prophylaxis (e.g., RhoGAM). The chance that this woman will develop $Rh_o(D)$ isoimmunization if she does not receive $Rh_o(D)$ immunoglobin for subsequent pregnancies with Rh-positive fetuses is 50%.

6. The answer is B [Chapter 4 II A 2 a (1)]. Approximately 85% of patients with acquired heart disease, which is usually rheumatic in origin, have mitral stenosis. The main risk to these patients, who need plenty of diastolic filling time for blood to flow from the left atrium to the left ventricle, is tachycardia, which decreases the diastolic filling time. This can result in pulmonary congestion and hypotension.

7. The answer is A [Chapter 11 VI A 1]. Excessive female body hair can be categorized by a number of diagnoses. This patient demonstrates the typical presentation of hypertrichosis, in which there is excessive growth of only nonsexual hair. Hirsutism consists of increased growth of male-like, pigmented terminal hairs on the body midline (i.e., face, chest, abdomen, inner thighs). Defeminization is associated with decreased breast size and female contours. Virilization involves hirsutism plus clitoromegaly, temporal balding, and deepening voice.

8. The answer is B [Chapter 7 III C 5 b (3)]. The scenario describes a case of postpartum endomyometritis. It is the most common cause of puerperal fever and classically develops on the third postpartum day. Parenteral antibiotics should be continued for 48 hours after the patient's temperature returns to normal. Endometrial cultures are not usually helpful with a polymicrobial spectrum of organisms that are usually normal genital flora involving both aerobic and anaerobic bacteria.

9. The answer is C [Chapter 13 II I]. The scenario represents a case of ovarian carcinoma. The most common method of ovarian carcinoma metastasis involves exfoliation of malignant cells that become implanted throughout the peritoneal cavity. Although lymphatic spread, direct extension, and hematogenous spread are also found in the spread of ovarian cancer, they are less likely.

10. The answer is A [Chapter 4 X F 2]. Untreated urinary tract infections (UTIs) in pregnancy are associated with preterm labor and subsequent preterm delivery. Asymptomatic bacteriuria occurs in approximately 8% of pregnancies. Hydrops fetalis, spontaneous premature rupture of membranes (PROM), intrauterine growth restriction (IUGR), and postpartum hemorrhage are not associated with UTIs in pregnancy.

11. The answer is B [Chapter 3 VII D 4 a]. The scenario describes gestational trophoblastic disease. Most cases are found histologically to be benign on uterine curettage. If they are malignant, however, metastasis can occur. Lung metastasis is common but is successfully treated. Patients with good prognostic findings are almost uniformly successfully treated with single-agent chemotherapy. Poor prognostic findings include choriocarcinoma after full-term pregnancy, brain or liver metastases, a β-human chorionic gonadotropin (β-hCG) level higher than 40,000 mIU/ml at onset of therapy, and failed response to single-agent chemotherapy. These patients require multiple-agent chemotherapy and do not respond as well as patients with good prognostic findings. Bone metastasis is not usually associated with choriocarcinoma.

12. The answer is A [Chapter 8 III G 4]. The case describes the colposcopic appearance of cervical neoplasia. One of the most significant risk factors for cervical dysplasia is cigarette smoking. The change from normal cells to dysplastic cells may require the presence of a carcinogen. It is probable that some of the smoke-related mutagens are secreted through the endocervical glandular mucus, providing the neoplastic stimulus for the dysplastic changes. Family history and race are not risk factors for dysplasia. Early age of sexual intercourse, not early menarche, is a risk factor. Use of barrier methods of contraception may be protective against cervical dysplasia.

13. The answer is D [Chapter 3 V C 3 c]. The scenario describes a twin pregnancy with monochorionic, diamnionic placentation. Multiple gestation pregnancy is clearly high-risk for many reasons, including both maternal and fetal/neonatal hazards. Approximately 50% of pregnancies end in preterm deliveries (before 36 weeks' gestation). Although postpartum uterine atony, spontaneous premature rupture of membranes (PROM), iron-deficiency anemia, and pregnancy-induced hypertension pose increased risks, they do not approach the high risk of preterm labor and birth.

14. The answer is A [Chapter 7 I D 7]. Patients should avoid becoming pregnant for 3 months after receiving a rubella immunization. Postpartum immunization of rubella-susceptible women is an important part of appropriate puerperal care. Lactation is not contraindicated following rubella immunization. The vaccine uses a live attenuated virus, not a killed virus. The immunization works by an active not passive mechanism. Freedom from side effects is incorrect because arthralgias or rash can be common side effects of postpartum rubella immunization.

15. The answer is D [Chapter 3 VII]. The finding of hypertension and proteinuria before 24 weeks, along with a fundus larger than dates and vaginal bleeding, should strongly suggest molar pregnancy. Only 10% of patients with molar pregnancy present with early preeclampsia, but it should be an indicator for trophoblastic disease. The next steps should be performing a pelvic ultrasound, obtaining the serum β-human chorionic gonadotropin (β-hCG) level, and obtaining a chest radiograph to look for pulmonary metastasis.

16. The answer is B [Chapter 3 IV A 1, 2 a]. Assessment of cardiac activity by a skilled sonographer is the most accurate method of confirming fetal demise. Although fetal demise is a rare event, it accounts for approximately 50% of the perinatal mortality rates. Although neonatal mortality rates have been decreasing, little change has occurred in the antenatal fetal mortality rates. Whereas absence of fetal movement by maternal report, absence of fetal cardiac activity by external sonocardiography, absence of fetal heart tones by Doppler auscultation, and absence of fetal movement by sonography are useful in assessing fetal demise, all but absence of fetal cardiac motion on sonography have a high rate of false-positives.

17. The answer is A [Chapter 8 V C 3, 4]. The histology of this lesion is consistent with carcinoma in situ (CIS), or stage 0 vulvar carinoma. Skinning vulvectomy, which removes only the epithelium, is the treatment of choice for vulvar CIS. Medical treatment for premalignant or malignant vulvar lesions is not indicated. The basic therapeutic modality is surgical. Simple vulvectomy, which resects deeper tissues, is the treatment of choice for Paget's disease. Radical vulvectomy and regional lymphadenectomy are recommended treatments for invasive vulvar carcinoma. Radiation therapy is of limited value in vulvar cancer.

18. The answer is D [Chapter 11 II C 3; Table 11–5]. The findings in this 15-year-old are characteristic of Turner's syndrome or gonadal dysgenesis. Gonadal dysgenesis is characteristic of an individual with a 45,X karyotype who has streak gonads. Because two normal active X chromosomes are needed for normal gonadal/follicle development, and this individual has only one X chromosome, she has no follicles to produce estrogen. Without estrogen, she has no breast development. Because she has no Y chromosome to produce müllerian inhibitory factor, she has a normal uterus, although it is infantile in size.

19. The answer is E [Chapter 13 I C 6 b]. This woman has a condition known as ovarian torsion, which occurs when an ovarian mass twists on its pedicle. This obstructs the blood supply and risks ischemic injury. Presenting findings are acute onset of pelvic pain, abdominal tenderness, and leukocytosis. Risk factors, which are the same regardless of the cause of the mass or sonographic appearance, are its mobility and size. The longer the mass has been present without torsion, the greater the possibility that it is not very mobile. However, duration of the mass is incorrect because duration is not directly identifiable. Patient age is not related to torsion per se.

20. The answer is A [Chapter 4 IX D 1]. The case describes the characteristic clinical findings of iron-deficiency anemia, which is the most common anemia in pregnancy. An increase in total iron-binding capacity is a normal change in pregnancy (due to an increase in all plasma carrier proteins), rather than a diagnostic factor of iron deficiency. Iron deficiency is associated with a decrease in both mean corpuscular volume (MCV) and mean corpuscular hemoglobin. Bone marrow iron stores are completely depleted before evidence of hemoglobin decrease. The first response parameter with iron therapy is the reticulocyte count, not an increasing level of hemoglobin.

21. The answer is E [Chapter 11 II E 4 a]. A positive progesterone challenge test means that some withdrawal uterine bleeding has occurred within 2–14 days of administering progesterone. The amount of bleeding is not as important as the fact that there was some bleeding. Progesterone withdrawal bleeding occurs only if the endometrium has had adequate estrogen priming to allow the progesterone to ripen it. If the ovarian follicles are exhausted, there would be insufficient estrogen priming, and the progesterone challenge would be negative. Marked follicle-stimulating hormone (FSH) increase would be a sign of menopause, which would also result in a negative challenge test. A negative gonadotropin-releasing hormone (GnRH) stimulation would suggest pituitary failure leading to a negative challenge test, as would hypothalamic failure.

22. The answer is E [Chapter 3 VI C, D]. The first question to be answered is whether the father's red blood cells (RBCs) are antigen-positive. Isoimmunization in pregnancy requires that the mother have a negative antigen and the father have a positive antigen. If both parents are negative for the RBC antigen, the only antigen status possible for the infant would also be negative. If this is the case, all the other questions are irrelevant because the baby is not at risk. The other questions are important only if the father is antigen-positive for the atypical antibody.

23. The answer is A [Chapter 7 III A 1]. The scenario describes a case of puerperal fever. The incidence of puerperal fever is lower than 5% with vaginal deliveries but up to 30% with cesarean deliveries, particularly emergency procedures performed during labor. Postpartum febrile morbidity is defined as a temperature of 100.4°F (38°C) occurring for longer than 2 days consecutively, excluding the first 24 hours postpartum. Manual placental removal, prolonged labor, anemia, and premature rupture of membranes (PROM) are all additional risk factors but not as prevalent as cesarean delivery.

24. The answer is A [Chapter 3 VII A 1]. Bleeding before 16 weeks' gestation is by far the most frequent sign leading to diagnosis of hydatidiform mole (it is found in 90% of cases). Passage of vesicles vaginally is the second most common clinical finding. Hyperthyroidism, preeclampsia before 24 weeks' gestation, and severe hyperemesis each occur in approximately 10% of patients with hydatidiform mole.

25. The answer is D [Chapter 11 IV F 6]. The definitive diagnosis for assessing abnormal menstrual bleeding (i.e., after ruling out lower genital tract lesions) is an endometrial sampling for histological examination, which may require dilation and curettage (D&C). Often, a hysteroscopy is performed along with the D&C to identify polyps or structural lesions. Although a Papanicolaou (Pap) smear is unchallenged as a screen for cervical dysplasia, it is unreliable for assessing endometrial pathology. Ultrasound can visualize excessive endometrial thickness, but it will not provide a definitive diagnosis. A hysterosalpingogram (HSG) can outline uterine cavity contours, but it cannot provide a definitive diagnosis. Laparoscopy allows visualization of the external uterine contours, but it does not assess the uterine cavity.

26. The answer is C [Chapter 7 III E 4 a]. Pulmonary exercise is the most appropriate management because the most likely cause of the fever is atelectasis. In addition to risk factors, the possible causes of postpartum fever must be considered in relation to the time since delivery. This scenario is that of a scheduled cesarean without significant risk factors except general anesthesia and the fever that developed within hours. A pelvic examination would provide little additional information because an abscess would not yet have had time to develop. Intravenous (IV) heparin for septic pelvic thrombophlebitis is a consideration most often at day 5 or 6 postdelivery, when spiking fevers are resistant to broad-spectrum antibiotic coverage. Thus, IV antibiotics and blood cultures are also inappropriate for a pulmonary etiology.

27. The answer is D [Chapter 13 IV C]. The scenario presented is that of acute pelvic inflammatory disease (PID). Inpatient treatment of acute PID is reserved for those patients in whom the infectious process has progressed from local involvement to systemic disease of such degree that oral treatment on an outpatient basis could jeopardize satisfactory recovery. The cornerstones of inpatient treatment are parenteral antibiotics with surgical intervention only if medical management is unsuccessful. Evidence of pelvic abscess is correct because oral antibiotics would not achieve a high enough tissue level to treat an abscess. Kidney infections, as evidenced by costovertebral angle tenderness, are not related to decisions regarding PID treatment. Cervical motion tenderness, positive cervical culture, and increased sedimentation rate are incorrect because they are common findings with localized, early disease that can be treated satisfactorily on an outpatient basis.

28. The answer is C [Chapter 11, Table 11–1]. This patient is experiencing infertility due to anovulatory cycles along with galactorrhea. An elevated prolactin level can be responsible for all of these clinical findings. Prolactin is an anterior pituitary hormone that is a known inhibitor of gonadotropin-releasing hormone (GnRH). Agents that increase the prolactin level suppress ovulation, whereas agents that decrease the prolactin level enhance ovulation. Bromocriptine stimulates dopamine receptors, which inhibit prolactin secretion (thus enhancing ovulation). Opiates, phenothiazines, butyrophenones, and methyldopa all increase prolactin secretion, and therefore would suppress ovulation.

29. The answer is A [Chapter 3 V B 2 b]. This scenario represents a dichorionic twin pregnancy. Examination of the placenta(s) of a twin pregnancy provides much useful information and should be a routine part of the management. However, not all questions regarding zygosity can be answered by inspecting the placenta(s). With two separate chorions and, therefore, two separate amnions, the dividing membrane between the two sacs would normally be four layers thick. One cannot assume that the twin girls are identical simply because the placentation of same-gender twins is dichorionic; the zygosity could be either monozygotic or dizygotic. Nor can one assume that the risk of birth defects/anomalies is high because the twins could be dizygotic with a low risk of anomalies. Zygote cleavage occurring on day 14 postconception only applies to conjoined twins. Assuming the pregnancy was a consequence of ovulation induction is incorrect because the twins could be either monozygotic or dizygotic. Ovulation induction results in dizygotic twins.

30. The answer is D [Chapter 13 V G 1, 2 a]. The general guidelines for surgical intervention with tubal ectopic pregnancy are to perform the least invasive procedure and leave the anatomy as intact as possible. Laparoscopic linear salpingostomy is correct for two reasons: (1) laparoscopy is less invasive than a laparotomy, and (2) the ampullary location allows a salpingostomy (i.e., opening the salpinx with a linear incision) and removal of the products of conception versus a salpingectomy or partial resection, which would be more appropriate for an isthmic pregnancy.

31. The answer is B [Chapter 6 I C]. The scenario presents a case of active phase arrest due to inadequate uterine contractions (UCs). The appropriate next step in management is to increase the strength of UCs. β-adrenergic agonists is the correct answer (but incorrect statement) because they inhibit, rather than enhance myometrial contractility. They are an important class of tocolytic agents (e.g., terbutaline, ritodrine). Induction of labor is a frequent obstetrical intervention performed for both maternal as well as fetal indications. Phosphorylation of myosin, activation of myosin light-chain kinase, prostaglandin $F_{2\alpha}$, and oxytocin do enhance myometrial contractility. Prostaglandin $F_{2\alpha}$ and oxytocin are specific agents used clinically to induce labor.

32. The answer is A [Chapter 4 VIII A 1]. The case presented describes gestational diabetes mellitus (GDM), with a positive 1-hour 50-gram diabetic screen with a value over 140 mg/dl followed by a positive 3-hour oral glucose tolerance test (OGTT). Because the 1-hour and 2-hour values exceed the upper limits of normal, the OGTT is consistent with GDM, the most common type of diabetes in pregnancy. Most patients with true GDM are diagnosed as glucose intolerant in the last half of a pregnancy. Glucose intolerance first diagnosed before 20 weeks' gestation is considered to be GDM for classification purposes. However, it is most likely to be either type I or type II diabetes mellitus (DM) that newly developed or that existed and was undiagnosed before pregnancy. A 75-g, 2-hour OGTT performed after 6 weeks postpartum yields normal findings. GDM is usually managed by diet therapy alone but may require insulin supplementation in a minority of cases.

33. The answer is A [Chapter 13 V F 4]. It is crucial that the diagnosis of ectopic pregnancy be ruled out in this case. Ectopic pregnancy has been called "the great imitator" because its findings can be subtle and vague. Because the purpose of culdocentesis is to identify a ruptured ectopic pregnancy, absence of free blood in the pouch of Douglas does not rule out the condition. A negative culdocentesis also does not rule out an ectopic pregnancy. Amenorrhea, vaginal bleeding, and abdominal pain are very helpful and constitute the classic triad for ectopic pregnancy. A β-human chorionic gonadotropin (β-hCG) test is a very useful test because it is almost always positive in women with an ectopic pregnancy.

34. The answer is A [Chapter 9 II A 5 a]. The scenario describes a lower reproductive tract infection. The absence of gram-negative diplococci suggests that the etiology is more likely chlamydial than gonococcal. Chlamydial infections in the female are frequently asymptomatic. Chlamydia does cause acute urethral syndrome, and it is associated with hypertrophic cervical inflammation and inflammatory changes in the oviduct. Infertility is a common sequelae of inadequate treatment of chlamydia.

35. The answer is A [Chapter 8 I A 3]. Identification of the number of confirmed pregnancies a patient has had is an important part of the reproductive history. The late onset of menses is not an adequate criterion for a pregnancy. It is essential to obtain verifying data to support that pregnancy did occur. A positive pregnancy test, sonographic demonstration of an embryo, passage of a fetus, and a positive pathology report are all corroborative evidence of a pregnancy.

36. The answer is B [Chapter 4 VIII A 3]. The scenario describes a case of gestational diabetes mellitus (GDM because the initial glucose screen is negative but becomes positive later in the pregnancy. In general, GDM is diagnosed in the latter half of the pregnancy. Although pancreatic islet cell insufficiency is the pathogenesis of type I diabetes mellitus (DM), it is not pathogenic of GDM. Human placental lactogen (hPL), placental insulinase, increased levels of free cortisol, and increased levels of progesterone are true factors in the pathogenesis of GDM.

37. The answer is A [Chapter 6 IV C 2, 3 c]. The scenario describes a case of possible preterm premature rupture of membranes (PPROM), which is the single most common diagnosis leading to neonatal intensive care unit admissions in the United States. A digital examination is not recommended in a patient with PPROM because of the increased risk of chorioamnionitis. A speculum examination should allow assessment of not only pooling but also advanced cervical dilation. Cultures for group B streptococcus are necessary because the premature infant is at greater risk for sepsis from this organism. Prophylactic antibiotics are started until negative cultures come back. Assessment of fetal and maternal well-being are important before embarking on a course of conservative management.

38. The answer is D [Chapter 7 II F 1, 2]. The scenario represents a case of postpartum bleeding due to a retained placenta. A placental abnormality (e.g., succenturiate lobed or bilobed placenta, in which the placenta is not a single disk) is often associated with a retained placenta. The abnormalities can be divided into two categories: gross anatomic abnormalities or an abnormality of trophoblastic invasion. Abnormalities of trophoblastic invasion are the least common general category. They result when the placental trophoblastic invasion has penetrated beyond normal limits because of the absence of Nitabuch's layer of the uterine wall. In patients with placenta percreta [which is very rare (5% of trophoblastic invasion abnormalities)], the villi penetrate the full thickness into the uterine serosa. More frequent manifestations are placenta increta, in which villi invade the myometrium (but not the full thickness), and placenta accreta, in which the villi invade the decidua basalis but not the myometrium.

39. The answer is C [Chapter 6 IV C 3 b (1)]. Conservative management of this pregnancy by attempting to stop contractions with terbutaline would jeopardize not only the mother but also the fetus. The clinical picture is one of preterm contractions with chorioamnionitis, probably from the premature membrane rupture. It makes good sense to attempt to induce fetal pulmonary maturity transplacentally through maternal steroid administration while initiating delivery. Obtaining cervical cultures is needed to identify any organism that might not be covered by the parental antibiotics, which are appropriately suggested. Continuous electronic fetal monitoring (EFM) is prudent to ensure fetal well-being during the period of time until delivery occurs.

40. The answer is A [Chapter 6 III B 5, 6]. The case describes a nonreassuring fetal monitor pattern with moderate variable decelerations occurring with contractions. The decelerations are consistent with increases in fetal vagal tone secondary to umbilical cord compression. All generic interventions seek to increase fetal oxygenation. An increase in intravenous (IV) infusion rate, not a decrease, is recommended to enhance maternal perfusion of the placenta. A change in maternal position attempts to displace the fetus from compressing a loop of umbilical cord. Decreasing uterine activity may increase intervals of blood flow by decreasing uterine contractions (UCs). Administering high-flow oxygen enhances the transfer of oxygen across the placenta by increasing the oxygen level in the maternal circulation. Vaginal examination identifies if the umbilical cord is being compressed by prolapsing through the cervix ahead of the presenting fetal part.

41. The answer is A [Chapter 6 VI A]. Unless the cervix is completely dilated, the use of forceps may cause extensive maternal lacerations. Obstetrical forceps are effective instruments for assisting in a vaginal delivery that otherwise might not occur. Conditions for their use are well defined and should be carefully followed to minimize injury to the mother or fetus. Prerequisites for forceps use include all of the following: the head must be engaged, the orientation of the head must be known, the membranes must be ruptured, and the bladder should be empty.

42. The answer is B [Chapter 11 V B]. The symptoms of premenstrual syndrome (PMS) are diverse, involving a variety of organ systems. Changes in the frequency, duration, and amount of menstrual flow are not typical findings in patients with PMS. Headache, nausea, breast tenderness, and mood changes are frequently found symptoms.

43. The answer is E [Chapter 8 VI B]. The scenario describes a number of features of pelvic relaxation such as first-degree uterine prolapse and cystocele. There is no relationship between endometriosis and pelvic relaxation. Ascites and chronic cough are risk factors because each increases intra-abdominal pressure. Genetic predisposition and previous pregnancies weaken the ligamentous support, which is also a risk factor for pelvic relaxation.

44. The answer is C [Chapter 6 III B 2 a (2)]. Fetal arrhythmia usually results in increased rather than decreased variability. Beat-to-beat variability, which refers to the small, rapid rhythmic fluctuations in the fetal heart rate (FHR), is a normal finding that is a reassuring sign of healthy interplay in the heart rate (HR) regulatory mechanism between the fetal sympathetic and parasympathetic nervous systems. Sedatives, chronic hypoxemia, fetal prematurity, and fetal sleep can all result in a decreased baseline FHR variability.

45. The answer is D [Chapter 13 II C]. The case presented is highly suggestive of ovarian carcinoma. Approximately 1% of American women eventually die of ovarian cancer, which is often undiagnosed until it reaches an advanced stage of spread. The use of oral contraceptives tends to decrease rather than increase the risk of ovarian carcinoma. Positive family history, Caucasian race, and late menopause are all known risk factors for ovarian cancer.

46. The answer is B [Chapter 6 III B 2 a]. The scenario describes fetal tachycardia. Maternal hyperglycemia has no relationship to fetal tachycardia. The baseline fetal heart rate (FHR) is the average rate between peaks and depressions. Normal baseline FHR is 120–160 beats/min. Moderate tachycardia is diagnosed when the baseline FHR is 160–180 beats/min. Maternal fever, fetal hypoxia, prematurity, and β-agonists can all result in baseline fetal tachycardia.

47–53. The answers are: 47-D [Chapter 2 III B 2 c (1)], **48-B** [Chapter 2 III B 2 b], **49-B** [Chapter 2 III B 2 b], **50-A** [Chapter 2 III B 2 a], **51-C** [Chapter 2 III B 2 c (1)], **52-A** [Chapter 2 III B 2 a], **53-E** [Chapter 2 III B 3]. Maternal age-related anomalies (usually trisomies 21 and 18) are cytogenetic. In autosomal recessive disorders, which include biochemical disorders, genes from both parents are typically required for expression. In autosomal dominant disorders, which include gross anatomic lesions, unaffected offspring are free from transmitting the disease. In sex-linked disorders, only the mother can pass on an affected X chromosome; a father cannot give it to his son. Polygenic or multifactorial etiologies have a 2% recurrence rate and are responsible for most newborn congenital malformations.

54–58. The answers are: 54-C [Chapter 8 VIII D 4 c (1)], **55-E** [Chapter 8 VIII D 1 d (1)], **56-B** [Chapter 8 VIII D 3 e (1)], **57-B** [Chapter 8 VIII D 2 e (4)], **58-A** [Chapter 8 VIII D 1 e]. Chronic, long-term intermittent catheterization may be necessary in patients with overflow incontinence secondary to permanent conditions such as lower motor neuron lesions. Estrogen replacement may improve pelvic tissue strength to relieve symptoms of genuine stress incontinence. Anticholinergic medications can inhibit excessive activity of the detrusor muscle in motor urge incontinence. Bladder retraining exercises, along with anticholinergics, may help to control the excessive detrusor muscle activity of motor urge incontinence. The incontinence of sensory irritation caused by acute cystitis is relieved by antibiotic treatment of the susceptible bacteria.

59–63. The answers are: 59-A, 60-C, 61-D, 62-A, 63-B [Chapter 6 III B 2 c (1)–(4); Table 6–7]. Accelerations mediated by sympathetic stimulation are always reassuring and are a response to fetal movement. Variable decelerations are vagally mediated often from cord compression. Late decelerations can be either vagally mediated or from myocardial depression due to hypoxia, and are never reassuring. Early decelerations are vagally mediated and result from fetal head compression.

64–66. The answers are: 64-C, 65-A, 66-B [Chapter 13 IV A 2; Table 13–5]. Chlamydial pelvic inflammatory disease (PID) results in purulent salpingitis. The route of dissemination is endometrial/salpingeal as the organisms ascend from the cervix attaching to columnar epithelium without deep invasion. Another organism that follows the same route is *Neisseria gonorrheae*. Postabortion *Escherichia coli* infections start from the endometrium involving sequentially the myometrium then the parametrium by using a lymphatic route of spread. There is deep invasion of the tissues through a cellulitis. Pelvic tuberculosis (TB) is carried from the lungs to the pelvic organs by hematogenous spread. It is a frequent cause of infertility in developing countries.

67–71. The answers are: 67-D, 68-E, 69-G, 70-F, 71-B [Chapter 3 IV D; Table 3–6]. The Kleihauer-Betke test uses differential staining of fetal red blood cells (RBCs) in the maternal circulation, and thus would be used to diagnose a fetomaternal bleed. Karyotyping identifies a fetal cytogenetic abnormality if present, and thus would be used to diagnose fetal aneuploidy. An atypical antibody titer identifies the presence of high antibody titers against foreign RBC antigens if present, suggesting isoimmunization as a factor. Therefore, the atypical antibody titer would be used to diagnose maternal isoimmunization. Total body radiograph shows abnormal skeletal anatomy or calcification if present. Therefore, it would be used to diagnose osteochondrodysplasia. A fetal autopsy provides information for identification of syndromes of anomalies such as gross anatomic anomalies.

72–76. The answers are: 72-B, 73-C, 74-C, 75-A, 76-E [Chapter 3 I C 2, D; Table 3–1]. Emptying the uterus with a missed abortion is not an urgency; therefore, an emergency dilation and curettage (D&C) is not required. A characteristic of a completed abortion is one in which all the products of conception have been expelled from the uterus. Observation and serial β-human chorionic gonadotropin (β-hCG) determinations are appropriate management for a completed abortion because they ensure that an ectopic pregnancy is not overlooked. Heavy bleeding, cramping, and a dilated internal cervical os with *no* passed tissue is the classic definition of an inevitable abortion. Heavy bleeding, cramping, and a dilated internal cervical os *with* tissue passed is the classic definition of an incomplete abortion.

77–88. The answers are: 77-B [Chapter 1 IV D 2 b; Table 1–2], **78-C** [Chapter 1 IV D 2 b; Table 1–2], **79-A** [Chapter 1 IV D 2 b; Table 1–2], **80-A** [Chapter 1 IV D 2 b; Table 1–2], **81-B** [Chapter 1 IV D 2 b; Table 1–2], **82-A** [Chapter 1 IV F 6 a (1), b], **83-B** [Chapter 1 IV F 6 b, 7 c (2)], **84-A** [Chapter 1 IV F 6 b, 7 c (3)], **85-C** [Chapter 1 IV F 6 b, 7 c (4)], **86-A** [Chapter 1 IV F 6 b], **87-C** [Chapter 1 IV F 6 b, 7 c (4)], **88-C** [Chapter 1 IV F 6 b]. Blood urea nitrogen (BUN) decreases during pregnancy because of the increased ability of the kidneys to clear metabolic wastes. Urine protein does not change significantly during pregnancy. The glomerular filtration rate (GFR) increases because of the increased renal blood flow during pregnancy. Creatinine clearance (CrCl) increases because of the increased renal blood flow during pregnancy. Uric acid decreases because of the increased ability of the kidneys to clear metabolic wastes in pregnancy.

89–94. The answers are: 89-A [Chapter 2 IV B 1], **90-A** [Chapter 2 IV B 1], **91-B** [Chapter 2 IV B], **92-C** [Chapter 2 IV B 1], **93-B** [Chapter 2 IV B 1], **94-C** [Chapter 2 IV B 1]. In symmetric intrauterine growth restriction (IUGR), placental perfusion (and thus fetal renal perfusion) is not usually impaired. Symmetric IUGR is mostly due to fetal infection, karyotype abnormality, or gross anatomic anomaly. Asymmetric IUGR is mostly due to late second- and third-trimester decrease in nutrient and blood flow. In both symmetric and asymmetric IUGR, fetal abdominal circumference (AC) is decreased but because of different mechanisms. In asymmetric IUGR, femur growth is spared despite decreased placental perfusion. Both symmetric and asymmetric IUGR are dependent on sonographic measurements for assessment.

95–100. The answers are: 95-C [Chapter 1 IV G 3 d (1)], **96-A** [Chapter 1 IV G 1 b], **97-C** [Chapter 1 IV G 3 d (2) (a)–(b)], **98-D** [Chapter 1 IV G 3 d (2) (b)], **99-B** [Chapter 1 IV G 3 d (2) (b)], **100-C** [Chapter 1 IV G 3 d (1)]. Insulin does not cross the placenta, perhaps because of the large size of the insulin molecule. Amino acids, the building blocks of body proteins, mostly cross the placenta via active transport, with differences found among the essential and nonessential ones. Thyroxine does not cross the placenta significantly although it is a small molecule. Glucose is essential for fetal survival; thus, it crosses the placenta by facilitated diffusion. Ketones cross the placenta by simple diffusion. Glucagon does not cross the placenta, possibly because it is also a large molecule.

ABBREVIATIONS

ΔOD_{450}	Optical density measured at 450 nm
AAS	Atypical antibody screen
ABG	Arterial blood gas
AC	Abdominal circumference
ACOG	American College of Obstetrics and Gynecology
ADA	American Diabetes Association
AF-AFP	Amniotic fluid α-fetoprotein
AFI	Amniotic fluid index
AIDS	Acquired immunodeficiency syndrome
ALT	Alanine aminotransferase
ASB	Asymptomatic bacteriuria
ASD	Atrial septal defect
AST	Aspartate aminotransferase
AZT	Azidothymidine
BBT	Basal body temperature
BP	Blood pressure
BPD	Biparietal diameter
BPD	Bronchopulmonary dysplasia
BPP	Biophysical profile
BSE	Breast self exam
BSO	Bilateral salpingo-oophorectomy
BUN	Blood urea nitrogen
BV	Bacterial vaginosis
BVOD	Biventricular outer end-diastolic
CA	Carcinoma
CA-125	Cancer antigen 125
CAH	Congenital adrenal hyperplasia
CDC	Centers for Disease Control and Prevention
CEA	Carcinoembryonic antigen
CIN	Cervical intraepithelial neoplasia
CIS	Carcinoma in situ
CMV	Cytomegalovirus
CNS	Central nervous system
CO	Cardiac output
CPD	Cephalopelvic disproportion
Cr cl	Creatinine clearance
CRL	Crown-rump length
CST	Contraction stress test
CT	Computerized tomography
CVS	Chorionic villus sampling
D&C	Dilation and curettage

D&E	Dilation and evacuation
DES	Diethylstilbestrol
DHEA	Dehydroepiandrosterone
DHEAS	Dehydroepiandrosterone sulfate
DHT	Dihydrotestosterone
DIC	Disseminated intravascular coagulation
DM	Diabetes mellitus
DMPA	Depomedroxyprogesterone acetate
DUB	Dysfunctional uterine bleeding
DVT	Deep venous thrombosis
ECC	Endocervical curettage
EDD	Estimated due date
EFM	Electronic fetal monitor
EKG	Electrocardiogram
ELISA	Enzyme-linked immunosorbent assay
ERT	Estrogen replacement therapy
ERV	Expiratory reserve volume
ESR	Erythrocyte sedimentation rate
FEV$_1$	Forced expiratory volume at 1 second
FHR	Fetal heart rate
FIGO	International Federation of Gynecologists and Obstetricians
FL	Femur length
FNA	Fine needle aspiration
FRC	Functional residual capacity
FSH	Follicle-stimulating hormone
FTA-ABS	Fluorescent antibody absorption test
GBBS	Group B β-hemolytic streptococcus
GDM	Gestational diabetes mellitus
GFR	Glomerular filtration rate
GGT	Gamma glutamyltransferase
GI	Gastrointestinal
GnRH	Gonadotropin releasing hormone
GTN	Gestational trophoblastic neoplasia
GU	Genitourinary
HAV	Hepatitis A virus
HBsAg	Hepatitis B surface antigen
HBV	Hepatitis B virus
HC	Head circumference
HCG	Human chorionic gonadotropin
HCV	Hepatitis C virus
HDL	High density lipoprotein
HDV	Hepatitis D virus
HEV	Hepatitis E virus
Hgb	Hemoglobin
HIV	Human immunodeficiency virus
HPL	Human placental lactogen
HPO axis	Hypothalamic-pituitary-ovarian axis
HPV	Human papilloma virus
HR	Heart rate
HSG	Hysterosalpingogram
HSV	Herpes simplex virus

IBW	Ideal body weight
IC	Inspiratory capacity
ICSI	Intracytoplasmic sperm injection
IFN-α	Interferon-α
IM	Intramuscular
IRP	International reference preparation
IRV	Inspiratory reserve volume
IUD	Intrauterine device
IUGR	Intrauterine growth restriction
IUI	Intrauterine insemination
IV	Intravenous
IVC	Inferior vena cava
IVF	Invitro fertilization
IVH	Intraventricular hemorrhage
IVP	Intravenous pyelogram
JVD	Jugular venous distention
KOH prep	Potassium hydroxide preparation
LDL	Low density lipoprotein
LEEP	Loop electrodiathermy excision procedure
LGV	Lymphogranuloma venereum
LH	Luteinizing hormone
LMP	Last menstrual period
MAO	Monoamine oxidase
MCHC	Mean corpuscular hemoglobin concentration
MCV	Mean corpuscular volume
MHA-TP	Microhemagglutination assay for T. pallidum
MIU	Milli-international units
MoM	Multiples of the median
MRI	Magnetic resonance imaging
MSAFP	Maternal serum α-fetoprotein
NEC	Necrotizing enterocolitis
NSAID	Nonsteroidal anti-inflammatory drug
NST	Nonstress test
OGTT	Oral glucose tolerance test
Pap	Papanicalaou
PAS	Para aminosalicylic acid
PCO	Polycystic ovarian syndrome
PCR	Polymerase chain reaction
PCT	Postcoital test
PDA	Patent ductus arteriosus
PE	Pulmonary embolus
PID	Pelvic inflammatory disease
PMS	Premenstrual syndrome
PPH	Postpartum hemorrhage
PPROM	Preterm premature rupture of membranes
PPW	Prepregnancy weight
PROM	Premature rupture of membranes
PT	Prothrombin time
PTT	Partial thromboplastin time
PTU	Propylthiouracil
PUBS	Percutaneous umbilical blood sampling

PUPPP	Pruritic urticarial papules and pustules of pregnancy
PVR	Peripheral vascular resistance
RBC	Red blood cell
RDW	Red cell distribution width
ROP	Retinopathy of prematurity
RPR test	Rapid plasma reagin test
RR	Respiratory rate
RV	Residual volume
SC	Squamocolumnar
SERM	Selective estrogen receptor modulator
SHBG	Sex hormone binding globulin
SIL	Squamous intraepithelial lesion
SPROM	Spontaneous premature rupture of membranes
SQ	Subcutaneous
SSRI	Selective serotonine reuptake inhibitors
STD	Sexually transmitted disease
SV	Stroke volume
SVC	Superior vena cava
T$_3$	Triiodothyronine
T$_4$	Thyroxine
TAH	Total abdominal hysterectomy
TAH-BSO	Total abdominal hysterectomy & bilateral salpingo-oophorectomy
TB	Tuberculosis
TBG	Thyroid-binding globulin
TLC	Total lung capacity
TOA	Tubo-ovarian abscess
TRH	Thyrotropin-releasing hormone
TSH	Thyroid-stimulating hormone
TSS	Toxic shock syndrome
TV	Tidal volume
T-Zone	Transformation zone
UCs	Uterine contractions
UTI	Urinary tract infection
V/Q scan	Ventilation-perfusion scan
VC	Vital capacity
VDRL test	Venereal disease research laboratory test
VIN	Vulvar intraepithelial neoplasia
VSD	Ventricular septal defect
VWD	Ventral wall defect
WBC	White blood cell

Index

References in *italics* indicate figures; those followed by "t" denote tables